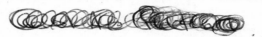

OXFORD MEDICAL PUBLICATIONS

THE COMPLETE RECOVERY ROOM BOOK

Second Edition

THE
COMPLETE RECOVERY
ROOM BOOK

SECOND EDITION

ANTHEA HATFIELD
Austin Hospital, Melbourne, Australia

and

MICHAEL TRONSON
Box Hill Hospital, Melbourne, Australia

Oxford   New York   Melbourne
OXFORD UNIVERSITY PRESS

Oxford University Press, Great Clarendon Street, Oxford OX2 6DP

Oxford   New York

Athens   Auckland   Bangkok   Bogota   Bombay   Buenos Aires
Calcutta   Cape Town   Dar es Salaam   Delhi   Florence   Hong Kong   Istanbul
Karachi   Kuala Lumpur   Madras   Madrid   Melbourne   Mexico City
Nairobi   Paris   Singapore   Taipei   Tokyo   Toronto   Warsaw
and associated companies in
Berlin   Ibadan

Oxford is a trade mark of Oxford University Press

Published in the United States
by Oxford University Press Inc., New York

Reprinted 1998

A catalogue for this book is available from the British Library

Library of Congress Cataloging in Publication Data
(Data available)
ISBN 019 262715 5 p/b
ISBN 019 262716 3 h/b

Printed and bound in Great Britain by
Biddles Ltd, Guildford and King's Lynn

FOREWORD

The recovery room is an essential part of anaesthesia. Not only does it ensure patients' safety in the intermediate stage between full anaesthesia and full consciousness, it also provides an opportunity for the stabilization of normal physiological processes.

Recovery from anaesthesia is taken for granted; it should not be. It requires skill and knowledge to make it safe and routine. Until now these attributes have been learned by practical experience and discussion.

Dr Hatfield and Dr Tronson have seen a need for a book bringing together all this knowledge. With the first edition of *The Complete Recovery Room Book* they covered all the areas of protocol, equipment, drug therapy and most important of all, patient care, that are necessary to establish, and run a successful recovery room. In this second edition they have expanded the sections on physiology and pharmacology, adding a new dimension to the understanding of patients' needs in the hours after anaesthesia.

The authors are experienced anaesthetists who have worked in a wide range of recovery rooms; in both sophisticated and simple environments and in many different countries. They have used this experience to write a book that covers the whole spectrum of recovery room activity.

John Ashton
Consultant Anaesthetist
Monash Medical Centre
Melbourne

PREFACE

This is a book for staff who, when alone and confronted with a problem in an *isolated hospital*, need practical advice on what to do. Its aim is to help you save lives. Saving lives includes preventing complications that may, at worst, permanently maim the patient, for example, brain damage; or less seriously, delay their discharge from hospital.

It is a practical book for those who are neither fully trained anaesthetists, nor specialist trained recovery room nursing staff. While the text is purposefully dogmatic and direct, the regimes described are effective under most circumstances. This book is not a substitute for personal instruction from an expert, nor an alternative for practical experience. It does not compare theories, or argue different points of view.

In the best of circumstances, in properly staffed teaching hospitals, the safety of about 30 per cent of patients is in jeopardy during the first postoperative hour, and up to 50 per cent of all postoperative deaths occur during this time [1,2]. The outcome of major complications is better if they occur during anaesthesia; than if they occur in the recovery period [3]. Our experience suggests that the death rate in the recovery room of an isolated hospital is higher than that at a major teaching hospital. Urban hospitals also have periods of isolation, for instance after-hours, at weekends, during holiday periods, and at night. At these times fully trained recovery staff may be unavailable, their places taken by part-time staff who are unfamiliar with routine procedures.

Recovery rooms are specialized intensive care units, where patients need frequent and careful observation. It is our opinion that the recovery room is the most important room in a hospital. It is here that a patient is at greatest risk, and it is here the staff need to give immediate and skilled attention to save lives.

Only a paradigm shift in the minds of anaesthetists, clinical staff, and administrators will further reduce perioperative mortality and morbidity. There have been astounding advances in anaesthesia in the past 25 years, the intraoperative death rate has fallen perhaps twenty-fold, and it is rare for a patient to suffer harm from the anaesthetic. The time has come to turn attention to the neglected first few hours after surgery. Clinical impressions, although statistically useless, are a good starting place to design trials. Clinical audit is essential, but impressions are needed to help guide what to audit. We believe that clinical research should now aim at

identifying factors that predict the outcome of events in the recovery room
For instance our own clinical impressions suggest that life-threatening
events take place during the physiological and biochemical, turmoil of the
first few hours after emergence from anaesthesia. It is at this time that
events such as deep vein thrombosis, postoperative hypoxaemia,
pneumonia, and cardiac problems begin. We believe that it is possible to
achieve a further reduction in postoperative morbidity and mortality, but to
achieve this, facts are needed; and as we have discovered, facts about the
recovery room are hard to find.

Melbourne   A.H.
March 1996   M.T.

1. Zelcer J., Wells D. G. (1987). *Anaesthesia and Intensive Care,* 15: 168-173
2. *Report on Deaths Associated with Anaesthesia in Australia* 1988-1990; National Health and
   Medical Research Council Document.
3. Tirets L., Desmont J. M. (1986). *Canadian Anaesthetists' Society Journal,* 33: 336-44

THE ISOLATED HOSPITAL AND DEDICATION TO THE SECOND EDITION

The difficulties encountered by an isolated hospital are different from those of large, busy urban hospitals. The staff of isolated hospitals have often spent years without contact with people of similar interests and with no chance to exchange ideas and experiences. New techniques are slow to arrive, and drugs and other essential items are scarce. Equipment fails, and no one knows how to repair it. These problems are exacerbated by local health authorities, who seem to neither understand the problems, nor care. The grind of constant work, and the battle for limited resources, exhausts enthusiasm and depresses the spirit. The result is intellectual burn out; the standard of care imperceptibly drops, and untoward incidents occur. Morale falls and a feeling of helplessness begins to seep into the soul of the staff. The difficulties soon come to be regarded as inevitable. This is made worse by visitors who tactlessly point out what is wrong, without having any idea of the cause, or of the constant struggle required to maintain standards.

We dedicate this second edition of *The Complete Recovery Room Book* to all the doctors and nurses who, each day, strive to maintain standards despite overwhelming difficulties, and especially those we have met in the hospitals of the South West Pacific.

FIRST EDITION DEDICATED TO

Pamela Deighton, Palega Vaeau, and Grant Scarf
- the first recovery room team to Samoa

CONTENTS

INTRODUCTION 1

1. GOLDEN RULES 5

2. ROUTINE RECOVERY ROOM PROCEDURES 10

3. DRAINS AND CATHETERS 27

4. INFECTION CONTROL 35

5. PHARMACOLOGY 41

6. INTRAVENOUS FLUIDS 50

7. DIFFERENT AGE GROUPS 62

8. DAY SURGERY 75

9. SURGICAL OPERATIONS 82

10. PRE-EXISTING DISEASE 117

11. DIFFICULTIES AND DISASTERS 140

12. PAIN CONTROL IN THE RECOVERY ROOM 182

13. POSTOPERATIVE NAUSEA AND VOMITING 221

14. THE CARDIOVASCULAR SYSTEM 233

15. HYPOXIA AND RESPIRATORY PHYSIOLOGY 301

16. RESPIRATORY PROBLEMS IN THE RECOVERY ROOM 322

17. THE KIDNEY 340

18. THE BLEEDING PATIENT 347

19. MONITORING 373

20. EQUIPMENT IN THE RECOVERY ROOM 393

21. PURCHASING EQUIPMENT AND SAFETY 417

22. DESIGN OF THE RECOVERY ROOM 423

23. STAFFING AND MANAGEMENT 432

24. DRUGS USED IN THE RECOVERY ROOM 438

25. USEFUL DATA 464

26. ABBREVIATIONS 467

INDEX 473

INTRODUCTION

Eternal vigilance is the price of safety.

It is a common belief that patients are *asleep* during their operation. They are not asleep. They are in a drug induced coma, and to metabolize and excrete these drugs takes time. During this time they gradually recover consciousness, but remain unable to care for themselves. They are at risk from a range of disasters as they emerge from the protection of the anaesthetic. Suddenly, they are exposed to extreme physiological disturbances, caused by pain, hypothermia, hypoxia and shifts in blood volume. Not only do the recovery room staff have to be adept at the management of a comatose, and physiologically unstable patient; but also in the care of a surgical patient with drains, drips and dressings.

Before recovery rooms were routinely available, almost half the deaths in the immediate postoperative period, such as airway obstruction or aspiration of stomach contents, were preventable.

The recovery room provides a way of smoothing the transition of patient care from the operating theatre to the wards. Its function is to safeguard the patient in the immediate postoperative period when he is least able to look after himself. It relieves the ward of the necessity to dedicate one nurse to one patient, and removes the need to duplicate equipment. It also enables staff with special training to be concentrated in one area so they can maintain their skills and train more junior staff.

Recovery rooms improve patient safety, save money,
and allow the wards to work more efficiently.

How To Use This Book

Use this book like an encyclopaedia to provide information quickly about an unfamiliar clinical problem, operative procedure, or an emergency. It is not intended to be read in one sitting. There are many cross references, and at times deliberate repetition of material to help you find answers to your questions easily and quickly.

Terminology

In recent years the term *post anaesthetic care unit* (with its acronym *PACU*) has become popular. *Recovery room,* is still the most common term in the village or district hospital. The word *recovery* emphasizes the function of this room; to safeguard patients recovering from the insults of surgery and anaesthesia; and for this reason we have retained it.

In the United Kingdom it has become customary to measure pressures in kilopascals (kPa); however, most other countries continue to measure pressures, especially blood pressures, in millimetres of mercury (mmHg). We have decided to stay with common usage in our region, so blood pressures are recorded in millimetres of mercury, with kilopascals quoted for blood gases. There is a conversion table on page 466.

In some parts of the world anaesthetists are not medically qualified, whereas anaesthesiologists are. In our region (and in our book) anaesthetists are medically qualified, and the term *anaesthetist* refers to both anaesthetist and anaesthesiologists.

Grammar

Most medical textbooks and journal articles are written in the past passive tense. This form is an academic convention and is sometimes ambiguous. It is also boring, and difficult to understand for those who do not speak English as their first language. With these readers in mind, we have tried to keep our writing as simple, and as graphic, as possible. We have deliberately written much of this text in direct active speech, a 'do this', 'do that' form, that we hope will link educational goals with service needs.

Drug Names

In the workplace, drug trade names are often more recognizable than generic names. Although this is theoretically undesirable, it is a fact, and for this reason the trade names of drugs are usually quoted after the generic names, for instance: propofol (Diprivan®). It is not feasible to quote all the trade names, so where relevant we have used the trade name of the company that first developed the drug. The appendix on drugs will help you convert generic names to trade names.

Aphorisms

We make no apology for these simple, direct and obvious catch phrases scattered throughout the book. They are there to jog the memory. Staff may not remember the physiological reasons for something, but they do remember the phrase.

Tables

Some of the tables and lists are designed to be photocopied as wall charts.

Gender

For the sake of simplicity in the text, nurses and paramedical staff are referred to as she, and doctors and patients as he. This is still the commonest configuration in most parts of the world and no offence is intended.

Abbreviations

The number and variety of abbreviations used in medicine is increasing at a bewildering rate. We have made up a list of the ones we have collected over the years, but it is far from complete.

References

In the previous edition we deliberately avoided references. This was to save space and reduce the cost of the book. Isolated hospitals commonly have difficulty obtaining journals. We have included references in this text, confining them mainly to articles from major journals. These articles have been chosen because they give a good up-to-date overview of the topic. Every fact is not referenced; however, where we feel we have departed from mainstream practice, or are dealing with new or controversial issues; we have documented the source.

Drugs

Drug schedules are continually revised, new side effects and hazards recognized and formulations changed. For this reason every reader is urged to consult the pharmaceutical company's printed instructions before administering any of the drugs recommended in this book.

Our Opinions

Medical knowledge is advancing rapidly. New ideas come, and concepts that have been worshipped as dogma for years are dropped. In an attempt to keep this edition simple, and practical; and the cost down, we have pruned and simplified the text. We have decided not to attempt to describe every disorder, but to devote most of the space usefully, to commonly encountered problems. This book is written forthrightly, and the opinions expressed are our own. We appreciate that there are many different points of view on what is, and what is not, the correct treatment of a particular clinical problem. This book tells the way we do it, and not everyone may agree. This book is a guide, not a rule book. It offers suggestions, not instructions. It is impossible to cover every clinical situation, and sometimes you will need common sense to modify treatment to fit the circumstances. Safety is our prime concern; if you have any doubts about what you are doing, we urge you to consult a colleague.

In medicine there are rarely absolutes; events and outcomes may, or may not happen. We have written this book to teach, and are purposely dogmatic. It is easier to remember that hypoxia is harmful, than hypoxia may be harmful under certain circumstances.

There are certain to be omissions of fact, and we would be grateful for suggestions on ways to improve this manual for a future edition.

Acknowledgements

We acknowledge thankfully all the people who have helped us, wittingly or unwittingly. Over the years we have accumulated notes, listened to presentations at conferences, read journals and texts, and absorbed large amounts of anecdotal data in operating theatre tea-rooms. Many of the sources of this information are lost, but to these our unknown teachers and advisers, we express our most grateful thanks.

Acknowledgements to the Second Edition

Peter McCall for reading the cardiac chapter. Peter Hatfield for reading the renal chapter. Ian Cobble for the information on fire safety.

Book Design and Illustrations

Inhouse Design Group Ltd., 4 Richbourne St., Auckland, New Zealand.

1. GOLDEN RULES

These rules were learned by experience. They seem simple, but it is attention to the simple things that improves patient care.

Ignorance can be lethal…
If you are in any doubt …ask somebody!

1. The confused, restless and agitated patient is hypoxic until proven otherwise.

There are many causes of confusion and agitation, but the most serious, hypoxia and hypoglycaemia irreversibly damage the brain within minutes. Initially, assume that all confusion and agitation is hypoxic; give oxygen and then look for other causes. Check diabetic and alcoholic patients' blood sugar when they are admitted to the recovery room. Never sedate or give analgesia to a confused patient until you are sure of the cause of the confusion.

2. Patients must never be left alone for any reason.

Patients can endanger themselves frighteningly fast. Unconscious patients may quickly and quietly suffocate. Conscious patients can fall off trolleys; or pull drips and drains out. Keep the trolley sides up, and use quick release restraining straps if need be.

3. The blood pressure does not necessarily fall in haemorrhagic shock.

With intense vasoconstriction, young people can compensate so well for a depleted blood volume that their blood pressure may not fall. Look for other signs of developing shock such as tachycardia, low urine output (less than 1 ml/kg/hour), and a poor perfusion status with cool hands.

4. Never ignore a tachycardia, find the cause.

A tachycardia is a non-specific warning sign that something is wrong. It is often accompanied by cool or cold hands. These are signs that the body's alarm mechanism, the sympathetic nervous system, has swung into action.

5. Postoperative hypertension is dangerous.

Blood oxygen saturations are often low following emergence from anaesthesia. Hypertension increases cardiac work and the heart's oxygen requirements; and a tachycardia reduces the time available for blood to flow through the coronary arteries. These three factors, hypertension, tachycardia and a low oxygen saturation combine to cause cellular hypoxia which may trigger arrhythmias, myocardial infarction or stroke. Monitor hypertensive patients with an ECG. Consider treating hypertension and tachycardia, particularly if arrhythmias occur.

6. Do not use a painful stimulus to rouse a patient.
If the pain of surgery will not rouse the patient from his coma, neither will applying a painful stimuli. The bruising caused by this sadistic manoeuvre may hurt for days. Furthermore, the pain may raise his blood pressure and pulse rate.

7. Noisy breathing is obstructed breathing; however, not all obstructed breathing is noisy.
No patient should snore in the recovery room, it is a sign of an obstructed airway. Although the obstruction is usually in the pharynx, it may be in the larynx or lower airway. If the patient has had an opioid drug he may not struggle against the obstruction, but stop breathing altogether. A patient with complete respiratory obstruction may move his chest up and down without moving air in or out.

8. Nurse comatose patients on their sides in the coma position.
Regrettably it is still common to see unconscious patients nursed on their backs. A wise old aphorism says that 'Those who look to heaven, are likely to go there'. Patients lying on their backs are at risk of upper airway obstruction. More insidiously, there is a risk of them silently aspirating material into their lower airways, and this predisposes to postoperative chest infections. Keep a high capacity sucker ready to aspirate secretions as soon as they form. Don't put the patient's head on a high pillow. Keep the head low so the saliva and mucus can drain downhill and out of the patient's mouth.

9. Let the patient take out his own airway.
It is an error to remove the pharyngeal airway before the patient is awake. He will always remove his own airway eventually, this demonstrates that he can co-ordinate his actions. A patient is unlikely to walk out of the hospital with his airway still in place. If the airway is removed too soon he may clench his jaws so tightly that it becomes impossible to reinsert it should it be needed. A patient with an unprotected airway is in danger of aspiration pneumonitis.

10. Patients must be able to lift their heads from the pillow, cough, and take deep breaths before being discharged from the recovery room.

Without doubt respiratory problems are the major cause of death in the immediate postoperative period. Inadequate breathing and ineffective coughing are the commonest cause of problems once the patient has returned to the ward. Following the use of muscle relaxants, a good test for the proper return of muscle power is to ask the patient to lift his head off the pillow for 5 seconds. The ability to cough confirms the patency of the upper and lower airway. Airway obstruction, or trunk pain, stops the patient coughing freely. During the cough you may hear a wheeze suggesting aspiration, asthma or cardiac failure. The ability to take a deep breath is a further test of respiratory fitness.

11. Treat the patient, not the monitor.

Many problems occur because staff believe what they see on the monitor, and ignore the clinical condition of the patient. If a patient looks cyanosed then he probably is, despite what the oximeter tells you. If the ECG shows a normal rhythm, and the non-invasive blood pressure is reporting a normal reading, but the patient appears to be hypotensive with poor perfusion, he probably is unstable. If a patient has a bradycardia, but is warm and well perfused with a good blood pressure, and appears to be clinically stable; he probably is. Do not treat the bradycardia.

12. The opioids do not cause a fall in blood pressure in stable patients.

Always look for another cause for hypotension. Occasionally opioids, particularly, pethidine, cause a small drop in blood pressure, but it is a mistake to assume that an opioid is the only cause of the hypotension. There is a risk of overlooking a more serious problem such as bleeding, cardiac failure, sepsis or hypoxia. Sometimes opioid analgesia is withheld because of the fear that it will drop the blood pressure. Even sick patients will tolerate small increments of morphine given slowly intravenously.

13. Pain prevention is easier than pain relief.

The emerging understanding of pain mechanisms has confirmed the clinical observation that preventing pain sensations reaching the brain is better than trying to relieve them once they have arrived. Use local anaesthesia where possible, and you will reap the benefits of decreased analgesic requirements and fewer distressed patients. Waking up in pain and without full control of his faculties is a horrible experience that reduces the patient's confidence in the nursing and medical staff.

14. Cuddle crying children.

Children waking from anaesthesia are often distressed, frightened, disoriented and in pain. Small children quickly respond to the warmth of a cuddle. It may not be possible to pick the child up, but touch is very reassuring. A toddler out of routine, is anxious and upset; but a toddler out of routine and in pain is inconsolable, and very, very angry. (see rule #13).

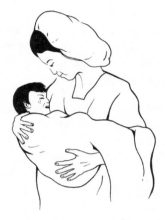

Fig 1.1 *Cuddle crying children*

15. Warm blood with an in-line blood warmer.

Blood is a living tissue transplant. Treat it with care, because the red cells can haemolyse, releasing haemoglobin into the circulation causing renal failure and coagulopathies. We have seen blood warmed in dangerous and bizarre ways: including a microwave oven, or slowly brought to body temperature by running under a tap or standing in a water bath.

16. Hypothermia is insidious and common.

Many patients will be cold on admission to the recovery room. This is a particular hazard in the very young, the elderly, or debilitated patient. It is responsible for a host of problems, including delayed recovery from anaesthesia, and poor tolerance of drugs. Do not discharge patients to the ward until their core temperature is above 36.5°C.

17. When giving drugs to the elderly, start by giving half as much, twice as slowly.

Although not an absolute rule, the sentiment behind this principle is a reminder that the elderly tolerate many drugs poorly. Benzodiazepines, and drugs used as anti-emetics such as the butyrephenones, and phenothiazines groups frequently have unpredictable and prolonged effects.

18. If you do not know the pharmacology of a drug, then do not give it.

In the recovery room drugs are usually given intravenously and adverse reactions are common. During the operation the patient will have received a number of different drugs, increasing the possibility of pharmacological interactions. Some of these interactions are obscure, and give rise to the temptation to use even more drugs to counteract their side effects. This may well make the problem even worse. Drug manufacturers produce detailed literature. Usually these are included in the packet with the drug, and are regularly updated with new facts. The correct dose of a drug is enough, and it is unwise to exceed the dose recommended by the manufacturer.

19. Thrombophlebitis is a sin, do not keep that IV in.

Painful, or inflamed veins are a potential hazard. Replace inflamed drips at another site with a new catheter, new giving set and fresh intravenous fluid. Insertion of drips is a sterile procedure. Wear gloves for the protection of both yourself and the patient.

20. If confused read rule #1.

Look after all patients as though they
are either your parents or your children.

2. ROUTINE RECOVERY ROOM PROCEDURES

This chapter follows the patient from the operating theatre, discusses his care in the recovery room and finally describes his discharge and transport to the ward.

PREPARATION BEFORE THE PATIENT'S ADMISSION

Make it a routine to check all equipment before receiving a patient. Fatalities can happen for lack of something simple like proper suction tubing, or because of a disconnected oxygen line.

Everything must be ready
before the patient comes from theatre.

At the beginning of each shift check that:
- the resuscitation trolley has been checked. Enter this fact in the trolley's maintenance book;
- the drug cupboard is restocked;
- disposable items have been replaced;
- sharps and rubbish containers are emptied and cleaned;
- suction bottles and tubing are clean and working;
- oxygen and suction supplies are adequate;
- a good supply of warm blankets and clean gowns is available;
- alarm bells are working.

Before each patient arrives check:
- a clean high capacity sucker is switched on and working;
- oxygen mask is connected and ready;
- if oxygen cylinders are being used then check there is sufficient oxygen in them;
- some means of assisting the patient's breathing, such as a Mapleson's C circuit, or an Ambu®, or Laerdal® bag with properly fitting mask is available;
- pulse oximeter is switched on and working;
- intravenous drip hangers are ready.

Transport to the Recovery Room

Moving the patient from the operating table to the special recovery room trolley requires skill and care. Lines, drains and monitors easily become disconnected at this stage.

Many hands make light work.

The anaesthetist, and a nurse must accompany the patient from the operating theatre to the recovery room.

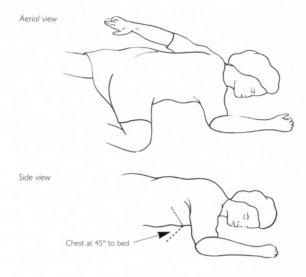

Fig 2.1 *Typical recovery position*

Wheel the patient from the operating theatre feet first. The anaesthetist walks forwards (never backwards) maintaining an airway. Generally the patient will lie in the left lateral or coma position.

Admission to the Recovery Room

This is a most important procedure because the responsibility for the immediate care of the patient is being handed from the medical staff to the recovery room nursing staff. (The medical staff still remain responsible for the overall medical care of the patient.) Both the anaesthetist and the nurse need to hand over separately, to a competent member of the recovery room staff.

Anaesthetic handover should include:
- checking the name of the patient against their notes and identity bracelet;
- age of the patient;
- significant medical conditions;
- procedure (this may differ from the scheduled operation) and the surgeon;
- details of vital signs: blood pressure, pulse, respiratory rate;
- untoward incidents during or before surgery;
- analgesia given and anticipated analgesic needs;
- blood loss;
- fluids given and future needs;
- antibiotics given, and when the next dose is due;
- urine output during the procedure, and expected output for the next few hours;
- the patient's anxiety level and preoperative psychological problems;
- monitoring required in the recovery room;
- investigations required.

The anaesthetist should also tell the nursing staff where he will be so that they may contact him quickly if the need arises. The anaesthetist should not be far away while the patient is still in the recovery room.

Maintain the patient's airway
during the handover.

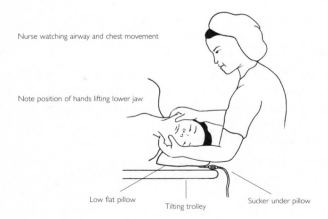

Nurse watching airway and chest movement

Note position of hands lifting lower jaw

Low flat pillow

Tilting trolley

Sucker under pillow

Fig 2.2 *Attention to the patient's airway*

Nursing staff handover includes:

- care and placement of drains;
- precautions about dressings;
- special nursing requirements, such as the position of the patient;
- nursing problems, such as pressure areas, and psychological status;
- organisation of the patient's notes;
- ensuring correct charts and x-rays accompany the patient;
- personal belongings, such as dentures and hearing aids.

Perceptions of Recovery Room

Staff perception of a patient's recovery

If still under the influence of the anaesthetic the airway will need support, and the pharynx and mouth kept clear of secretions. At this stage the patient may not respond to any stimuli. Plantar reflexes may not react, or if the patient is lightening will show an upgoing response, the pupils may not react to light. As the patient lightens, his gaze becomes divergent and the pupils constrict in reaction to light. A few moments before awakening pupils dilate and the patient starts to move his limbs and perhaps shiver or shake. His pulse and blood pressure often rise. He then usually takes a big breath; or sighs just before opening his eyes. Although awake the patient may have clouded consciousness for 5 to 10 minutes. He probably will have no memory of this stage.

Occasionally the patient is confused, restless, disoriented and possibly fearful. You will not be able to reason with him. This period of delirium, is sometimes called an *acute brain syndrome* (see page 153).

Exclude hypoxia and hypoglycaemia
as a cause of postoperative restlessness.

Patient's perception of their own recovery

Hearing is the first sense to return. Voices are very loud, distorted and sometimes frightening. Even the sound of a telephone ringing can be alarming. Lights seem unduly bright hurting the eyes. Vision is blurred. Arms and legs feel heavy. Pain may be unbelievable and is often described as the worst the patient has ever experienced. Finally sense of locality and memory return. The patient feels disoriented and giddy, and often asks 'Where am I?'

Visitors

Apart from mothers of children it is probably unwise to allow visitors to see patients who are recovering from anaesthesia. Visitors can become distressed if they see a loved one disoriented, vomiting, or in pain.

Initial Assessment

On admission to the recovery room immediately check in the following order the A,B,C,D and Es:

A = Airway

• Make sure the patient has a clear airway, is breathing and the air is moving freely and quietly in and out of the chest.
• If necessary gently suck out the patient's mouth and pharynx. If he is still unconscious make sure an oral airway is properly located between his teeth and tongue and lips are in no danger of being bitten.
• Administer oxygen with a mask. Begin with a flow rate of 6 litres of oxygen per minute. Attach a pulse oximeter.

B = Breathing

• Check his chest is moving and you can feel air flowing in and out of his mouth.
• Look for any sign of cyanosis and note the reading on the pulse oximeter. If it is reading less than 97%, then search for the reason. (See hypoxia page 324.)

C = Circulation

• Only then measure the blood pressure, pulse rate and rhythm and record these observations on the chart.
• Note his *perfusion status* (see page 236) and record this in the notes.

D = Drugs, Drips and Drains

• Note drugs given in theatre, particularly analgesics, that may affect the patient's breathing. Check whether the patient has any allergies, and what drugs he will require while in the recovery room.
• Note intravenous fluids in progress, how much fluid and what type have been given during the operation. Check that the drip is running freely, and is well sited. Make sure that no pieces of tape encircle the arm, replace these if necessary. Tape encircling the arm might cause distal ischaemia if the arm swells for any reason. Splint the infusion site if the cannula lies across the wrist or elbow joint.
• Note drain tubes; with what and how fast they are draining. Make sure the urinary catheter is not obstructed, note the contents of the collecting bag.

E = Extras
- If the patient is a diabetic measure his blood glucose or urinary sugars.
- Check the patient's history to see whether there are any risk factors that predispose to hypoglycaemia.
- Plaster checks.
- Check pulses following arterial surgery.
- Check circulation of graft sites.

CONTINUING CARE IN RECOVERY ROOM

Phases in Recovery[1]

Phase 1

The patient returns to consciousness with intact protective reflexes. (If this takes longer than 10 minutes then see page 152). He should be able to sustain a head lift for 5 seconds, deep breathe, and cough effectively.

Phase 2

During this phase the patient recovers the ability to think clearly and movement returns. At the end of this phase the patient can return to the ward.

Phase 3

At the end of this phase all the effects of the anaesthetic should be gone. It can take 48 hours or more before the patient feels 'normal' again.

Monitoring after Admission

Monitors have two functions, firstly to alert you to life-threatening situations, and secondly to allow you to more easily follow trends in the patient's physiological variables, such as blood pressure, pulse, and oxygenation.

Treat the patient not the monitor.

Blood pressure

Take the blood pressure on admission, then at 5 minute intervals for 15 minutes, and then every ten minutes thereafter. If a patient has had intravenous drugs measure the blood pressure more frequently. A non-invasive blood pressure (NBP) monitor is useful for patients with cardiovascular instability, following major blood or fluid loss, and in head injured patients. The NBP monitor is subject to errors, and is especially inaccurate if the pulse is irregular. Always check the first one or two readings with a manual blood pressure machine.

Pulse

Record the pulse rate, rhythm and volume. If the pulse rate is irregular, suspect an arrhythmia. The most common cause of an irregular pulse is sinus arrhythmia, a normal variation in young people where the pulse rises and falls with respiration. More insidious are atrial fibrillation or ventricular premature beats (see page 259).

If you detect an irregular pulse
monitor with an ECG.

Respiratory rate

Causes for a rising respiratory rate include sputum retention, developing heart failure rising temperature or a change in intracranial pressure. The commonest reason for a falling respiratory rate is opioid overdose.

Temperature

Put your hand on the patient's chest to gauge the temperature. If he feels hot, cold or is sweating, measure his temperature.

Pulse oximeter

All patients need access to this facility. If you only have one pulse oximeter, share it between patients.

ECG

Monitor with an ECG, any patient who is at risk of cardiac arrhythmias, or ischaemic heart disease. There is a list of major risk factors on page 385.

RECOVERY ROOM SCORING SYSTEMS

The recovery room records are a continuation of the anaesthetic record. It is better to keep them on the same chart, with the anaesthetic record on the left of the chart, and the recovery room record on the right side.

Many recovery rooms have a scoring system for assessing, and monitoring their patients' and to ensure they are safe and comfortable for discharge. For analysis data can be entered on a standard spread sheet computer program and presented every month at the recovery room meeting. There have been many different proposed scoring systems, however the one shown below is useful. With some score systems the patient can be hypertensive, hypoxic and at risk of myocardial infarction or ischaemia, yet scored as fit for discharge from the recovery room.

In using these scores consider two separate issues. Firstly, is the patient safe to discharge from the recovery room; and secondly is he comfortable?

PATIENT ADMISSION ASSESSMENT

SAFETY CRITERIA

Respiration	0	Needs assisted ventilation.
	1	Laboured or > 20 or < 10 breaths/minute.
	2	Normal rate 12–15 breaths/minute. Can take deep breaths and cough.
Perfusion	0	Cyanotic or dusky colour.
	1	Pale with cold hands.
	2	Warm and pink.
Power	0	Unable to lift head or move limbs on command.
	1	Moves limbs but unable to sustain head lift.
	2	Sustains head lift for full 5 seconds.
Circulation	0	Blood pressure increased or decreased by 50% of preoperative level; or pulse >150 or <45.
	1	Blood pressure 20% above or below preoperative level.
	2	Stable blood pressure and pulse with no significant changes for 3 sets of quarter hourly readings.
Sedation	0	Does not respond to shaking by shoulder.
	1	Rouses only on stimulation.
	2	Awake communicating and seldom drowses.
Temperature	0	Axillary temperature < 35°C.
	1	Axillary temperature 35–36°C.
	2	Axillary temperature > 36°C.

Score out of 12

COMFORT CRITERIA

Nausea	0	Nauseated and vomiting.
	1	Nauseated only.
	2	Neither nauseated nor vomiting.
Pain	0	Severe distressing pain.
	1	Uncomfortable.
	2	Pain free.

Score out of 4

These scores are simple to use and they provide objective evidence on which to base quality assessment and educational programs. They enable statistics to be gathered, workloads assessed, and staff deployed for maximum efficiency. The use of a scoring system is good for the morale of the recovery room staff. It gives them feedback on specific areas of their work, and makes potential problems more easily defined. For instance, any patient who does not score at least 10 out of 12 within the first 30 minutes should be reported to the anaesthetist.

PROCEDURES

Stir-up Exercises for the Emerging Patient

Once the patient is awake encourage him to do a number of simple exercises to reduce the chance of postoperative pneumonia and deep vein thrombosis. The exercises are sometimes referred to as *stir-up exercises*.

Deep breathing exercises

The aim is to inflate segments of lung that inevitably collapse during general anaesthesia. Encourage the patient to take 2–3 very deep breaths every 5 minutes.

Coughing exercises

These clear the airways of mucus and dried secretions. Sit the patient up if possible. If he has an abdominal wound, then show him how to hold it when he coughs. Coughing exercises must not be done after open eye, middle ear, intracranial, facial or plastic surgery.

Leg exercises

These prevent a deep vein thrombosis forming. Get the patient to move their feet up and down, and to bend their legs at the knees. Fit anti-embolic stockings to patients at risk from thromboembolism.

Most deep vein thrombosis
starts in the recovery room.

Pressure Care

Check the patient's body for pressure areas. Make sure the patient is lying on a soft smooth surface. If areas of redness are still present when the patient is ready to leave recovery room, point them out to the ward staff. Do not rub red areas, they are already traumatized enough, just pad them, and remove the weight from the area.

Beware of red areas in elderly,
thin and malnourished patients.

Suction

Pharyngeal suction

Keep a high flow, high capacity suction under each patient's pillow. Unconscious patients are unable to cope with their secretions and need to be nursed in the standard coma position.

If necessary clear the mouth and pharynx with a dental sucker. Do not force the sucker between the teeth or you may damage the delicate mucosal lining of the mouth and pharynx, dislodge restorative dental caps or loose teeth. If the sucker touches the posterior pharyngeal wall or the soft palate, it can make the patient gag or vomit. Patients recovering from a halothane or enflurane anaesthetic sometimes clench their teeth tightly making it difficult to pass the sucker into their mouth. In these cases pass a soft 16 G plastic Y-suction catheter down along the floor of their nose into their pharynx. Remember the floor of the nose runs straight back, and not upwards. Frequently the patient will respond by tossing his head from side to side, and opening his mouth enabling you to insert an oropharyngeal airway.

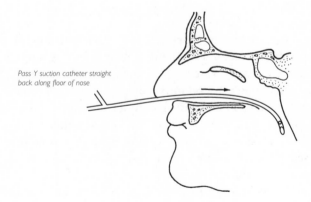

Pass Y suction catheter straight back along floor of nose

Fig 2.3 *Transnasal suction of nasopharynx*

Tracheobronchial suction[2] (*sucking out*)

Occasionally patients are intubated or have a tracheostomy when they return to the recovery room. Their endotracheal tubes need to be aspirated at intervals to clear the accumulating sputum. Smokers produce more sputum than a normal patient, and need more nursing care.

Excessive mucus in the airways can be heard as a harsh rattling sound during breathing. This is a sign the patient requires sucking out. Palpation of the chest will reveal a coarse vibration as air gurgles past the mucus in the trachea or major bronchi.

Suction is not necessary in every patient.

USEFUL TIPS

- To obtund the violent responses and patient distress to this unpleasant procedure use 1% lignocaine 0.1 ml/kg down the tracheal tube, and repeat after one minute.
- Explain to the patient what is to happen.
- For unstable patients get an assistant to help you.
- Pre-oxygenate on 100% oxygen for at least a minute.
- It is a sterile procedure, so wear gloves.
- Hold your own breath while you a sucking the patient out to remind you how long the patient is holding his breath.
- Gently and slowly withdraw the catheter, watching for secretions.
- If the sputum is tenacious, try instilling 2–3 ml of 0.9% saline down the tube.
- Turning the head to one side often allows the sucker to go down the opposite bronchus.

Tracheobronchial suction is not a procedure to be undertaken lightly. It is distressing and painful for an awake patient, similar to having a lump of food 'go down the wrong way'. Vigorous coughing sharply raises the blood pressure, intracranial pressure, and intraocular pressure, and causes venous congestion in the head and neck. Hypoxia is a constant risk; reflex bradycardia or tachycardia can occur. A dangerous, and sometimes fatal, decrease in intrathoracic pressure can rupture lung tissue if too large a suction catheter is used. Take care to use a catheter that is less than half the diameter of the lumen of the endotracheal tube[3].

Many patients who have heart disease, with unstable circulations, are at risk from arrhythmias and hypoxia. To prevent endotracheal suction causing a sharp rise in blood pressure, with the risk of aggravating bleeding, or causing other complications, instill lignocaine 1 mg/kg down the endotracheal tube. Similarly, use lignocaine in patients with the following risk factors:
- head injury;
- eye surgery;

- ear surgery;
- neurosurgery;
- plastic surgery on the head or neck;
- hypertension;
- ischaemic heart disease.

Intubated Patients

Occasionally the anaesthetist will bring a patient to the recovery room still intubated. Reasons for this include, a prolonged operation, poor respiratory function, elderly patients, sicker patients, difficulty reversing the muscle relaxants, hypothermia. Usually these patients will be extubated in the recovery room before they are returned to the ward. They may or may not need ventilating during this period.

Extubation[4]

TEN STEPS IN EXTUBATION

1. Put the patient on high inspired concentration of oxygen for 3 minutes before proceeding. Bring the resuscitation trolley to the bedside. Attach a pulse oximeter and an ECG.
2. Check the pharynx with a laryngoscope making sure there is no foreign material, such as a throat pack present, if so remove it.
3. Under direct vision suck out the pharynx to remove all secretions and blood. Remember to check the nasopharynx behind and above the soft palate for blood clot, secretions and foreign material. A clot forming in the nasopharynx cannot be seen by merely looking in the pharynx. In the past these clots have fallen into the larynx, or have been aspirated into the trachea obstructing it suddenly. It may be the coroner who finds this on post mortem, hence its name.
4. Lay the patient on his left side.
5. Remove the ties and tapes securing the endotracheal tube, and deflate the cuff slowly with a 20 ml syringe.
6. Disconnect the catheter mount. If the patient has audible secretions in their chest pass a soft suction catheter down the endotracheal tube. While applying suction ask the patient to take a big breath in. At the end of inspiration with one smooth movement withdraw the tube together with the suction catheter. The patient will now have a lung full of air and will cough.
7. Put the patient on an oxygen mask with a 6 litre per minute flow.
8. Encourage a few deep breaths and coughs to reassure both the patient and yourself.
9. Watch the oximeter to check the patient's saturation remains good.
10. Watch for signs of postoperative hypoxia or hypercarbia. Encourage the patient to deep breathe and cough.

About 5 per cent of patients will require extubation in the recovery room. Before this can be safely performed the patient must fulfil three criteria.
1. They must be able to breath adequately.
2. They must not be unduly depressed by narcotic drugs.
3. They must be able to protect their own airway against accidental aspiration of material in the pharynx.

1. Can the patient breathe adequately?
    It is probably safe to extubate:
- If the patient has normal lungs and can take deep breaths on command through the endotracheal tube;
- If you are uncertain whether the tidal volume is adequate, measure it for one minute with a Dragermeter®, or Wright's Respirometer®. Before extubation the patient's tidal volume needs to be 5–7 ml/kg with a respiratory rate greater than 10 breaths per minute;
- If you do not have either of these instruments, then prime an anaesthetic machine with oxygen and attach the patient. When the patient takes a deep breath the black reservoir bag should deflate by 800 ml or more. To gauge the volume it is useful to remember the volume of a normal adult clenched fist is about 350–400 ml.

2. Is the patient unduly depressed by narcotic drugs or are their lungs affected in other ways?
- Attach the patient to a 'T-piece' and observe their ventilatory rate. If it is less than 8 breaths per minute do not attempt extubation. If it is less than 5 breaths a minute, then assist the patient's breathing and assume that his respiration is depressed by narcotics. Unless the patient is distressed, delay extubation if the arterial PCO_2 is greater than 50 mmHg (6.6 kPa) or the arterial PO_2 is less than 100 mmHg (13 kPa) while breathing 35% oxygen.
- The oxygen saturation meter can help you make a decision about whether the PaO_2 is high enough to extubate the patient. See the table on page 389.

3. Can the patient protect his own airway?
- Unless the patient is fully conscious it is unwise to extubate the patient if there is a suspicion that he may have a full stomach.
- Delay extubation until the patient is conscious if the intubation was difficult, or the patient has an abnormal upper airway.
- Do not extubate a patient, unless, on command, he can sustain a 5 second head lift from the pillow; and touch the tip of his nose with his finger.

• If a restless patient is co-ordinated enough to reach up and grab his own endotracheal tube, he will be conscious enough to guard his airway.

DISCHARGE AND TRANSPORT

Length of Stay in the Recovery Room

Adults

Ideally patients stay in the recovery room for at least an hour after general anaesthesia and half an hour after local anaesthesia. Each hospital has its own protocols, but the following guidelines are widely accepted. Patients with regional anaesthetic blocks, such as spinal and epidural anaesthesia stay at least an hour after the blood pressure becomes stable. Patients stay 30 minutes after an intramuscular dose of opioid.

Children

Observe healthy children for at least 30 minutes if they have received inhalational anaesthesia by mask or laryngeal mask. Observe healthy children who have been intubated for at least an hour, because laryngeal oedema may take this long to become obvious. Following tonsillectomy, adenoidectomy, cleft palate repair, pharyngeal or other major intra-oral procedures observe the patient for at least 90 minutes. Infants less than 12 months of age, and those who have received naloxone are best observed for a minimum of two hours.

The anaesthetist, or a member of the medical staff, should review the patient's status before discharge, and make an appropriate note on the patient's chart. The anaesthetist must be certain that the patient is safe to leave his immediate care, and that some other member of the medical staff is available, and properly instructed, to take over responsibility for the patient's welfare.

Discharge to the Ward

1. Minimum criteria for discharge to the ward are:
   • the patient has a stable pulse rate, rhythm and blood pressure;
   • the patient is conscious and able to lift head clear of the pillow on demand;
   • the patient is able to take a deep breath on command;
   • the patient is able to touch tip of his nose with his forefinger;
   • pain has been relieved;
   • there is no excessive loss from drains or bleeding from wound sites;
   • observation charts are completed;
   • patient is clean, dry, warm and comfortable.

2. Remove all unnecessary intravenous lines.
3. Remove ECG dots, and check the diathermy pad is not still attached.
4. Check that the medical and nursing staff have completed all the charts and notes and send them back to the ward with the patient.
5. Ensure the patient's recovery room record is. clear and concise. The ward staff will need an accurate record to quickly identify any deterioration.
6. Allow thirty minutes to elapse between the last dose of analgesia and the patient's discharge from the recovery room.

PROTOCOL
CARE OF THE PATIENT AFTER SPINAL ANAESTHESIA

OBSERVATIONS
Standard post-anaesthetic observations.
Sensation should return within 4 hours. If after 4 hours the patient remains numb, and there is no 'pins-and-needles' sensation, notify the anaesthetist.

ANALGESIA
Severe pain may return suddenly once the spinal block has worn off. Give analgesia at the first complaint of pain.

FASTING
Fasting is not necessary unless it is a surgical requirement, such as after abdominal operations.

POSTURE
It is not necessary to lie the patient flat for 24 hours. The patient should be able to sit up as soon as the analgesia has worn off.

AMBULATION
If not surgically contraindicated the patient may get out of bed 2 hours after the return of normal sensation, but only with assistance. Before getting the patient out of bed sit him up slowly, and check his blood pressure. If the systolic blood pressure falls more than 20 mmHg, or if the patient feels faint, dizzy or nauseated, then lie the patient down, and notify the anaesthetist.

POTENTIAL COMPLICATIONS

POSTURAL HYPOTENSION
Lie the patient in bed, and notify the anaesthetic registrar on duty who will increase the fluid intake, or will order vasopressors.

URINARY RETENTION
Encourage the patient to void when sensation returns. If the patient has not voided within 4 hours, or his bladder can be palpated, he will require a catheter.

Please report any abnormalities
or concerns to the anaesthetist immediately

Fig 2.4 Example of postoperative care protocol that would accompany the patient to the ward.

Handover to Ward Staff

The recovery room staff must be certain that the ward nurse understands the patient's problems, and is willing and competent to accept responsibility for the patient's care. This fact should be noted on the patient's chart.

Transport

A nurse and an orderly should always accompany the patient when they return to the ward. Every trolley needs to carry portable oxygen and suction. Good combination units are commercially available. Keep an emergency box containing a self-inflating resuscitation bag, airways and a range of masks on the trolley.

Transport patients facing forward and semi-sitting.

Discharge to the Intensive Care Unit

If the patient is going to the intensive care unit send for the bed, and check it has the following equipment with it:
• a full cylinder of oxygen with flow meter;
• a portable battery powered ECG monitor and defibrillator;
• a pulse oximeter;
• suction;
• emergency drugs, syringes, and needles in a closed sealed carrying box;
• an anaesthetist, or member of the medical staff, should accompany patients returning to the intensive care unit.

If recovery rooms are properly staffed and equipped sick patients can be held overnight instead of discharging them to intensive care. This may be an economical option.

Patients who need admission to intensive care postoperatively include:
• those who are already in ICU but are having an operative procedure, such as a tracheostomy;
• those patients having uncomplicated surgery, but with severe intercurrent medical conditions, such as diabetes, myasthenia gravis or unstable angina;
• those patients having a big operation, such as oesophagogastrectomy, liver or pancreatic surgery or prolonged plastic surgery;
• those patients where it may be reasonably anticipated that complications

will arise, such as the head injured multiple trauma patient who is unable to protect his airway.

It is better to plan an elective admission to the intensive care unit, than to attempt an operation and find that the patient is too unstable to transfer back to the ordinary surgical ward. This is largely a matter of common sense, and a properly run audit will identify potential problems.

1. Adams A. P. (1994). *Recent Advances in Anaesthesia and Analgesia,* 18: 123-43. Published; Churchill Livingstone, London, England.
2. Voss T. J. (1994). *Australian Anaesthesia 1994,* pp115-25. Published by Australian and New Zealand College of Anaesthetists, Melbourne, Australia.
3. Rosen M., Hillard E. K. (1960). *British Journal of Anaesthesia,* 32: 486-504
4. Hartley H., Vaughan R. S. (1993). *British Journal of Anaesthesia,* 71: 561-8

3. DRAINS AND CATHETERS

DRAINS

Surgical drains allow body secretions and tissue debris to flow away from the surgical site, where, if they accumulated they could:
- become contaminated with bacteria and be a source of infection;
- distend hollow cavities; and tear the sutures;
- allow secretions, such as pancreatic juice, to accumulate and delay healing;
- exert undesirable pressure, for example in the pericardial sac, pleura, or inside the skull.

Principles of Care

- Fluids drain with gravity, so keep the collecting containers below the level of the patient at all times.
- Do not apply high pressure suction to any drain; not even for a moment.

A routine drain check includes patency of the tubing, the amount of drainage, the colour of the drainage, and its character.

The main types of drains are:
1. Simple drains that are open to the dressings.
2. Closed drains that flow into a container.
3. Sump drains
4. Pleural drains

1. Simple drains

Examples of the open type are: Yates, Penrose, corrugated rubber, wicks, and ribbon drains. Simple drains are usually covered by a pad. Once the pad becomes soaked, replace it. If the loss becomes excessive tell the surgeon. To prevent bacterial contamination keep the outside of the pad dry.

2. Closed drains

Examples of the closed type are free drainage tubes and vacuum suction tubes. Commercially available ones include Redivac®, Manovac® or Haemovac®. Vacuum drains must have their concertinas collapsed to function correctly.

3. Sump drains

A *sump drain* is sometimes used in bowel surgery. It consists of two tubes one used to flush the wound, and one to remove fluid, clots and debris. Low pressure continuous suction can be applied to drains from special suction devices. Do not attach them to high pressure suction inlets on the wall suction, because serious tissue damage can occur.

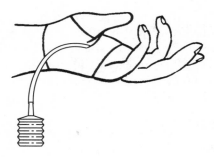

Fig 3.1 Concertina drain

4. Pleural drains[1]

Pleural drains remove fluid, or air from the pleural space, and allow low pressure, low flow suction to be applied to aid re-expansion of the lung; but special safeguards have to be used to avoid accidental damage to the lungs, or to prevent a pneumothorax occurring.

Following cardiothoracic surgery two chest tubes are often used. One is placed high and anteriorly within the thoracic cavity to drain air, and the other low and posteriorly to drain fluid. Do not use Y-connector links tubes when fluid is being drained from two or more tubes; because it makes it difficult to account for, and localize excessive drainage. You can use a Y-connector if one of the drains is primarily for air and the other for fluid. This minimizes the number of bottles around the bedside.

Pleural drains, sometimes, have to be inserted as an urgent procedure. Keep a sterile thoracic drainage tray set up ready.

There are three forms of closed chest drainage:
• water seal (one bottle) drainage;
• water seal (two bottle) drainage;
• suction (three bottle) drainage.

While these glass bottle systems are a bit cumbersome they are effective, and it is easy to see how they work. Once you understand the principles, you can apply them to set up any of the commercially available disposable plastic systems. They all work on the principle of either, water seal, or suction drainage.

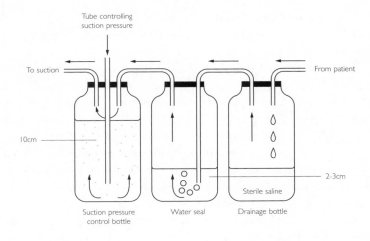

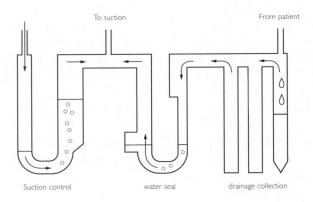

Fig 3.2 *Set up for continuous three bottle low pressure drainage of the thoracic cavity. Notice how the prinicple of the three bottle drainage is incorporated into a modern plastic drainage system molded to form three chambers*

Water seal drainage. One bottle acts as a trap to collect pleural fluid. This is kept sterile. It is connected to an underwater tube which allows air to escape whenever the pressure within the chest and the trap rises above one or two centimetres of water pressure, but prevents air leaking into the system whenever the pressure falls.

Keep the stoppers tightly secured in their bottles. Check the tips of the long glass tubes (straws) are 2-3 cm below the fluid surface. Make sure the short glass straw is not obstructed, and is serving properly as an air vent.

Note that without suction, bubbles from a pleural air leak occur only during expiration, or when the patient coughs, but with suction it occurs continuously.

Suction drainage exerts a continuous negative pressure. It is the most common form of drainage used. The first bottle acts as a trap for pleural fluids. If the tube entering it from the pleural space is just below the fluid level in the trap it will detect any air leak. The first bottle serves as a water seal, in case the system is disconnected from the source of suction.

The centre bottle acts as a break in the system. It allows air to enter if the suction pressure exceeds a set limit. This pressure limit is determined by depth the tip of the centre straw extends below the surface of the liquid. The third bottle serves as a fluid trap.

Make sure the level of water in the tube swings with respiration. It may bubble at first, but once the air is removed from the pleural space, and the lung is fully expanded the bubbling will stop. The glass tube in the suction control bottle is usually 10 cm below the fluid level, but it may be increased to 20 cm or more should the surgeon require stronger suction. If the suction pump stops or becomes disconnected the system reverts to a gravity drainage system. If this occurs pressure will build up in the system unless it is able to vent to the air. If the pump fails, disconnect the tube leading to it so the system can vent to the air.

If the patient is moved, clamp the tubes first. Do not leave the tubes clamped. Do not lift the bottles above the level of the bed without first clamping the tubing, or fluid will run back into the chest. Do not clamp the drains if the patient is being ventilated, because of the risk of a tension pneumothorax. Two rubber tipped clamps should accompany the patient to the ward; this precaution is taken in case the water seals become disconnected during transport.

Never *milk* pleural drains with a roller clamp. These archaic devices generate enormous pressures, and can damage lungs tissue. Avoid dependent loops in the tubes, because fluid will collect in the loops and interfere with the drainage.

Secure the tubing to the bed, leaving plenty of slack, to prevent it being accidentally pulled out. A large rubber band attached to a strong safety pin is useful for this purpose. Whenever the patient is moved check the security of the tubing, and make sure the patient is not lying on it. To stop the tube kinking as it comes out of the drain bottle, it is sometimes helpful to tape a small tongue depressor to the point where it goes through the rubber stopper.

EMERGENCY INSERTION OF A PLEURAL DRAIN

The commonest reason to insert a pleural drain in the recovery room is to manage a pneumothorax, if it exceeds 20% of the pleural volume; or if the patient is dyspnoeic with a pneumothorax that is less than 20% as may be the case in a patient with emphysema.

If the patient is not in danger, get an erect chest x-ray before proceeding. Keep the film where you can see it as you insert the catheter.

Distrust anything other than an erect chest x-ray,
when assessing a pneumo- or haemothorax.

Check the side is correct, and that there are no underlying abnormalities. Use intercostal catheters (Argyle®) size 20 G, 22 G, for draining gas, and 32 G for draining fluid or blood. Use the size 16 G in prepubertal children.

Have the erect chest x-ray on view when inserting intercostal catheters.

THE AXILLARY APPROACH
This is preferable for draining fluid and air collections. Using pillows or towels to lie the patient comfortably in a supine position, but slightly on their side. The catheter is inserted in the 4th or 5th intercostal space, just posterior to the midaxillary line just above the rib.

THE ANTERIOR APPROACH
Here the catheter is inserted in the second intercostal space just lateral to the midclavicular line. Have the patient sitting comfortably in bed propped up at 45° on three or four pillows. Use ample local anaesthetic.

Use blunt dissection when inserting intercostal catheters.

CAUTIONS
Never insert an axillary catheter, unless you have previously detected air or fluid with a small 19 G aspirating needle.

• To avoid damaging the heart, never angle the catheter anteromedially when inserting it on the left side.
• Never insert a catheter anterior to the mid-axillary line.
• Always check the size and site of the heart shadow.
• To avoid damage to the liver or spleen, never go below the level of 6th intercostal space in the mid axillary line.
• Never push hard to pass the trocar through the thoracic wall. If you are pushing then your technique is wrong. Use gentle blunt dissection to find your way through the tissue planes and follow the hole you have made with the catheter. Enlarge the hole with your finger.

UNEXPECTED HAEMORRHAGE
A serious error is to go too low, or anterior to the mid-axillary line. If by mischance, you enter the heart, or the great vessels with the trocar, and blood gushes out from the catheter, clamp the catheter. Do not attempt to take the catheter out. Call a thoracic surgeon, and lots of help as quickly as possible. Set up for a massive blood transfusion.

Chest drains are painful when the patient deep breathes or coughs. Give effective analgesia, preferably with intercostal or paravertebral blocks, or a thoracic epidural. Intrapleural analgesia does not work as well as might be expected.

Nasogastric Tubes

Nasogastric tubes stop the stomach from distending with gas or fluid. They are used after bowel surgery, or whenever it is thought the patient might develop a paralytic ileus. Take care not to displace them. In some operations (such as after an oesphagectomy or gastrectomy) the nasogastric tube lies across the surgical suture lines. This is to prevent distension of the bowel that would tear the stitches. If the nasogastric tube is accidentally pulled out, it is impossible to reinsert it safely. Some anaesthetists suture them into the frenulum of the nose so that they cannot be accidentally pulled out. In any case nasogastric tubes should be guarded well, and firmly taped into position.

Check with the surgeon, whether to clamp them, or leave them on free drainage.

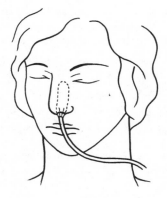

Fig 3.3 Fastening of nasogastric tubes

Aspirate nasogastric tubes gently. Do not suck hard with a syringe, because the soft mucosal folds of the stomach will wrap around the tip of the tube. If nothing comes back after gentle suction on the tube, blow 10-20 ml of air down it to free the tip from the folds of the fragile gastric mucosa, and attempt to aspirate gently again. If there is still no aspirate then the stomach is probably empty. Do not kink off the tube to prevent air going down to the stomach. Air will not rush down the tube to fill up the stomach.

Never aspirate nasogastric tubes using the unmodified suction from the wall suction point, because it will severely damage the delicate mucosa making it bleed.

Before the patient leaves the recovery room, check inside his mouth to make sure the nasogastric tube is not coiled up there, or in his pharynx. Check there are written orders for the nursing staff in the ward about the care of the tube.

URINARY CATHETERS

If the patient already has a urinary catheter in when they arrive in the recovery room then check that:
• urine flows freely;
• the bladder is not distended;
• the male foreskin is covering the tip of the penis;
and record the urine output.

Urinary catheters are prophylactically inserted:
• after surgery or trauma;
• before pelvic surgery;
• to measure urine output accurately;
• to distinguish between retention and anuria;
• to manage shock, and impending renal failure;
• to provide access to the bladder;
• in patients who have epidural catheters for pain relief.

HINTS FOR INSERTION OF URINARY CATHETERS

1. Use plenty of lignocaine lubricating gel.
2. Small catheters sometimes buckle in the urethra, try a larger one.
3. Do not try to force the insertion of a urinary catheter, the urethra is easily damaged. If you have difficulty call for expert help.

Males insert the catheter all the way to the Y- junction before inflating the balloon, then pull back gently. The catheter will have the volume needed to inflate the balloon printed on it. Replace the foreskin over the tip of the penis, otherwise it may form a constrictive band (a paraphimosis) around the penis. This causes pain, and can be difficult to pull down at a later time.

Females check the catheter actually enters the urethra, and not the vagina.

Catheter Care
• Connect the catheter to a closed sterile collecting system.

- Strap the catheter over (not under) the patient's thigh to minimize the risk of faecal soiling.
- Do not strap the catheter to the bed or the bed linen.
    If urine will not flow:
- Try pressing gently on the suprapubic area.
- The catheter may not be in far enough or be wrongly positioned.
- The catheter may be blocked. Irrigate it gently with saline using a 50 ml syringe.
- Check the bladder is empty by palpating above the pubic symphysis. If it is empty, irrigate the catheter with 50 ml of sterile saline; all this saline should come back again. If the saline goes in, but does not return, the catheter is either blocked, or not in the bladder.

Blocked Catheters

Patients who have had bladder surgery will pass clots through the catheter. Gently milk the tube from time to time to ensure free flow. If the catheter seems to be blocked by clots, take a 60 ml syringe, and using a sterile technique wash it out with water or saline. Gently instil 30 ml then ask the patient if he is in pain. Pain is a sign of an over-filled bladder. Aspirate, if this is successful instil 30 ml quickly and aspirate. Repeat this several times to break up the clots. If you are unsuccessful in relieving the obstruction call the surgeon.

Continuous Irrigation

This is a technique for washing out the bladder, to stop clots forming. Make sure fluid is continuously draining out, and the bladder is not distended. If the outlet is blocked with clots, and fluid continues to go in, there is danger of rupturing the bladder or disrupting the surgery.

Suprapubic Catheterization

It may be necessary to insert a suprapubic catheter if urethral catheterization is unsuccessful; or is contraindicated. Use an Argyle® or Ingram® 12–16 F trocar catheter, or an equivalent. A suprapubic catheter is safer for the patient if there is any suggestion of urethral stricture.
    Contraindications to suprapubic catheters are:
- a bladder that is not easy to define by palpation or percussion;
- a lower midline abdominal scar warning of the danger of puncturing adherent bowel.

1. Kam A. C. O'Brien M. *et al.* (1993) *Anaesthesia*, 48: 154-61

4. INFECTION CONTROL

INFECTIONS AND YOU

While AIDS is on everyone's mind, the chance of transmission of HIV from an HIV positive patient by needlestick injury appears to be about 1:200–400. The risk of contracting one of the hepatitis viruses is much greater. The risk of transmission to non-immune staff after accidental needle stick injury with a hepatitis B contaminated needle carries a 3–35 per cent risk of infection. Everyone working in the recovery room should be immunized against Hepatitis B with the safe and effective genetically engineered vaccine. Five to ten per cent of recipients of the vaccine do not develop protective antibodies after the completion of the course, and remain at risk. Test for Hepatitis B antibody two months after completion of the initial three dose course. Repeat the course if needed. At this time there is no vaccine for Hepatitis C.

If you are ill stay at home until you are better. Do not come to work with a cold, influenza or other infectious diseases. The fact that you are sick testifies to the virulence of the organism. Patients recovering from anaesthesia are particularly likely to catch airborne viruses that can cause major complications such as pneumonia. You may also infect other staff. One person with a cold who spreads it around can cause havoc with the rosters.

If you are sick
stay at home.

Working in the recovery room demands concentration and vigilance. Ill people cannot perform their jobs properly, and are more likely to make mistakes.

UNIVERSAL PRECAUTIONS

With the advent of AIDS and the growing prevalence of the Hepatitis B and C and its newly discovered cousins Hepatitis D and E all of which are most unpleasant, every recovery room should have written protocols for infection control. The aim is to minimize hospital cross infection and the risk of patients or staff acquiring Hepatitis or HIV.

All patients are potentially infectious.

Some patients carry diseases such as HIV, viral hepatitis, or TB but have no symptoms or signs of the disease. It is impracticable to test every patient for these diseases, and furthermore there is an inevitable delay in laboratory processing and reporting. Some common illness not considered to be dangerous may in fact be so, for instance, pneumonia that turns out to be open tuberculosis. For these reasons many hospitals have adopted the principle that *all patients are potentially carrying an infectious disease and have adopted Universal Precautions* to prevent their transmission.

Universal precautions include

1. Handwashing. Wash your hands after any patient contact to remove transient surface organisms. Make this a habit.
2. Gloves. Use gloves if you anticipate contact with blood or body secretions. Dispose of them after use.
3. Gowns. Plastic aprons and goggles are recommended if you anticipate that blood or other body secretions are likely to splash on to your face or clothing.
4. Place soiled linen in leak proof bags for transport and disposal. If the outside of the bag becomes moist with blood or faeces place it inside a big stout plastic bag for transport. Clearly label this linen as infectious.
5. Treat all waste contaminated with blood or body secretions as potentially infectious.
6. Tightly seal specimens for laboratory investigations in stout containers to prevent leakage during transport.
7. Do not share items for individual use among patients. This includes inhalers, creams and ointments.
8. Cleaning. Routine cleaning with neutral detergent is sufficient to make surfaces microbiologically safe. Wipe up spills as soon as they occur.
   - wear gloves;
   - mop up the bulk of the spill using absorbent towel;
   - apply hypochlorite (5000 ppm) and leave to dry for 5 minutes;
   - rinse off with clean water and leave to dry;
9. Avoid injury from contaminated sharps.
   - do not recap needles;
   - do not remove needles from syringes, discard them in one piece;
   - discard all sharps into sharps containers;
   - do not leave sharps in the drapes;
   - never pass an unguarded needle to another person;
   - ensure that others cannot be jabbed at any stage while assisting you, cleaning up afterwards or transporting the sharps;

Table 4.1

SOURCES OF INFECTION

POTENTIALLY INFECTIOUS BODY FLUIDS

MAJOR:
- blood;
- serous ooze;
- pus;
- faeces;
- sputum;
- saliva.

MINOR:
- urine;
- nasal secretions;
- gastric secretions;
- peritoneal dialysis fluid;
- ascitic fluid;
- pleural and pericardial fluid.

POTENTIALLY INFECTIOUS BODY SITES.

MAJOR:
- wounds;
- skin lesions;
- drainage sites;
- perianal area.

MINOR:
- nasal passages;
- mouth;
- intravascular access sites.

STAFF EXPOSED TO CONTAMINATION WITH POTENTIAL PATHOGENS

Report all injuries or accidents involving blood or blood-stained body fluids. Each hospital will need to develop a policy of how to manage and counsel staff who have had a needlestick injury, or accidental exposure to potentially contaminated substances.

If a member of the staff has been exposed to blood-borne pathogens:
- Wash the affected area well with soap and water.
- If the eyes are contaminated rinse gently with normal saline while the eyes are open.
- If blood gets in the mouth, spit it out and then rinse the mouth with water several times.
- Apply an antiseptic solution such as 0.5% chlorhexidine in 70% alcohol, or a povidone iodine solution such as Betadine® to skin wounds. Do not use these solutions on mucosal surfaces or the eyes.
- Seek immediate medical attention. Decisions about treatment options need to be made within two hours of exposure.

Do not recap needles.

Principles for Preventing Cross Infection

1. Set up an Infection Subcommittee as part of the organization of your operating theatres. Its duty is to set standards, and write protocols for the prevention of cross infection.
2. Every one in recovery room needs proper protective clothing. Staff should not wear street dress, or their normal uniforms while attending patients.
3. When working in the recovery room do not wear wedding rings, and hand jewellery.
4. Design the recovery room to prevent dust from accumulating. Keep your recovery room as tidy as possible. Do not use it as a general storage area for bulky equipment. Put these things away somewhere else.
5. Keep to a regular cleaning schedule.
6. Place contaminated material in leak-proof sealed containers which must be removed at scheduled intervals, and not just when they are full.
7. The most important point for the prevention of cross infection is proper hand washing. Use liquid soap from squirt containers. Do not use bar soap. Wet bar soap is a good growing medium for some bacteria. Use disposable, preferably paper, towels. Hot-air hand driers are noisy and slow and blow skin squames and dust into the air. They are not suitable for recovery room.

> *Germs don't fly—they hitch hike.*
> *Wash your hands properly before,*
> *and after touching a patient.*

8. Disposable gloves should be freely available throughout the recovery room.
9. Use single-use sterile needles and syringes. Use these only once and then discard them. If you use pins for neurological testing then use once only.

Principles for Cleaning and Sterilizing Equipment

Cleaning is a process which removes micro-organisms and biohazardous materials from the surface of an object.

Disinfection is a process eliminating all micro-organisms except bacterial spores.

Sterilization is a process intended to eliminate or destroy all forms of microbial life including viruses and bacterial spores.

Practical Points

1. If possible have a qualified person to supervise cleaning and sterilization of equipment.
2. Physically clean the equipment thoroughly before sterilization to remove blood and other debris. First rinse the instruments under cold running water. Do not use hot water, because it coagulates proteins which stick to the equipment offering shelter to micro-organisms.
3. Initial cleaning reduces the risk of infecting the staff handling the dirty instruments. Wear heavy duty gloves, and goggles, or preferably visors to protect face, eyes and mouth from contaminated aerosols. Do not clean or wash instruments in hand basins.
4. Steam under pressure (autoclave) is the best method of sterilization. Heat destroys bacteria by coagulating protein in the cells. Boiling will disinfect but not sterilize instruments. Metal instruments (non-porous) require surface sterilization. Rubber, towels, hollow items and plastic (porous) require penetrating sterilization. To be effective autoclaves must meet one of the following criteria:[1]

Gravity displacement sterilizers
- non-porous items 3 minutes at (or above) 132°C
- porous items 10 minutes at (or above) 132°C

Prevacuum or high vacuum sterilizers
- non-porous items 3 minutes at (or above) 132°C
- porous items 4 minutes at (or above) 132°C

5. Chemical sterilization is best avoided. However, some items are not suitable to be autoclaved. Ethylene oxide is useful to sterilize heat sensitive materials such as plastic, electrical apparatus, endoscopes and sphygmomanometers. Some equipment will need to be sterilized by soaking in gluteraldehyde.
6. Review sterilization procedures regularly. Check the steam penetration of each load with a Bowie-Dick type test paper (Incheque™) which turns black after being exposed to steam. Autoclave tapes only show that items have been exposed to steam, but not if satisfactory sterilization conditions were met. For this reason use a spore strip of Bacillus stearothermophilus to monitor the autoclaves at least once a week.
7. Keep sterilizers in top working condition. Ensure regular maintenance

by the hospital engineers. Ask the manufacturers to inspect, and submit, a report on the condition of the equipment each year.

8. Stamp the shelf life showing a use-by date on the outside of packs.

9. Store sterile stock in dust-free drawers or cupboards with doors.

1. Fogg D. M. (1989). *AORN Journal*, 50: 888-92

5. PHARMACOLOGY

A wide range of drugs are needed in the recovery room, sometimes urgently. It is wise to have them near by. If you only have limited stocks of drugs in your hospital, then keep them in the recovery room rather than in the pharmacy. Having to send to the pharmacy when an emergency occurs, causes dangerous delays.

Many drugs are chemically incompatible with each other, and strange things can happen if you mix drugs, or dilute them with the wrong fluid. Most, but not all, drugs are stable in 0.9% saline or 5% dextrose. Never add drugs to blood, blood products, fat emulsions, parenteral nutrition fluids or sodium bicarbonate. Read the manufacturer's recommendations, or check with your hospital pharmacist if you are in doubt. It is useful to save the drug manufacturer's package inserts and paste them in a book as a study guide and for reference. These inserts are updated regularly with new information.

HOW TO PREVENT ACCIDENTS WITH DRUGS

The commonest errors are:
- overdosage;
- under dosage;
- not anticipating side effects;
- the wrong drug or dose is accidentally given, because a syringe or an ampoule is swapped, or confused; so label them clearly;
- an allergic response;
- using an inappropriate drug;
- staff being unaware of drug interactions;
- nerve damage, because the injection was given in the wrong place.

FORMULARY
Get a good reference book about drugs, and keep it available. Tie it down if necessary. One of the best references is the excellent and cheap British National Formulary which is jointly published by the British Medical Association and the Royal Pharmaceutical Society of Great Britain. Copies can be obtained from the British Medical Association, Tavistock Square, London WC1H 9JP, England. Other countries have their own formularies. Check your local medical authority. You will also need a drug interaction and compatibility guide.

Patient Factors:

- Do not use a drug unless there is a clear reason to do so.
- If a patient is pregnant do not use any drug unless it is absolutely necessary.
- Check the patient's notes, and his *alert bracelet* for allergies and sensitivities.
- If the patient is hypersensitive to a drug never give it, and avoid other members of the same group of drugs.
- Check if the patient has been taking any prescription drugs, or medicine that he has bought for himself (especially aspirin).
- Use smaller doses in the elderly, or if the patient has liver or renal disease.
- Prescribe as few drugs as possible.
- Where possible use a drug that you are familiar with.

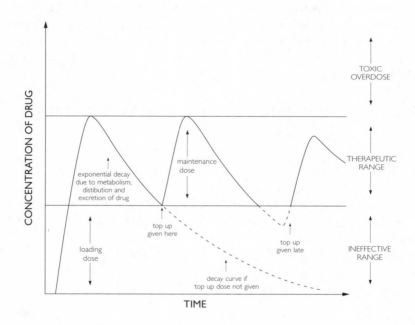

Fig 5.1 *Effect of drug dosing and its exponential decay*

Staff Factors:

- Most accidents happen because people make mistakes.
- Never accept an illegible, altered or doubtful order for drugs.
- Always check the dose and calculations with a second qualified person.

- Discourage telephone orders for drugs. If this is unavoidable a second person should independently check the order.
- Write the word *units* in full on a separate line for drugs such as insulin or heparin. Many disasters have occurred because a simple 'U' has been mistaken for '0', leading to ten times the dose being administered.
- Some doctors' writing is barely legible. Drug orders must be printed in block capital letters, but even then it is sometimes difficult to tell whether IM or IV has been written. Intravenous orders should be written IV and intramuscular orders I/M.
- It is an unfortunate fact that the wrong drug given to the wrong patient is a very common error. Check that the patient's identity bands, and drug sensitivity labels correspond with the name on the drug order sheet. Make sure that the drug is the correct drug, the strength is correct, the drug has not expired and confirm the route of administration.

THE BASICS OF PHARMACOLOGY

Pharmacokinetics is the study of drug absorption, distribution, metabolism, and excretion. Pharmacodynamics is the study of the effects of drugs, whether these be wanted (therapeutic) or unwanted and harmful (side effects).

Pharmacokinetics is how the body handles the drug.
Pharmocodynamics is what the drug does to the body.

PHARMACOKINETICS

Absorption
In the recovery room most drugs are injected either intramuscularly, where they are absorbed and released slowly into the blood stream, or intravenously where they are quickly carried to every tissue in the body.

Distribution
Some drugs soak into the tissues (especially fat or muscle tissue). This means there is only a small amount of drug left in the blood stream, and its concentration is low. If the concentration of drug in the blood is now measured, it appears as if the drug has been diluted in a bigger volume than would otherwise be expected. This calculated volume, which may vary from a few litres to many hundreds of litres, is called the volume of distribution. Cardiac failure will also slow the distribution of a drug.

Once the body has been given a proper loading dose; repeated smaller amounts will maintain the drug at a therapeutic level. The dose of drug needed to keep a constant therapeutic level is called the maintenance dose. A constant drug level and its clinical effect, can only be sustained if the maintenance dose is given at the same rate as the body removes the drug.

Elimination and Excretion

The body immediately starts eliminating the drug by:

- metabolizing it in the liver or;
- excreting it through the kidneys, or;
- using enzymes to break it down, or;
- storing it.

The time taken to eliminate drugs varies from a second or two, to months. The time taken to eliminate half the dose given is called the elimination half life. Clearance is that volume of plasma from which the drug is completely removed in a given time.

Clinical factors altering the pharmacokinetics and pharmacodynamics of a drug given in the recovery room are:

- Cardiac failure delays their distribution.
- Bleeding, or shocked patients have reduced tissue distribution.
- Interaction with residual anaesthetic drugs.
- Hypothermia will delay their metabolism and elimination.

PHARMACODYNAMICS

When the drug reaches its site of action it causes an effect. It may act on special structures called *receptors*, either on the cell membrane, or within the cell. The effect depends on how much of the drug is given. All drugs are *toxic* if given in too great a dose, and ineffective if given in too small a dose. The right dose is called the *therapeutic dose*. With many drugs it is necessary to build up the concentration of the drug in the body to achieve its desired effect. The dose of drug needed to do this is called the loading dose. The dose range between the ineffective dose and the toxic dose is called the therapeutic margin. Safe drugs have a wide therapeutic margin.

The *potency* of a drug is the amount of drug needed to achieve a given effect. For instance one-thousandth of the amount of fentanyl is required to achieve the same level of analgesia as pethidine. Fentanyl is 1000 times more potent than pethidine.

Sometimes, despite a therapeutic level of a drug in the blood, the clinical effect begins to wear off. This phenomenon is called *tachyphylaxis* if it occurs over minutes or hours; or *tolerance* if it occurs over days or weeks.

Injections

Give deep intramuscular injections only into the upper (outer) lateral quadrant of the thigh. Adults of normal weight and muscle mass can tolerate a maximum of 5 ml of injection. Patients weighing less than 45 kg can tolerate no more than 2 ml injections into their muscles. Make sure the needle is long enough to deposit the drug into the muscle, and not into the fat covering it because fat is poorly perfused and the drug absorption will be delayed. Wait until the prep is dry. Grasp the injection site firmly, and insert the needle at 90°. Dart the needle in, and press the plunger slowly to avoid sudden painful distension of the muscle. Do not massage the injection site, but encourage the patient to move his leg around.

Intramuscular injections should never be given into the buttocks of children. Sometimes drugs have been accidentally injected into the sciatic nerve; permanently damaging it, and causing the leg to become paralysed.

In children, and thin adults avoid injections into the deltoid muscle because this can injure the circumflex nerve. The upper outer lateral aspect of the thigh is the only safe intramuscular injection site in children.

Table 5.1

SUGGESTED NEEDLE SIZES		
PATIENT SIZE	**NEEDLE SIZE (inches)**	**NEEDLE SIZE (mm)**
Obese adult	21 G x 1.50	0.80 x 38
Average adult	23 G x 1.25	0.63 x 32
Thin or emaciated adult	25 G x 1.25	0.50 x 25
Child	25 G x 1.00	0.50 x 22

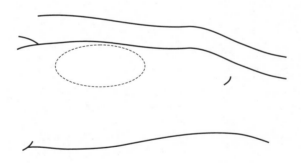

Fig 5.2 *Safe area for intramuscular injections in children on the upper outer lateral quadrant of the thigh*

DRUGS, AGE AND BODY BUILD

Drug Doses in Paediatrics

Children under 12 years do not respond to drugs like small adults; this particularly applies to neonates. Children's doses may be calculated from adult doses by body weight; or more reliably, by body surface area.

It is still common practice to give drugs to children based on their body weight. This may cause unexpected reactions; for instance, a fat child would receive a higher than appropriate dose. In such a case the dose should be calculated from an ideal weight based on height and age. If you need to calculate doses on weight alone, never give more than you would to a 50 kg adult. Be careful of sedatives (hallucinations), and antiemetics (dystonic reactions).

It is better to use a table such as the one below to calculate approximate drug doses. Even using this table does not guarantee safety, because some drugs have a small margin between the therapeutic dose and the toxic dose. If you have any doubts about the safety of a drug, or how to use it in children, then consult the literature, or a paediatric specialist. Be especially careful when giving drugs to babies in their first thirty days of life.

The age of premature babies is calculated in post-conceptual weeks. A baby born at 28 weeks and now 4 weeks old is 32 weeks' post conception.

Table 5.2

PAEDIATRIC DRUG DOSES		
AGE	AVERAGE BODY WEIGHT (kg)	PERCENTAGE OF ADULT DOSE
Neonate*	3.5	12.5
1 month*	4.2	14.5
3 months*	5.6	18
6 months	7.7	22
1 year	10	25
2 years	12	28
3 years	14	33
4 years	16	35
5 years	18	40
6 years	20	46
7 years	22	50
8 years	25	54
9 years	28	59
10 years	31	66
11 years	35	70
12 years	39	75
13 years	43	80
14 years	50	100

* Applies to full term, but not to premature infants.

IDEAL BODY WEIGHT IN CHILDREN

A well nourished child's approximate ideal weight

Age less than 9 years Weight in kg $= (2 \times \text{age}) + 9$

Age more than 9 years Weight in kg $= \text{age} \times 3$

Approximate dose for a child $= \dfrac{\text{surface area of patient (m}^2) \times \text{adult dose}}{1.8}$

Drugs Doses in the Obese Patient

When calculating the dose of a drug in an obese adult, estimate what their body weight would be if they were not fat. This is called the *expected lean body mass*. A guide to their lean body mass can be obtained from their height and by feeling the diameter of their clavicle, which will help you estimate whether their body build is slight, average, or heavy. From a pharmacokinetic point of view, fat people are just thinner people covered with a layer of poorly perfused adipose tissue.

Drug Doses in the Elderly

It is generally accepted that, *elderly* people are over the age of 65 and the *aged* are over 80 years. However, the physiological age of their kidneys, muscle, brain and liver varies enormously, as do their response to drugs.

Much of the body's mass in young people is muscle that has a high water content. As the body ages, muscle is progressively replaced with fat, with a low water content; therefore the elderly have proportionately less body water than young people. A water-soluble drug injected into an elderly person will have less water to dissolve in and is therefore more concentrated. In other words the drug's volume of distribution will be smaller. This is one reason why the elderly need smaller doses of drugs.

Many drugs are transported around the circulation partly bound to plasma proteins and partly free in the plasma. It is only the free drug that is available for action. For instance, normally, fentanyl is transported 70% bound to plasma protein and 30% is free to act. If nutrition is poor, as it often is in the elderly, or the liver is not manufacturing sufficient plasma proteins, there will be less protein available to bind the drug. This means there will be more active drug in the circulation, and the potency of a given dose of drug will be increased. Fentanyl is thought to be bound to skeletal muscle protein. In the recovery room the elderly tend not to move about much; however once back in the ward, when they start to move their limbs, the increased muscle blood flow washes the fentanyl back into the circulation. This sudden rush of fentanyl is thought to be the cause of the delayed respiratory depression sometimes seen many hours after the last dose.

When using drugs in the elderly,
give half as much,
twice as slowly.

A useful guide in the elderly, but particularly in the aged, is to start with half the dose and give it twice as slowly. The elderly have a slow circulation time and drugs take longer to reach their target. This means that the onset of even fast-acting drugs is delayed, for instance naloxone may

---

PHARMACOLOGY IN THE ELDERLY

Much of the body's mass in young people is muscle with a high water content. As the body ages muscle is progressively replaced by fat, with a low water content. Therefore the elderly have proportionately less body water than young people. A drug injected into an older person will have less water to dissolve in and is therefore more concentrated. This is the main reason the elderly require smaller doses of drugs to achieve the same effect.

Many drugs are transported partly bound to plasma proteins and partly free in the plasma. For example, fentanyl is 70% bound to protein and 30% is carried free in the plasma. Only the free portion is available to act on the receptors. If nutrition is poor there is less plasma protein available to bind the drug. This means there is more active drug free in the plasma which increases the potency of a given dose.

Liver and renal function decline, delaying the rate of metabolism and excretion of drugs and prolonging their action.

The elderly are often on multiple medications increasing the risk of adverse interactions and unwanted effects.

If the operation has lasted more than an hour, many elderly patients will be hypothermic. This delays the enzymatic degradation of drugs.

Fentanyl is thought to be bound to skeletal muscle protein. In the recovery room the elderly tend not to move about much; however, once back in the ward, when they start to move their limbs, the increased muscle blood flow washes the fentanyl back into the circulation. This sudden rush of fentanyl is thought to be the cause of the delayed respiratory depression sometimes seen many hours after the last dose.

take 3 minutes or more to work; whereas in a young person the effect may be seen in less than 90 seconds. It is easy to give an overdose when titrating a rapidly acting drug, if this point is not understood.

When prescribing drugs for the elderly
ask yourself 'Is this drug indicated at all ?'

Liver, and especially renal function decline with age, and this delays the elimination of drugs and prolongs their effects.

The elderly cool down quickly on the operating tables. Hypothermia delays the metabolism and excretion of drugs. This is a big factor if the operation has lasted more than an hour.

Bleeding associated with aspirin and other NSAIDs is more common in the elderly, and the consequences more severe.

The elderly are often on many drugs, and this increases their chance of drug interactions causing unwanted effects.

For a list of drugs see Chapter 24.

6. INTRAVENOUS FLUIDS

PHYSIOLOGY OF BODY FLUIDS

For practical purposes the body is divided into two fluid compartments separated by a semi-permeable *cell membrane*. These are the *extracellular* compartment and the *intracellular* compartments.

There are also two types of fluid, water which contains no ions; and isotonic fluids, which have the same ionic concentration as the extracellular fluid.

Blood, a complex colloid solution, is confined inside the blood vessels (the *intravascular space*). In a hypovolaemic patient, first give either blood or another colloid to provide sufficient intravascular volume to perfuse the heart, lungs, liver and kidney.

The body has two sensor receptor systems that recognize the two types of fluids. These are *volume receptors* and *osmoreceptors*. Volume receptors recognize isotonic fluids and colloids. Osmoreceptors recognize pure water containing no dissolved ions.

Table 6.1

FLUID SPACES		
	EXTRACELLULAR FLUID	**INTRACELLULAR FLUID**
Volume	15 litres	30 litres
Sodium	140 mmol/litre	2 mmol/litre
Potassium	4 mmol/litre	140 mmol/litre
Other cations	3 mmol/litre	5 mmol/litre
Osmols*	294 mosmol	294 mosmol
Sensing mechanism	volume receptors	osmoreceptors

An osmol is a unit of osmotic pressure. It is the osmotic pressure generated by one mol of a substance. 1 osmol = 1000 milli osmols (mosmol)

Normal blood volume is 70 – 80 ml/kg.
A newborn baby has a blood volume of 100 ml/kg.

Physiology of the Distribution of Fluids

Water load

Giving 5% dextrose is a way of giving water. The water spreads through the 45 litres of body fluids, moving freely both into the intracellular fluid (ICF) and through the extracellular fluid (ECF). In doing so water dilutes the extracellular sodium ion. A water overload shows up as a falling serum sodium, and water deficit as a rising serum sodium. A simple proportion calculation will reveal that in an adult a rise of 3 mmol of sodium (say from 140 mmol/litre to 143 mmol/litre) indicates a deficit of one litre of water. The body's osmoreceptors detect this change, and antidiuretic hormone adjusts the kidney tubules to reabsorb water.

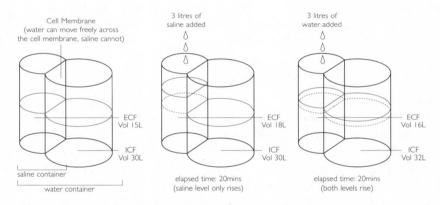

Fig 6.1 *Distribution of body fluids*

Saline load

For convenience, let us call these isotonic saline-like solutions, saline. Unlike water, saline does not move into cells. Saline is confined to the 15 litres of extracellular fluid. Once a bolus of saline enters the circulation it equilibrates, within about 10–15 minutes, throughout the extracellular fluid volume. If infused quickly, the blood volume initially rises and then falls again as the saline seeps into the extracellular fluid space. It does not dilute the extracellular sodium, so the measured plasma sodium concentration remains unaltered. Volume receptors in the right atria and great veins detect the saline's presence. These receptors respond in a variety of ways involving atrial naturetic peptide, blood pressure, and other mechanisms, to prompt the kidneys to excrete the equivalent amount of near isotonic urine. Given a mean blood pressure above 75 mmHg, a normal well oxygenated kidney will competently adjust the extracellular volume.

Other fluids

Blood and the colloids are confined to the 5 litres of vascular space, and do not spread right through the extracellular fluid. Protein solutions take about 18 hours to clear from the circulation, and polygeline about 8 hours.

Apart from the special case of blood and colloids, all the fluids we use in clinical practice are variations on water or isotonic fluids. The sensor systems recognize mixtures of water and isotonic fluids as being a certain proportion of isotonic fluid, and a certain proportion of water. For instance the body regards 1000 ml of the commonly used 4% dextrose and $^1/_5$ normal saline as 800 ml of water, and 200 ml of isotonic fluid.

Hypertonic fluids that contain levels of sodium ion higher than in the extracellular fluid will 'suck' water from the cells to dilute the ions. In this way they steal from the intracellular volume to expand the extracellular volume. This may not be a good thing.

DISORDERED FLUID BALANCE

Depleted blood volume

Patients who have lost a lot of blood during the operation often come to the recovery room haemodynamically unstable. At the end of the operation the patient may deceptively have a good blood pressure, good perfusion and stable pulse rate. Moving the patient from theatre to the recovery room can cause a dramatic fall in blood pressure; this is frequently seen after major vascular surgery. They may need a litre, or more, of colloid to restore the blood volume. The reasons for this fall are unclear.

The signs are:
• tachycardia;
• urine output of less than 0.5 ml/kg/hour;
• pallor;
• cold hands and feet;
• hypotension may or may not be present

Water depletion

Signs indicating 5% dextrose (water) is needed are:
• high serum sodium;
• concentrated urine with a urine osmolarity greater than 1000 mosmols;
• evidence of water loss such as sweating;

A normal sized adult, needs an extra litre of water for each 3 mmol/litre rise in the serum sodium above the normal value of 140 mmol/litre. Replace these deficits over 36 hours, or more slowly if the deficit is severe. For instance, a serum sodium of 145 mmol/litre would indicate a water deficit of about 1750 ml. This can be given as 5% dextrose over the next 36 hours.

Water overload

A serum sodium of less than 135 mmol/litre is a sign that too much water or 5% dextrose has been administered. This problem is usually iatrogenic.

Acute water overload is a complication of bladder or prostate surgery. The signs may present in the recovery room (see page 110).

Fitting and coma may occur if the water overload drops the serum sodium from 140 mmol/l to less than 125 mmol/litre in 24 hours or less. Often the water overload upsets tubular function, and renal failure can make the problem worse.

Treat mild water overload (serum sodium 130–135 mmol/litre) by restricting 5% dextrose and free water. Do not simply fluid restrict the patient as he still may, or may not, need saline. To deprive a water overloaded patient of saline will cause acute renal failure.

If the patient is confused, or the serum sodium ion is less than 120 mmol per litre, then consider using hypertonic 3 normal saline (3N saline) to correct the water overload. Each litre of 3N saline will convert 2 litres of water overload to 2 litres of saline overload. Frusemide will remove the excess saline. Readjust the fluids very slowly because it is easy to precipitate cardiac failure with this regime.

Some urological surgeons use prophylactic gentamicin to prevent infection. Keep in mind that the combination of gentamicin and frusemide is both nephrotoxic and ototoxic in the dehydrated patient. Ringing in the ears is an early sign of this problem, and it may first occur in recovery room. Unfortunately the damage is irreversible, and deafness may occur.

Rarely the *Syndrome of inappropriate antidiuretic hormone secretion* (SIADH) occurs, but this is only seen in patients who were very sick preoperatively. Consider the diagnosis if the urinary sodium concentration is higher than the serum sodium concentration.

Saline depletion

Signs indicating that 0.9% saline is needed are:
• urine output less than 60 ml per hour;
• postural drop in systolic blood pressure of more than 20 mmHg when the patient is sat up;
• tachycardia with a pulse rate > 100 per minute;
• low jugular (central) venous pressure;

• evidence of extracellular fluid loss such as: nasogastric loss, vomiting, burns, fistulae, bowel obstruction, and diarrhoea.

Saline overload

Raised jugular pressure, added heart sounds, creps in the lungs, peripheral pitting oedema and pulmonary oedema are signs of saline overload. In effect these signs mean the heart is unable to cope with the extra saline load, and is failing. Treat saline overload with frusemide.

AN ANALOGY FOR TERMINOLOGY

A useful analogy is to consider a car. It has a petrol tank and a water tank. If you put water in the petrol tank, the car will not run. Similarly, the body has two *tanks*, a *saline tank* and a *water tank*. These two tanks or compartments; have two sets of 'gauges' or receptors that enable us to tell how full or empty each tank is. We can read the water gauge easily, by measuring the serum sodium. The saline gauge requires us to look at all those variables listed above; of which (in a normal patient) urine output, and postural drop are the most useful.

We have purposely used the words *water overload*, and *water depletion*, instead of the terms *hyponatraemia* and *hypernatraemia*. Try to avoid these latter terms because they cause confusion. Hyponatraemia suggests that there is not enough salt, which may prompt the wrong response; that is, to give saline. There is no point filling up the saline tank, if the problem is that the water tank is overflowing. The term water overload, implies that it would be folly to give more water, and water depletion suggests that the proper response would be to give water. *Saline overload* implies too much saline, and *saline deficit* begs to be treated with saline; all of which are appropriate responses.

Dehydration is a non-specific term meaning the patient is fluid deplete, that is either saline or water deplete; or both.

Blood volume overload

If the patient has received too much blood or colloid during the operation, he will present with signs of left ventricular failure. The treatment is the same as for saline overload, although occasionally he may need phlebotomy.

Blood volume deficit

This presents as hypovolaemic shock, and usually occurs after blood loss. There is much heated controversy about whether these losses should initially be replaced by crystalloid or colloid, or a mixture of both. As a general rule in the recovery room, we feel it is best to replace what the patient has lost; so give blood, or colloid if the patient has lost blood. Your immediate aim is to preserve circulating volume, and protect the perfusion and oxygenation of the kidneys.

Potassium Disturbances

Hypokalaemia may aggravate residual paralysis following the use of muscle relaxant drugs. The patient will have a weak hand grip and be unable to sustain a 5 second head lift from the pillow. Rarely, it is a cause of muscle breakdown (rhabdomyolysis) that turns the urine brown. Suspect this problem if the ECG shows flattened or inverted T waves, increasing prominence of the U wave, and sagging of the ST segment. Treat hypokalaemia by adding 2 grams (26.8 mmol) of potassium chloride to 1000 ml of dextrose or saline, and give it at a rate of not more than 2 grams per hour, and then only with ECG control. If extrasystoles occur, slow the infusion rate.

Hyperkalaemia

Patients, particularly those with renal failure, may come to the operating theatre with a high serum potassium. Others at risk from hyperkalaemia are patients with: burns, severe crush injuries, established paralysis, incompatible blood transfusions or where haemolysis has occurred. In the recovery room the ECG shows high peaked T waves, especially in the precordial leads, but there should be no prolongation of the QT interval. Later there will be prolongation of the PR interval, progressing to heart block, with widening of the QRS interval and finally asystole. Should arrhythmias become a problem give calcium gluconate 1 gram intravenously over two minutes, which may be repeated if needed. Acute hyperkalaemia is treated with insulin and a glucose infusion which moves the potassium into the cells. Slower control can be gained by a calcium resonium enema; other options are peritoneal or haemodialysis.

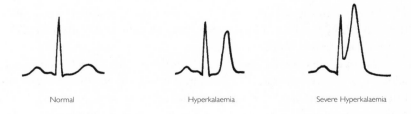

Normal   Hyperkalaemia   Severe Hyperkalaemia

Fig 6.2 ECG changes in potassium disturbance

How to correct electrolyte disorders

1. First determine if the circulation is overloaded. Signs of an overloaded circulation are raised JVP, added heart sounds, and pulmonary oedema. A chest x-ray may show pulmonary venous engorgement, or even frank interstitial or alveolar oedema. Signs of a depleted circulating volume are the signs of shock (see page 236).
2. Now assess the patient's water status using the serum sodium. Adjust the amount of 5% dextrose accordingly.
3. Next assess the saline status. This involves assessment of urine output, pulse rate, postural drop, and blood pressure, and the presence or absence of pulmonary or peripheral oedema.
4. Finally add potassium if necessary. The daily maintenance requirement of potassium is 1 mmol/kg. One gram of potassium chloride contains 13.4 mmol of potassium. Concentrated potassium ions will damage veins and cause severe thrombophlebitis and tissue necrosis. Never give more than 2 grams of potassium chloride per litre of saline or dextrose through a peripheral drip. If the patient complains of pain, then re-site the catheter, and use a more dilute solution.

PROCEDURES

Some Practical Points About Fluid Therapy

Always use a burette when putting additives into a flask or bag. Check the order is written in full, because using abbreviations or symbols may cause errors. The order should state:

- flask or bag number;
- substance to be added;
- dose;
- time to start;
- duration of infusion;
- route; that is whether the additive is added to the flask or to the burette;
- dilution;

Always use an additive label. These are usually coloured red to signal that something has been added to the flask. Mix the added drug well, or it will pool at the bottom of the bag.

Two persons should check and sign the additive label. Commercial additive labels are available. Before adding any substance to an intravenous infusion check that the drug and the solution are compatible. The necessary information should be on the drug information leaflet packed with the drug. If you have doubts about compatibility, then contact your pharmacy.

Patient's name............................ Unit record number ....

Ward .... Date .... Time prepared ....

Prepared by. .... Checked by ....

DRUG AND DOSE ADDED

Concentration .... Duration of infusion ....

Time started .... Time to finish ....

Fig 6.3 Adhesive patient additive label—to be attached to intravenous fluid container.

Sometimes lines are flushed with heparinized saline. This can cause bruising and haemorrhage if it extravasates into the tissues. Apart from arterial cannulae it is not necessary to use heparinized saline; instead, flush the lines with normal saline every 4 hours.

For safety, never mix additives with blood.

Intravenous Cannula and Their Insertion

1. The chosen cannula should be appropriate to the task.
   • Blood transfusion size 14 to 16 G.
   • Electrolyte solutions size 18 to 20 G.
   • Drug administration size 22–24 G
2. If you are inserting a cannula larger than size 22, then use a 30 G needle to raise a skin bleb with local anaesthetic. An alternative is to use an *insulin syringe*, its tiny needle can barely be felt as it enters the skin.
3. Choose a vein on the forearm well away from the elbows
4. Do not put cannulas in veins near flexures such as the elbow or wrist joint, because as the joint moves the cannula will abrade the inside of the vein causing inflammation. They are also likely to kink off. If you insert a drip near a joint, then use a splint.
5. Use a sterile technique for insertion. Use gloves and allow enough time (about 90 seconds) for the skin prep to dry.
6. A transparent dressing is useful to protect the insertion site. If these are not available, use a small adhesive dressing over the puncture wound and fix the cannula with tape on top of this.
7. Cannula should be replaced within 48 hours.

8. Fluids will flow faster if the cannula is short with a wide bore and the flask is hung on a high drip stand.
9. Cut downs on to the saphenous veins or cubital are rarely used now. A valuable approach in an emergency is to insert a large bore cannula into the femoral vein using a Seldinger wire technique.
10.   In the complete absence of veins in children an intramedullary or intraosseous infusion can be used[1]. Insert a large bore, short bevelled needle into marrow of the sternum or preferably the tibia taking care to avoid the epiphysial plates. Use an infusion pressure of up to 300 mmHg.

Thrombophlebitis[2]

In some cases patients will come to theatre with established intravenous lines. Check them on admission to recovery room. Thrombophlebitis is potentially lethal. It can lead to septicaemia. If there is any sign of thrombophlebitis, re-site the cannula, and put up a new infusion and giving set.

There are many causes of thrombophlebitis.

• If the antiseptic skin prep is not properly dry, it can be dragged into the vein as the cannula is inserted and irritate the endothelium.
• Improper aseptic technique is another potent cause. Always use a sterile technique and wear gloves when inserting a drip.
• Movement of the cannula in the vein.
• Hypertonic fluids such as 50% dextrose or intravenous parenteral feeding formulas.
• Drugs, many of which are irritant. Check the manufacturer's recommendations.

Table 6.2

ISOTONIC SOLUTIONS					
Solution	Na+	K+	Lactate	Cl-	Ca^{2+}
Saline 0.9%	150			150	
Hartmann's solution*	131	5	29	111	2
Ringer's lactate	131	5	29	111	2
Ringer's solution	147	4		156	2.2

*Hartmann's solution is the name used in Australia, New Zealand and Oceania for Ringer's solution. Hartmann's solution (Ringer's lactate), Ringer's solution and 0.9% saline are isotonic solutions.

Maintenance Fluid Requirements

Types of fluid

1. Crystalloids:
   - 5% dextrose also known as dextrose or glucose, or D5W.
   - 0.9% physiological saline also known as saline;
   - Hartmann's solution (Ringer's lactate);
   - Ringer's solution
   - 4% dextrose + 1/5th saline.
2. Blood:
   - whole blood;
   - packed cells;
   - blood products.
3. Colloids:
   - polygeline, which is gelatin polymers in saline, (Haemaccel®; Gelofusin®);
   - esterified starch (Hetastarch);
   - plasma protein fraction (PPF);
   - human albumin solution;
   - plasma;
   - dextrans (Macrodex®, Reomacrodex®);

Daily maintenance

Postoperative fluid therapy is often planned by agreement between the anaesthetist, surgeon and the recovery room nursing staff. Often the first 24 hours of fluid therapy are organized at this time. An understanding of the physiology involved enables sensible planning.

Adult maintenance

Adult maintenance fluids = 40 ml + 1 ml/kg each hour.

A 70 kg man will require 40 +(70 x 1) = 110 ml/hour. This is 2640 ml/day. Add 13.4 (1 gram) mmol of potassium per litre. For a routine adult patient who is expected to drink within a few hours maintenance fluids would be 1 litre of saline and 2 litres of 5% dextrose daily. Give each litre over 8 hours.

Child maintenance

A solution of 1/5 saline and 4% dextrose is a commonly used fluid for small children.

For the first 10 kg give 4 ml/kg/hour
Add a further 2 ml/kg/hour for children weighing 10–20 kg
Add a further 1 ml/kg/hour for children over 20 kg

Examples:
- 5 kg infant would require 5 × 4 = 20 ml/hour or 480 ml/day
- 15 kg child would require:

for the first 10 kg give 4 ml/kg/hour	=	10 × 4	=	40 ml
add 2 ml/kg/hour for the next 5 kg	=	5 × 2	=	10 ml
total requirements	=	50 ml/hour or 1200 ml/day		

- 28 kg child would require:

for the first 10 kg give 4 ml/kg/hour	=	10 × 4	=	40 ml
add 2 ml/kg/hour for next 10 kg	=	10 × 2	=	20 ml
then add 1 ml/kg/hour for next 8 kg	=	8 × 1	=	8 ml
total requirements	=	68 ml/hour or 1632 ml/day		

Consider putting these formulas on a wall chart in the recovery room.

Fluids after surgery

For some days after bowel surgery isotonic fluid transudates into the gut. The atonic bowel may contain 6 litres or more. As this fluid is lost from the extracellular space and is unavailable to interchange with the circulation it is sometimes called the *third space loss*. It takes up to 6 or more days for the bowel to recover its function. If the patient drinks fluids he runs the risk of acute gastric distension and vomiting. Replace 4/5ths of the fluid requirements with isotonic solutions, such as saline or Hartmann's solution. The patient will need additional potassium supplements. The basic potassium requirements is 1.0 mmol/kg/day. Adult patients may require up to a litre more than the basic fluid replacement determined by the formula above. Other guides to fluid status are: urine output, pulse rate, perfusion status, jugular venous pressure and auscultation of the chest.

Following urinary tract surgery more fluids are necessary to maintain a high urine output to flush the blood away. In this case, give a normal adult about 3000 ml per day.

Many neurosurgeons prefer to keep their patients water deplete, with their serum sodium ion concentration higher than normal. There is little evidence that this exercise reduces the incidence of cerebral oedema. Indiscriminate fluid restriction may cause saline depletion, and jeopardize the patient's kidney perfusion resulting in renal failure. Remember these patients still require saline to preserve renal function, even if they need less water.

In patients with renal failure it is better to leave their fluid management to the renal physicians. Their problems can be complex. If in doubt, give 5% dextrose 700 ml per day in addition to their urine output. Monitor their electrolytes daily. Watch to see they do not become saline overloaded with peripheral oedema or worse still pulmonary oedema.

Patients with cardiac failure need frequent attention to the balance of the fluid given and the urine produced. Listen to their chests for the fine moist sounds, and added heart sounds (see page 283) which indicate fluid overload. Recovery room staff should be alert for a rising respiratory rate, wheezing or signs of confusion or alteration in conscious state that warn of hypoxia.

Patients with temperature greater than 39°C need an additional 500 ml of saline daily to make up for their sweat loss. Sweat is about half saline and half water.

1. Fisher D. H. (1990). *New England Journal of Medicine,* 322: 1579–81
2. Elliot T. S., Faroqui M. H. (1992). *British Journal of Hospital Medicine,* 48: 496–503

7. DIFFERENT AGE GROUPS

Every patient is an individual with different needs. This chapter deals with the special needs for different age groups.

PAEDIATRICS

Children mature at different rates, but for the purposes of this book:
• Premature babies are those born before 37 weeks of gestation.
• Neonates are babies in the first month of life.
• Infants are under the age of two years.
• Babies include neonates and infants.
• Children are between the age of one year and twelve years.
• Adolescents are between the age of 13 and 16 years.

The anatomy and physiology of childhood poses special problems in the recovery room.

Respiratory System

Although neonates, (and to a lesser degree, infants) have pliant chest walls, their lungs are stiffer (less compliant) than an adult's. Events, such as pneumonia, or neonatal respiratory distress syndrome, make the lungs even stiffer. So when the neonate attempts to breathe in, instead of the lungs filling with air, the chest wall caves in. This results in scarcely any air entering the lungs. Furthermore at the end of expiration there is proportionately less air left in their lungs, than in an adult. This means neonates do not have a big reservoir of air (*functional residual capacity*) left in their lungs at the end of expiration, and without this store they become hypoxic very quickly. Neonates have a high metabolic rate. Their oxygen consumption is about 7 ml/kg per minute. This is twice that of an adult's 3.5 ml/kg/minute, and is another reason why neonates desaturate more rapidly than adult. The dead space volume of the neonatal airways is proportionally the same as in an adult, so they must breathe twice as quickly to meet their high oxygen demands.

Children become hypoxic and cyanosed frighteningly fast. Although their hearts are relatively resistant to hypoxia, their brains are not.

Airway obstruction

Factors that contribute to an obstructed airway in infants and children are:

- big floppy tongues;
- large tonsils and adenoids;
- a large epiglottis;
- a high larynx, with a small opening which is prone to oedema if it is traumatized or the infant is over hydrated; the narrowest part of a child's airway is at the cricoid cartilage;
- the ribs are flexible, making forceful coughing difficult;
- neonates, and infants less 2–3 months old, cannot breath through their mouths.

Airway problems seen in the first postoperative hour include:
- airway obstruction caused by the tongue obstructing the pharynx;
- laryngeal spasm;
- croup following extubation;
- respiratory depression;
- aspiration;
- apnoea.

Signs of an obstructed airway in an infant or child are:
- supracostal, intercostal, and subcostal retraction;
- inspiratory stridor or crowing;
- nasal flaring;
- decreased, or absent air entry.

Prevent airway obstruction, caused by the tongue falling back into the pharynx, by routinely nursing children in the coma position. If this fails, gently extend the neck to relieve the obstruction. If the obstruction is still not relieved then insert a nasal airway. Nasal airways are better than oral airways in children because they are less likely to stimulate gagging, vomiting or laryngospasm. Give 100% oxygen until the airway is completely clear.

Keep nasal airways available
when recovering children.

Laryngeal spasm[1]

This is caused by spasm of the intrinsic muscles of the larynx. The glottis reflexly closes in response to stimulation of the pharynx. Laryngeal spasm is the body's emergency response to prevent foreign material entering the lower respiratory tract. Spasm can be triggered by mucus, blood or other material in the pharynx; and sometimes just by suction of the upper airway. Be gentle when using a sucker.

The incidence of laryngeal spasm is higher in children under the age of 9 years, and reaches a maximum between the ages of 1–3 months. If the child has a respiratory tract infection the problem is more likely to occur. Laryngeal spasm is a frightening event. It may not resolve spontaneously, until the child has become deeply and dangerously hypoxic. Seek help early, and have your protocols on how to manage it worked out, and practised beforehand.

Acute pulmonary oedema is an uncommon complication of laryngospasm[2]. It is probably caused by the violent swings in intrathoracic pressure generated as the child attempts to overcome the obstruction. In young children the oedema responds to oxygen and diuretics, but older children may require assisted ventilation for some hours.

INITIAL MANAGEMENT
1. Give oxygen by mask.
2. Call for help.
3. Bring the emergency paediatric trolley to the bedside.
4. Attach a pulse oximeter.
5. Attach an ECG monitor and non-invasive blood pressure monitor.
6. Relieve the spasm by firm pressure applied behind the angles of the jaw which lifts it forward. Initially try ventilating the child using firm positive pressure from a mask. This may fail. Attempts to strenuously ventilate the patient by forcing air into the pharynx will worsen the obstruction.

MEDICAL MANAGEMENT
1. If the above measure fails to relieve the obstruction within 30 seconds, then an anaesthetist should give a small dose of suxamethonium 0.5–1 mg/kg intravenously together with atropine 20 micrograms/kg. You may need to intubate the patient and support his breathing until he is able to look after his own airway.
2. In older children, providing the airway obstruction is not complete, you could first try lignocaine 1.5 mg/kg intravenously[3].

Croup
Croup is due to oedema of the airway just below the larynx. The incidence is about 1–6 per cent of children who have been intubated. Oedema fluid easily accumulates in the loose submucosal tissue, where the cricoid cartilage forms a complete ring around the trachea. Intubation is the most probable cause immediately postoperatively. Infants are more susceptible than older children, because they have a smaller larynx (4 mm in diameter compared with 8 mm in an adult). A hoarse voice, or a barking

cough are signs of croup. These signs tend to resolve spontaneously. Rarely, it progresses to stridor that is a far more serious problem.

The signs of croup or stridor usually occur within the first hour (but it can be much later).

The signs are:

- stridor;
- rib and subcostal retraction;
- hoarseness;
- croupy cough;
- distress.

MANAGEMENT

1. Sit the patient up, give humidified oxygen, and nebulized adrenaline.
2. Take 2 ml of 1:1000 solution of adrenaline and make it up to a total of 5 ml in normal saline[4]. Give it by a nebulizer using a flow rate of oxygen of 5 litres/minute. It is believed to act by inducing vasoconstriction in the inflamed mucosa thus reducing oedema. The effects are short lived, and last about 2 hours. Admit the child to hospital for observation. The problem usually resolves within 24 hours.

Respiratory depression

Respiratory depression is commonly caused by residual effects of muscle relaxants. It is difficult to test for this, but an infant who pulls his legs up when he cries is unlikely to have residual muscle relaxants as the cause of his respiratory depression. Hypothermia, hypocalcaemia, or acidosis are common reasons for a delayed recovery from muscle relaxants. Do not hesitate to reintubate the infant and transfer him to intensive care for observation and ventilation. Another cause of respiratory depression is opioids. Naloxone can be used to reverse the effects of the opioids, but it only lasts for 30–60 minutes, and when it wears off the respiratory depression may recur. Fentanyl is very slowly metabolized and should not be used in the recovery room in infants.

Aspiration

Suspect aspiration if the child suddenly develops a wheeze or a cough. Infants are more susceptible to aspiration because they have a shorter oesophagus, their cough reflex is not well developed, and their laryngeal competence is decreased for 6–8 hours following extubation[5]. Atropine used during the procedure relaxes the cardiac sphincter allowing regurgitation of stomach contents.

ASSISTED VENTILATION IN THE NEONATE
AND INFANT < 10 kg

Aim for:

- respiratory rate 30–40 per minute;
- inflation pressure of up to 25 cm H_2O;
- fresh gas flows of 4 litres per minute;
- positive end expiratory pressures of 5 cm H_2O.

Apnoea in the newborn

Aponea in the newborn and premature infant is defined as a respiratory pause of 20 seconds or longer, or a briefer episode if it is associated with bradycardia, cyanosis, or pallor[6].

Infants who have been born prematurely, or have a history of respiratory distress syndrome or bronchopulmonary dysplasia, are susceptible to apnoea following anaesthetics even after minor operations, such as hernia repairs. This susceptibility persists for the six months of life and usually occurs within 12 hours of surgery. It is more common if muscle relaxants have been used. For this reason all infants who have been premature babies, and all infants who are less than three months (52 postconceptual weeks) are unsuitable for day case surgery. They need hospital admission and respiratory monitoring for the first 24 hours. Monitor infants of less than 45 conceptual weeks for 18 hours post anaesthesia. Monitor all infants under 6 months of age (64 postconceptual weeks) with a pulse oximeter, and if possible a respiratory monitor for at least two hours postoperatively.

Factors contributing to episodes of apnoea in the recovery room are:
- immaturity of the central nervous respiratory control centres;
- depression of the chemoreceptor response to hypoxia by residual anaesthetic agents;
- and residual effects of muscle relaxants.

Pneumothorax in infants

Pneumothorax occurs if their little lungs are over inflated. This easily happens if the baby coughs during intubation or extubation. Physical signs, such as absence of breath sounds, are difficult to detect, but the apex beat may be displaced with the shift in the mediastinum. Cyanosis and bradycardia are late signs. Think of pneumothorax if there is any sudden deterioration in a baby postoperatively. Have the necessary equipment sterilized, and ready to drain a pneumothorax.

The Cardiovascular System

The cardiac output in children is rate dependent. This means a bradycardia will cause hypotension. The heart's sympathetic innervation is not as well developed as its parasympathetic (vagus) nerve supply. This makes children prone to bradycardia which is not as well tolerated as a tachycardia. Bradycardia and apnoea may follow suctioning the pharynx. In a child the heart is relatively resistant to hypoxia, so by the time hypoxia is severe enough to cause a bradycardia cardiac arrest is near and severe brain damage will have already occurred.

Hypoxic bradycardia in children is a grave sign.

Table 7.1

NORMAL PAEDIATRIC HEART RATES AND BLOOD VOLUMES		
AGE	**HEART RATE beats/min**	**BLOOD VOLUME ml/kg**
I day	95–150	100
I week	90–160	90
I month	120–180	85
6 months	110170	80
12 months	90–150	75
6 years	70–135	70

Hypovolaemia

Hypovolaemia is a grave threat to neonates and infants. While an adult can lose 10 per cent of his blood volume without noticeable effect, a 10 per cent loss in a neonate is life threatening. A 2.5 kg neonate, with a normal a blood volume of about 250 ml, is severely shocked by a blood loss of only 20–25 ml.

Hypotension in older children is a disastrously late sign of hypovolaemia. It only becomes evident when the blood loss is more than 30 ml/kg. To test this diagnosis give a fluid challenge of 10 ml/kg of saline or a colloid. If the blood pressure rises, hypovolaemia is the probable cause of the hypotension.

Other useful signs are:
• a falling systolic pressure with a rising diastolic pressure;

- a muffled apex beat when you listen with a stethoscope;
- and a rising pulse rate (but, small infants may not get a tachycardia);
- a mottled blue appearance of the skin.

Transfusion in infants

Blood volume is higher in the neonate (90–100 ml/kg compared with the 70–80 ml/kg in the adult). Note the blood loss and blood replacement. The replacement should be to the nearest 10 ml above the loss. It is safer to slightly overload neonates and infants than to have them plasma volume deplete.

Arrhthymias

Abnormal arrhythmias are uncommon in children. If a child has had a recent respiratory tract infection, even if it had resolved before they came to theatre, then check their pulse rhythm. Viral respiratory tract infections are not uncommonly associated with mild viral myocarditis. Children with this problem may die suddenly during or after anaesthesia.

Intracranial haemorrhage

Intubation of a neonate without an anaesthetic causes a sudden surge in blood pressure. This may rupture intracranial (especially intra-ventricular) vessels. If a neonate deteriorates for no obvious reason in the recovery room, consider this factor.

Never turn your back on a child.
They get in trouble quickly.

Metabolic Problems

Drugs

Infants and neonates do not respond to drugs like small adults. Nevertheless drugs are usually prescribed on the basis of dose per kilogram body weight. Keep a *weight-for-age nomogram* available in case you do not know the child's weight. Having determined the correct dose of a drug you may need to convert this into millilitres of drug as supplied by the maker. Under a stressful situation it is easy to make mistakes. So make up some charts to convert directly from body weight to millilitres of solution. Tie these charts to your paediatric resuscitation trolley.

Hypoglycaemia

Babies are often hypoglycaemic after operations that involve periods of starvation. Hypoglycaemia is difficult to diagnose as signs and symptoms vary. It is defined as a blood glucose of less than 2.2 mmol/litre, at a level of 1.7 mmol/litre brain damage is imminent. Hypoglycaemia usually presents as muscle twitching, an obtunded conscious state, convulsions or just a reluctance to breathe. Most at risk are patients under the age of 4 years, or those weighing less than 15 kg. Hypoglycaemia is more likely if the child has been fasted for more than 6 hours. Children who go to bed at 18.00 hours will be starved for as long as 14–16 hours by the time they reach the recovery room next morning. If hypoglycaemia occurs give 0.5 ml/kg of 50% dextrose IV.

Hypocalcaemia

Although much less common than hypoglycaemia, the signs are similar. Measure the serum calcium levels after major surgery in neonates and infants. If the serum calcium is less than 1.75 mmol/litre, treat it by a slow intravenous injection of 15 mg/kg of **calcium gluconate** into a large vein. Do not use **calcium chloride**, because it causes tissue necrosis and severe thrombophlebitis in small veins; and is three times as potent.

Hyperthermia

Hyperthermia can occur.

Consider the following causes:

• an overdose of atropine, the baby looks red; and has a racing pulse;
• an infection;
• CO_2 retention.

Hypothermia

Compared with an adult, infants have a much bigger surface area in relation to their body weight. Work out ways of preventing hypothermia, consider the factors that would aggravate heat loss through each of the processes of convection, conduction, radiation and evaporation and try to reduce them.

Neonates lose heat faster, because they do not have much subcutaneous fat to insulate them. Considerable amounts of heat can be conducted to cold mattresses and blankets. Infants under the age of about 6 months do not shiver. If there is sufficient oxygen available babies generate heat by metabolizing specialized fatty tissue called *brown fat*. Brown fat can, at the best, only provide energy for a few hours. Once used, it is gone and it is not replaced.

Keep small infants warm. Cover their heads with a woollen hat, because they lose heat through their bald heads quickly. Ideally they should go straight into an incubator after surgery. To prevent heat loss, and provide a neutral thermal environment, full-term babies require an incubator temperature of 32.5°C, and premature babies require 35°C. Their oxygen requirement is high; so make sure that 28% oxygen flows into the incubator. Babies should be completely awake before the anaesthetist leaves them.

In small infants hypoventilation and hypothermia cause drowsiness. If the infant becomes lethargic and floppy, and its respiration, and pulse rate slow, then assist his breathing with a Cardiff Bag, and summon someone to help you. You will need to warm the baby, and check his blood sugar.

Nausea and Vomiting. See page 225.

Oxygen Toxicity in the Newborn. See page 313

Salivary Gland Enlargement[7]

Sometimes acute engorgement of the parotid, submaxillary or sublingual glands occurs during anaesthesia and persists during the recovery room stay. The face appears to be bloated (as if the child has mumps), and the glands are felt as firm masses. It usually subsides with an hour, and is not dangerous unless it causes airway obstruction.

Visitors for Children

A child is comforted by seeing his mother as he emerges from the anaesthetic. Thoroughly brief the mother on what to expect beforehand, so that she does not convey her anxiety to the child. It is wise to keep other visitors and relatives away from patients who are recovering from anaesthesia. They may become upset to see someone vomiting or in pain.

ADOLESCENTS AND YOUNG ADULTS

Teenagers and young adult patients can become very restless while waking up. They roll about, and may try to climb off the trolley before they can be reasoned with. Make sure the trolley sides are raised, and there is a strong person to help restrain the patient. Secure the intravenous lines, nasogastric tubes and other drains, otherwise they may be pulled out during this restless phase.

When emerging from any of the volatile agents, younger patients may get the *halothane* shakes with muscle rigidity, and violent shaking (see page 174).

From early teens through young adulthood, many patients seem surprisingly resistant to sedative and analgesic drugs. An alarmed young person will divert most of his blood supply to his muscles, (a part of the fight of flight response). When drugs are given intravenously they are more likely to be pumped to his muscle, rather than to his brain.

ELDERLY PATIENTS

It is generally accepted that *elderly* patients are those of 65 years or older. The *aged* are elderly patients of 80 years or older.

Ageing leads to a progressive impairment of all body functions. However, age alone cannot be used as the sole predictor for the outcome of surgery, or the likelihood of problems in the recovery room.

The three factors, which warn us to expect problems in the recovery room, are:
• surgery of over 45 minutes in duration;
• obesity;
• age greater than 70 years.

Anatomy and Physiology of Elderly

Respiratory system

In the elderly the lungs are less elastic, the chest wall is stiff, the respiratory muscles are weaker, airways are floppy and collapse easily; and the alveolar surface area is reduced. This means gas exchange is less efficient. For these reasons the elderly rapidly become hypoxic, and are slow to respond to oxygen therapy. They are likely to develop sputum retention, and their floppy airways and muscle weakness make it difficult for them to cough effectively.

Oxygen and the elderly

The arterial PaO_2 falls with age from around 100 mmHg (13.3 kPa) in a fit young person to about 80 mmHg (10.5 kPa) in an 80-year-old. This fall is aggravated by smoking or lung disease.

Diffusion hypoxia is a significant problem in the elderly. For about 10 minutes after the end of the anaesthetic, nitrous oxide seeps out of the blood and enters the lungs. This nitrous oxide occupies lung space normally available for oxygen resulting in persistent hypoxia in the early recovery period.

After operations, such as hip replacements, haemoglobin oxygen saturations below 85% may persist for up to a week[8]. If this hypoxia is untreated, particularly in conjunction with a low haemoglobin, it will result in confusion, delirium, cardiac failure, infarction or death.

Oxygen is necessary, even after local or regional anaesthesia. Regional anaesthesia causes vasodilation which requires the heart to increase its output in order to maintain a blood pressure. This extra work increases the cardiac oxygen demands. If the oxygen supply is not adequate the heart either fails, or becomes ischaemic.

Oxygen demand is highest when the patient wakes up with severe pain, and is further aggravated if there has been a major blood loss. Here, a rise in cardiac output and respiratory effort cannot meet the oxygen demand of the tissues. Some anaesthetists prefer to extubate their elderly patients in the recovery room, rather than risk hypoxia during the transfer from the operating theatre to the recovery room.

Cardiovascular system

All forms of cardiovascular disease are more common in the elderly. Circulation time is slower; and the vascular system is more rigid, being unable to compensate quickly, for sudden changes in blood pressure or blood volume.

Renal function

Kidney function declines in the elderly. By the time a patient is 70 years old, up to half his nephrons may not be functioning. This delays the excretion of water soluble drugs and may delay recovery. The glomerular filtration rate declines by 10 ml per minute every decade after 30 years of age, but the serum creatinine does not rise because there is a decline in muscle mass.

*The ageing kidney is susceptible
to drug induced renal damage.*

Liver function

Intestinal absorption and liver metabolism are altered, and there is a fall in serum albumin and other drug carrier proteins. that alter the availability of free drug.

Hypothermia

The elderly have a poor tolerance to heat loss. During and after their operations they have a greater fall in body temperature than younger patients. This loss is even worse if they are thin as well as old, because they have little subcutaneous fat to help conserve heat.

See also page 165.

Drugs, see page 47.

Joints
Elderly patients have stiff and easily damaged joints, be careful how you position them. Take care not to injure stiff backs and hips. The recovering patient cannot report pain that would normally warn them that their joints are over-stretched. Also they are unable to manoeuvre themselves around to relieve uncomfortable positions.

Skin
Skin is often very fragile and easily torn by simple things, such as turning the patient, or even removing the sticky ECG dots.

Confusion and Postoperative Delirium
Confusion is common postoperatively and approaches 50 per cent after fractured femurs[9]. Hypoxia, as always, must be the first suspect; and it comes in many disguises. Apart from obvious lung problems, heart failure is the major cause of hypoxia. The heart just cannot pump the blood around fast enough to deliver the oxygen to the tissues. This is made worse by anaemia (see page 310). It is difficult to over-emphasize the importance of proper oxygenation in the elderly. Once an old person has been hypoxic, even for a few minutes, their brain is damaged. Confusion, restlessness, agitation and aggression are difficult to manage. Even if proper tissue oxygenation is restored promptly, it takes, at best many hours, and probably days to resolve the delirium. It is a far, far better thing, to prevent hypoxic brain damage, than to have to treat it.

Always look for hypoxia as the cause of confusion.

Other causes of postoperative confusion include:
- preoperative dementia;
- hypotension during the anaesthetic;
- anticholinergic medication;
- stroke;
- depression;
- hypothyroidism;
- hypoglycaemia.

Poor eyesight and hearing add to an elderly person's disorientation. Despite their confusion they have an accurate perception of hurt and insult. Courtesy and respect for their dignity helps reduce feelings of alienation.

1. Roy W. L., Lerman J. (1988). *Canadian Journal of Anaesthesia,* 35: 93–8
2. Leek W., Downes J. J. (1983). *Anaesthesiology,* 59: 347–9
3. Baraka A. (1978). *Anaesthesia and Analgesia,* 57: 506–7
4. Child C. S. (1987). *Anaesthesia,* 42: 322–35
5. Burgess G. E., Cooper J. R., *et al.* (1979). *Anaesthesiology,* 51: 73–7
6. American Academy of Pediatrics Task Force, *Pediatrics,* (1985) 76: 129–31
7. Bonchek L. I. (1969). *Journal of the American Medical Association, (JAMA)* 209: 1716–8
8. Fugere F., Owen H., *et al.* (1994). *Anaesthesia and Intensive Care,* 22: 724–8
9. Berggren D., Gustafson Y., *et al.* (1987). *Anaesthesia and Analgesia,* 66: 497–500

8. Day Surgery

Introduction

Day surgery is popular with hospital management, and the authorities who finance them. It is cheaper to treat day patients, than have them stay overnight, or longer in hospital[1]. Many patients prefer to go home, even if it means a certain amount of discomfort.

With the growing confidence of medical and nursing staff, sicker patients are undergoing day surgery. The American Society of Anesthesiologists (ASA) physical status III, (see page 117) is now regarded, in some units, as acceptable fitness for day surgery, provided the disease is medically stable, and the anaesthetist agrees the risks are acceptable[2].

Problems in day surgery arise because of:
- the difficulty of patient selection;
- pre-existing disease;
- the difficulty of proper preoperative evaluation, and explanation about the procedure to the patient;
- it cannot be assumed that the patient is reliably fasted;
- difficulty in explaining postoperative instructions;
- the possibility that if the patient's condition deteriorates following his return home, he must rely on family and friends to get the medical attention he needs;
- drugs that the patient may already be taking, such as diazepam, can prolong the effect of anaesthesia, or have untoward effects once he arrives home.

Plan of Day Surgery Recovery Room

Recovery from anaesthesia must be as well supervised as in-patient surgery. Plan for the day surgery recovery room to be close to the operating theatre. You will need full recovery room facilities with the same equipment, monitoring, supervision and management as a normal recovery room. There should be an area set aside, where a patient, having recovered consciousness, can sit and comfortably complete his recovery. This area is the *step down bay*. No patient should leave this area unless he is in the company of a responsible adult. Recovery room staff requirements, and duties are similar to a normal recovery room; however, the need for a receptionist-secretary is greater.

ORGANIZATION

Some points to consider:

1. It is better to have operations under general anaesthesia only in the mornings. Afternoon surgery should be done under local anaesthesia.
2. It is useful to employ a community liaison sister. She needs a car to visit the patients in their homes. Her duties include changes of dressings, removal of sutures, and to treat postoperative pain, nausea, vomiting and headaches.
3. About 25 per cent of day cases suffer from nausea, headache and excessive drowsiness after their discharge from the hospital. Up to 20 per cent of patients do not go to work the following day.
4. About 0.2–3 per cent of the patients are unfit to go home, and need admission to hospital overnight. The most common causes for admission are haemorrhage, nausea and vomiting, and uncontrolled pain.

Written protocols should cover:

- admission and discharge;
- routines for checking equipment and drugs;
- the duties of all medical, nursing and paramedical staff;
- problems and how to handle them;
- lines of communication.

Responsibilities

Work these protocols out carefully, and write them down so everyone is clear about what their duties are. Many units use the following criteria.

Responsibilities of the anaesthetist are:

- supervising the recovery period;
- authorizing the patient's discharge;
- accompanying the patient to the recovery room;
- proper hand over to the nursing staff;
- providing written and verbal instructions to the recovery room staff;
- specifying the requirements for oxygen supplements;
- remaining close by until the patient is safe to leave in the care of the nursing staff.

*Postanaesthetic assessment is usually
the responsibility of the anaesthetist.*

Responsibilities of the surgeon are:
- authorizing the discharge of a patient from the recovery room when it depends on a surgical decision;
- being available to consult with the anaesthetist about the patient's welfare.

CLINICAL ASPECTS

Before transport from theatre patients must have:
- regained consciousness;
- a stable arterial blood pressure;
- be in control of their airway;
- be breathing adequately.

Occasionally a patient who has received propofol will, on awakening, become amorous. It would seem prudent for staff not to be alone in the recovery room[3].

Once awake, the patient will appear to be lucid and able to carry on an intelligent co-ordinated conversation. However, instructions given, or conversations held at this point are often forgotten, and the patient may have no recall whatsoever of the conversation. Occasionally after returning home, a patient will deny that he has even had a procedure. This profound amnesia occurs more frequently if midazolam has been used during the procedure.

Step Down Procedure

Recovery in day patients is usually a two step procedure.

Step 1. The patient recovers on the trolley, lying in the coma position until they are awake. After about fifteen minutes, providing their blood pressure is stable, the patient can be moved into a sitting position. If the patient has been intubated they should remain, for at least a full hour, in the recovery room before being discharged to the step down area.

Step 2. After an hour or more, the patient is encouraged to get up, and walk to an armchair. During this stage, providing nausea is not a problem, he can be offered fluids, and something light to eat.

Pain Relief

Analgesia for day surgery has its own requirements[4]. Simple oral analgesics, such as paracetamol or paracetamol–codeine compounds are usually sufficient to control pain. If a nerve block has been used, give the patient oral analgesia before it wears off. Opioids used, either during, or after the procedure increase nausea and vomiting.

Reversal of Drug Effects

Many patients are sedated with midazolam for a minor procedure. This drug impairs the patient's memory of both the procedure, and things you tell him before and afterwards. Although the sedative effects of the midazolam or diazepam are dramatically reversed by flumazenil (it works for about 30 minutes), often the amnesia persists. We recall a case where a 35-year-old man was discharged home after a day case gastroscopy. He later denied ever having had the procedure, and had no recollection of his stay in the day centre.

Naloxone too, which is used to reverse the effects of the opioids, has a short clinical effect of about 25 to 30 minutes. A patient who is sedated with opioids, and reversed with naloxone, may become re-narcotized later when the naloxone wears off.

Nausea and Vomiting

From the patient's point of view, nausea and vomiting is a disaster; but over 50 per cent of day patients will suffer from it when they get home. In adults it is more likely after ear surgery, laparoscopy, eye surgery and orthopaedic surgery. In children, operations for orchidopexy, squints, and tonsillectomy have a high incidence of postoperative nausea and vomiting. Check the notes, because a history of motion sickness, or vomiting after previous anaesthetics increases the risk. (For treatment of nausea and vomiting see page 221.)

Discharge Precautions

It is difficult to tell how well a patient has recovered following anaesthesia. No single test can demonstrate a patient is free from the effects of the anaesthetic, and is safe to leave the hospital. There is no substitute for clinical evaluation by the anaesthetist before a patient is discharged. Have an alternative arrangement for patients who are not ready to leave when you want to close down the facility for the night.

All patients must be 'street fit' before discharge.

Street Fitness

Street fitness is a useful, but not a well defined concept.
The criteria for street fitness include:
• the patient is awake and fully oriented;

- there are no active surgical complications;
- the dressings have been checked;
- there are no anaesthetic complications such as nausea or giddiness;
- no unsteadiness when standing.
- The patient is able to go to the bathroom to void without feeling faint;
- stable vital signs for 30 to 60 minutes.
- The patient has preferably eaten, and had a drink without feeling nauseated.
- Pain is controlled;
- absence of breathing problems.

Ruler Test

A simple test we have found useful to determine street fitness is to sit the patient on a chair, and rest the wrist of his dominant hand over the edge of a table. Suspend a 30 cm ruler between his forefinger and thumb. Tell him to grab it as it falls. If the distance the ruler falls is 50 per cent more than the pre-anaesthetic value his reflexes are still impaired and he should remain another half an hour for observation.

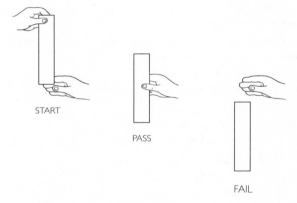

Fig 8.1 Ruler test

In some hospitals, patients for day case surgery go home from the recovery room. If this is so make sure they have written orders describing in detail, the medication they are to take, what the effects of the procedure are likely to be, and what to do if any problems arise. Have the responsible adult, who is to care for the patient, present while you tell them the instruction. Give them both a copy of the written instructions. If you just tell the patient, most will forget what you have said.

Also make sure that:

- they will be escorted by a competent adult;
- they have access to a telephone at home, and they have the phone numbers of the doctor, the hospital, and other support staff;
- they have a follow up appointment.

Immediately before discharge:

- check their blood pressure and pulse rate while sitting and then standing;
- stand them up and ask them to close their eyes to check they are steady on their feet (be prepared to steady them if necessary);
- check their dressings for ooze or haemorrhage;
- ask about pain;
- ask about nausea;
- make sure they have their medication;
- make sure they have all their belongings.

Tell them to expect for 24 hours:

- a mildly sore throat, especially if they have been intubated;
- perhaps some nausea and vomiting especially after the car journey home;
- mild headache for 12 hours which will be relieved by simple analgesia;
- possibly some muscular aches;
- mild to moderate pain;
- a blood stained weepy ooze from wound.

For the first 48 hours following general anaesthesia patients must be formally warned:

- not to drive a motor vehicle;
- not to use machinery that requires judgement or skill;
- not to drink alcohol;
- not to cook (because of the risk of burns);
- not to take medication unless prescribed by a doctor;
- not to sign any legal documents;
- not to make major financial decisions;
- not to be the only person in charge of children, or other dependent individuals.

In 1992 the Royal College of Surgeons of England issued a policy statement that the time limit for these precautions should be extended from 24 to 48 hours[5]. One survey showed that nearly 10 per cent of patients drove themselves home after day surgery, and 30 per cent of these had driven within 12 hours of their anaesthetic[6].

1. Kitz D. S., Lecky J. H., *et al*. (1987). *Anaesthesia and Analgesia*, 66: 97
2. Parness S. M. (1990). *Anesthesiology Clinics of North America*, Vol 8. No. 2 pages 399–421
3. Smith P. G., Collins Hogwill P. J. (1988). *Anaesthesia*, 43: 170–1
4. Baker A. B. (1992) *Medical Journal of Anaesthesia*, 156: 274–280
5. *Guidelines for Day Surgery Cases*. Royal College of Surgeons of England, London 1992.
6. Ogg T. W. (1985). *Anaesthesia Rounds*, No. 18 Imperial Chemical Industries (Pharmaceutical Division) Macclesfield, England.

9. Surgical Operations

Abdominal Surgery

Abdominal surgery is associated with prolonged postoperative hypoxaemia, because pain inhibits deep breathing and coughing, and general anaesthesia compromises lung function. Patients need good pain relief, and supplemental oxygen in the recovery room. If possible monitor all patients with a pulse oximeter. If you cannot dedicate a pulse oximeter monitor to each patient, then check their oxygen saturation intermittently.

Never ignore a falling oxygen saturation.

Intercostal blocks, or a thoracic epidural will help with most, but not all, of the pain. Encourage deep breathing, and coughing while supporting the wound. After major surgery on the lower abdomen, such as a total hysterectomy, or abdominoperineal resection patients usually need a urinary catheter to prevent retention.

Abdominal Lipectomy

Abdominal lipectomy (*apronectomy*) is a traumatic operation. The incision traverses the abdomen, and is sometimes closed under tension.

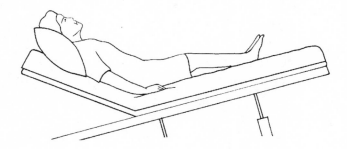

Fig 9.1 Banana position for recovering after abdominal lipectomy
(cot sides would normally be in place)

Blood loss is sometimes considerable. Many of the problems are similar to those of the obese patient (see page 129). Transfer the patient to her bed as soon as possible. Keep her knees bent, and upper body leaning forward like a banana, to prevent traction on the wound. Check that there is no swelling or wound ooze before giving analgesia. Pain is often the first sign of a developing haematoma. If she wishes to sit up, raise the foot of the bed into the *banana position.*

AORTIC SURGERY (See page 114)

BREAST SURGERY

Nurse mastectomy patients on their back with their heads turned to one side in case they vomit. If they are obese, sit them up as soon as they are fully conscious. As the dressings are often bulky and tight, check that the patient can breathe properly.

Elevate the arm (on the operative side) on two pillows. If the surgery has involved the axilla the venous drainage of the area may be impeded, causing the arm to become congested. If the arm is blue, or otherwise discoloured notify the surgeon. If the patient is uncomfortable help her to change her position, so that she does not hurt her arm, or put tension on the sutures. Before discharging the patient to the ward, check the drainage bottles for excessive bleeding.

Postoperatively breast binders are still occasionally used, in an optimistic attempt to reduce postoperative bruising. They seriously impede deep breathing and coughing.

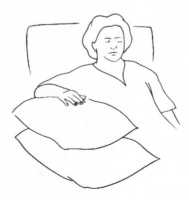

Fig 9.2 Patient after right sided breast surgery

BRONCHOSCOPY

Patients often cough uncontrollably after a bronchoscopy. The anaesthetist will have probably sprayed the throat, and larynx with lignocaine before the patient comes to the recovery room, but despite this they may cough violently becoming hypoxic and distressed. Sit the patient up, and support him on two or three pillows. This will make him more comfortable. If coughing is excessive, then give lignocaine 1.5 mg/kg intravenously[1].

Occasionally, a bronchoscopy is urgently needed for a postoperative patient. Keep a sterile bronchoscopy tray available.

BURNS

Patients with burns are physiologically unstable after surgery, so assign your most experienced staff to look after them.

Airway obstruction

Patients with facial burns have airway burns too, and probably smoke damage to bronchi and lung tissue as well. The airway becomes progressively oedematous and swollen. Wheezing, or noisy breathing will warn you of impending airway obstruction. Watch for agitation, or restlessness heralding hypoxia.

If the lips and tongue swell to close the airway you may need to gently insert a soft nasopharyngeal airway as a temporary measure. Lubricate it well with 2% lignocaine gel. These airways are well tolerated, even in a conscious patient. Avoid rigid plastic, or red rubber tubes that can damage tissues, rupture nasal cartilages, and introduce infection into the paranasal sinuses.

Monitoring

It can be difficult to find somewhere to put the ECG dots, or blood pressure cuffs. The ECG dots can go anywhere on the limbs, and they can even be put on the head if necessary. All you need to do, is place them, so they form the corners of triangle around the heart. You can use sterile subcutaneous needle electrodes, but check with the surgeon or anaesthetist first because of the danger of introducing subcutaneous infection. If necessary use a large blood pressure cuff on the thigh to measure blood pressure.

Pain

In full thickness burnt skin the nerve endings are destroyed, and the burn is painless. However, after debridement, burns, especially of the hands and feet, are very painful. Donor sites are more painful than the grafted area. Regional blocks are impractical if the debrided areas are extensive.

The pain of burns has a strong psychological element. Understandably the patient dreads the disfigurement, and in the recovery room may become very distressed. If high doses of opioids are ineffective, or only give short periods of pain relief, try ketamine. Use a loading dose of ketamine 0.1 mg/kg followed by an infusion of 1–4 mg/kg/hour. Use the larger dose in a young person, and lower in the elderly. To reduce the chance of hallucinations, keep the environment quiet, and do not disturb the patient. Use a small dose of diazepam or diazamuls to reduce the chance of hallucinations; midazolam is too short acting to be useful.

Hypothermia

Hypothermia is a serious problem[2], especially in the operating theatre where the ambient temperature is low and the evaporative losses are high. Burnt patients are invariably hypothermic on their return to the recovery room. To minimize further heat loss, increase the air temperature to above 30°C. Cover the patient with a warm air blanket, space blanket and warm towels. Warm all intravenous, or dialysate fluids. Heat and humidify the inspired air if possible. Monitor the patient's core temperature with a rectal thermistor probe, or tympanic membrane sensor.

Fluid balance

Monitor central venous pressure and urinary output. It is well known that patients with burns lose a lot of fluid but there is a risk of over-enthusiastic resuscitation causing pulmonary oedema. On the other hand there are risks of renal failure, and shock if fluid replacement is not adequate. Maintain the central venous pressure 9–12 cm of water above the level of the right atrium. Use a dopamine infusion of 3–5 microgram kg per minute to preserve renal function, and try to keep the urine output greater than 60 ml an hour. If possible avoid diuretics, because the hourly urine output is a useful guide to volume replacement in the early stages of burns resuscitation.

Burns oedema and limb ischaemia

About 18 hours after a burn the patient will become oedematous. Circumferential burns on a limb act like a nonflexible tourniquet as the oedema develops. Regularly check peripheral capillary return, because if a limb becomes congested, or white, an escharotomy is urgently needed. This involves cutting the tight band of dead tissue strangling the limb. It is a relatively painless procedure, and does not require an anaesthetic, but it may bleed vigorously so be prepared to give a rapid transfusion.

Bleeding

Grafted, and donor sites can bleed extensively. Watch the bandages carefully for signs of further blood or fluid loss. Monitor the patient for signs of impending hypovolaemia: tachycardia, a urine output less than 30 ml/hour, and poor peripheral circulation.

Septicaemia

All burns are potentially infected, and may release septicaemic showers during manipulation. If this happens the patient will become sweaty and hypotensive. Use large bore intravenous cannulae for all fluids so you can resuscitate him quickly if necessary.

If a burnt patient becomes sweaty and hypotensive consider either septicemia or hypovolaemia.

CAROTID SURGERY (See page 115)

CLEFT PALATE

A tongue suture enables the tongue to be pulled forward to clear the airway. Leave the suture in place for 36 hours until the risk of swelling in the mouth subsides. Keep the face clean, and watch for oozing from the nose or mouth. Notify the surgeon if this ooze does not slow and stop.

Splint the arms of children so that they cannot suck their fingers. To minimize distress, give analgesia early. Monitor the child's oxygenation with a pulse oximeter. Never turn your back on children, because respiratory obstruction occurs quickly, and without warning. You will find it easier to measure a child's pulse rate by feeling his apex beat, or brachial artery, rather than the radial or carotid pulse.

Never turn your back on a child.

DENTAL SURGERY

Many of the problems are similar to those of tonsillectomy. Recover the patient in the lateral position, without a pillow under his head, until he is conscious. Hypoxaemia is a risk in these patients[3]. All should receive oxygen until they are able to sit up and breathe deeply. Dental patients are often day patients, and despite their emphatic denial, may have had food or drink before the procedure, so keep a watch for regurgitation or vomiting. Never leave the patient unattended until he is able to lift his head, cough, and spit out blood and secretions on command. Pain may be severe and cause restlessness. Once conscious he will be more comfortable sitting up.

EAR SURGERY

Giddiness, vomiting, and nausea are common after operations on the ear. Anti-emetics like prochlorperazine (Stemetil®) or thiethylperazine (Torecan®) are usually given by the anaesthetist, before the patient leaves the operating theatre. Do not let the patient lie on his affected side. After major surgery transfer the patient directly from the operating table to his bed. Remember to ask the orderly, in ample time, to fetch the bed from the ward.

Following ear operations coughing or straining may disrupt the surgery especially if the tympanic membrane has been opened or grafted. For the management of coughing see page 149.

EYE SURGERY

Cataract

Cataract surgery is usually done under local anaesthetic so the patients are oriented when they come out of theatre. Patients are usually elderly and often have diabetes.

Do not let these patients cough vigorously, because of the risk that the iris may prolapse through the wound. Use a bolus dose of lignocaine 1 mg/kg intravenously to alleviate coughing if it becomes a problem.

Nausea

This is a difficult and persistent problem following eye surgery. Tell the patient to warn the nursing staff if he feels nauseated, so that anti-emetics can be given before vomiting becomes a problem. These patients are often more comfortable sitting up once they are awake. (See Chapter 13 for control of nausea and vomiting.)

Squints

These operations are usually done on young children, commonly as day surgery. There is a high incidence of nausea, and vomiting postoperatively. The incidence of postoperative and nausea can be reduced by keeping the child well hydrated, using droperidol 20 micrograms/kg intravenously before emergence, and avoiding the use of suxamethonium at induction[18].

FACIAL SURGERY

Following blephoroplasty, or meloplasty (face lift) sit the patient up. The eyes are usually covered with tight bandages. If the patient complains of pain, it may mean a haematoma is developing beneath the dressings, so inform the surgeon.

Iced water soaked gauze pads will help reduce the swelling after blephoroplasty. Do not encourage these patients to cough. Let them recover quietly. Before discharging the patient from the recovery room check that there is no double vision, which is another sign of a developing haematoma.

FACIO-MAXILLARY PROCEDURES

The operations are frequently long, and the patient may still be intubated on admission to the recovery room. These patients have had a deep anaesthetic, and take some time to wake up. The anaesthetist will not extubate them until they are sufficiently awake to look after their own airway. Rubber bands are sometimes used to stabilize the jaws, because these are easy to remove in an emergency. Modern bone plates allow stabilization of the jaw without the need to fasten the jaws together. Occasionally wires are still used, in this case make sure the anaesthetist has inserted a nasogastric tube, and keep wire cutters within reach. Vomiting with the teeth banded together can drown the patient. If he shows signs of vomiting, immediately, lie the patient down, call for help, start nasapharyngeal suction, and cut the wires, or rubber bands holding the jaw together. Do not worry they can easily be replaced later. Send the wire, or rubber band cutters to the ward with the patient. Leave them in a clear plastic bag taped to the top of the bed until the jaw is released.

Tongue sutures

When the patient comes to the recovery room there may be tongue suture protruding from his mouth. This allows the staff to pull his tongue forward if it swells to obstruct his pharynx and airway.

GYNAECOLOGY

Patients sometimes have psychosocial problems, becoming distressed and tearful especially after termination of pregnancy. For a short time after wakening they may become disinhibited, and talk or swear in an embarrassing way. Do your best to preserve their dignity.

Analgesia

Although lower abdominal operations are less painful than upper abdominal operations, patients still need good analgesia, and there will be a number of patients who require opioids.

Initially try to manage pain in day patients without opioids. The NSAIDs, particularly mefenamic acid, and tenoxicam are effective for uterine cramps following curettage[4]. The onset of pain relief with NSAIDs is slow, so they should be started preoperatively. If they are not working yet, use panadol suppositories, or try a glyceryl trinitrate skin patch.

Vaginal surgery

Vaginal surgery is performed with the legs in lithotomy position. Check for pressure areas, and numbness or tingling in the feet. Hip pain or back pain can be caused by over extension of the legs during the operation. If this occurs, note it in the history, and inform the surgeon. Patients who have been in lithotomy position with their legs up in stirrups during the operation may be hypotensive when they come to the recovery room. Nurse them with their legs elevated on pillows for the first hour following surgery. Check their pads for continuing vaginal bleeding. Some patients need urinary catheters to prevent postoperative retention. Check with the surgeon if a catheter is necessary, before sending the patient to the ward.

Laparoscopy

Laparoscopy is less painful than open surgery. NSAIDs given preoperatively, or during the operation help with postoperative pain relief. In spite of this, opioids may still be required to control the pain; especially if the Fallopian tubes have been cauterized. Some surgeons drip 0.5% bupivacaine 5 ml with 1:200 000 adrenaline on the cut end of the fallopian tubes at the end of the procedure[5]. This provides excellent pain relief for the first postoperative hour. Shoulder tip pain is a common complaint, probably due to gas accumulating under the diaphragm. It resolves quickly, but can be distressing while it lasts; sitting the patient up helps. Many of these patients want to go home on the same day as their surgery, but occasionally they are detained because of uncontrollable pain or postoperative nausea and vomiting.

HAND SURGERY

Most hand surgery is done under regional blockade. Since the arm is both numb and paralysed, warn the patient not to try to move his arm, because it may fly about uncontrollably. Patients have hit themselves in the face while attempting to investigate their new plaster, risking black eyes, or even fractured noses. Following hand surgery the arm is usually splinted with at least a plaster back slab. Elevate the arm in a *box sling* to reduce the swelling, and make sure it is comfortably positioned. Report to the surgeon, any problems with the perfusion of the arm.

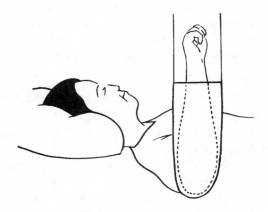

Fig 9.3 Position of the arm after hand surgery

LIPOSUCTION

Liposuction is a procedure for removing unwanted fat. It is frequently performed as day surgery, often under local anaesthesia. Large volumes of fluid containing local anaesthetic are injected into the fat and a lot of fluid is absorbed resulting in a diuresis. Check the patient's bladder as soon as she reaches recovery room. The combined effect of hypothermia, and the adrenaline used in the subcutaneous fluid causes the patients to become shaky after the procedure. Many suffer from headaches[6], which can be controlled with paracetamol. Toxicity from the absorption of the local anaesthetic does not appear to be a problem.

MALAR FRACTURE

Malar fracures, even after surgical reduction, are unstable. To prevent the pillow displacing the fracture, lie the patient with their fractured side uppermost. Mark the affected cheek with an ink cross, so that everyone knows it is an unstable fracture. Before the patient is discharged to the ward, check he does not have double vision, that would indicate that the fracture has become displaced.

MAMMOPLASTY

A developing haematoma following augmentation mammoplasty is usually painful. Check for swelling before prescribing analgesia.

More than 1500 ml of blood can be lost during reduction mammoplasty. Check the patient's perfusion status, and be prepared to replace the losses.

MEDIASTINOSCOPY

Patients come to the recovery room with a small wound, and no drainage tubes. Major complications can occur during the procedure, such as, bleeding, or tearing of the lungs or airways. Pneumothorax is the main complication. Watch for signs of airway obstruction, deviation of the trachea, and progressive dyspnoea. Consider a chest x-ray if there is any deterioration in the patient's condition. Look for widening of the mediastinum, pneumothorax, and pneumomediastinum. Air can track into the neck, so feel for crepitus (crackling under the skin), especially at the sternal notch.

If problems arise give high flow oxygen, and send for the surgeon. Prepare to insert a chest drain (see page 31). The patient may need to return to theatre if complications do not resolve.

NASAL SURGERY

Following nasal surgery the nose is usually packed with stuffed glove fingers, gauze, silk, or yellow BIP. A partially conscious patient finds it difficult to breathe through his mouth, and is distressed at having his airway blocked, he may become restless and thrash about. The anaesthetist should remain with the patient until he is fully conscious. Sit him up as soon as possible. This helps reduce venous bleeding into the soft tissues around the eyes, and prevents postoperative facial swelling.

Pain relief

Opioids are best given as premedication for nasal surgery and NSAIDS postoperatively. If the pain is severe and an opioid is used, give it cautiously.

Blood clots

Sometimes a piece of tissue, or blood clot will fall on to the vocal cords causing laryngospasm, coughing or a hoarse voice. If you suspect this has happened check the larynx, and pharynx with a laryngoscope.

A large blood clot can easily be hidden in the nasal pharynx where it cannot be seen. This *coroner's clot* (see page 334) can be aspirated without warning into the trachea, to totally block the airway. After surgery on the upper airway gently use a dental sucker to explore the nasopharynx.

An excessively dry throat may make the patient restless. Once he is fully conscious, give him a piece of wet gauze to suck or little sips of water.

Eye irritation

Sometimes small bits of plaster get into the eyes and irritate them. If this happens, notify the surgeon, and record the fact in the history. Irrigate the eyes with sterile normal saline. Check the eyes are not red before discharging the patient to the ward. Cold wet swabs to their eyes are comforting, and help prevent peri-orbital bruising.

NEUROSURGERY

Postoperative care after intracranial surgery requires close monitoring of the conscious state. Record the patient's pupils, state of consciousness, respiratory rate, and best reactions to stimuli on a *head injury chart*.

Sometimes the *Glasgow Coma Scale* is used to record the depth of coma. The lower the score the more deeply unconscious is the patient. With a score less than 8 the patient will be comatose and need his airway protected.

Never do anything to cause pain to a comatose neurosurgical patient, because there is a risk that it will raise intracranial pressure. Those who have just had intracranial operations, must be moved carefully, and not jolted, or handled roughly.

Signs of rising intracranial pressure are:
• deterioration of conscious state;
• decreased movement, and muscle power on one side of the body;
• a dilated, or oval pupil indicating transtentorial herniation of brain.

If any of these occur notify the neurosurgeon, and the anaesthetist immediately.

Beware of the unilateral dilating pupil.
Report it straight away, don't delay!

Most neurosurgical patients are extubated before returning to the recovery room. If the patient coughs vigorously his intracranial pressure will rise. So if he is still intubated consider using lignocaine 1.5 mg/kg intravenously slowly before aspirating the trachea which will lesson, but not abolish, the risk of coughing.

Table 9.1

GLASGOW COMA SCALE		
	RESPONSE	**SCORE**
Eyes open	Spontaneously	4
	To command	3
	To pain	2
	No response	1
Best motor response	Obeys	6
to command	Localizes	5
to pain	Flexion: non-localizing	4
	Flexion; decorticate	3
	Extension: decerebrate	2
	No response	1
Best verbal response	Oriented and converses	5
	Disoriented and converses	4
	Inappropriate words	3
	Incomprehensible sounds	2
	No response	1
	Score 3–15	

Hypotension

A fall in mean blood pressure will decrease cerebral blood flow, and can lead to hypoxia and fitting. Likely causes include:
• decreased blood volume;
• intraoperative diuretics;
• drug reactions, or interactions;
• adrenal cortical failure;
• decreased cardiac contractility.

(For diagnosis and management of hypotension see page 237.)

Hypertension

A rise in blood pressure increases intracranial pressure, increases the risk of haemorrhage at the operation site, and aggravates oedema formation. If the blood volume has been kept up during surgery, the blood pressure will rise once vascular tone returns. Hypertension may be a protective reflex to maintain cerebral blood flow. Eliminate hypoxia and hypercarbia as a cause. Aim to decrease the blood pressure slowly, watching carefully for signs of deteriorating conscious state.

(For management of hypertension see page 239.)

Head injuries

Head injured patients are likely to progressively develop cerebral oedema for the first 48 hours. Cerebral oedema may cause brainstem compression. An early sign of brainstem compression is a change in respiratory rate. Typically, it first rises then falls. A change of as little as 3 breaths a minute can be significant, so it is important to measure the respiratory rate for a full minute, noting rate, depth, and rhythm.

A change in respiratory pattern, or rate
indicates a change in conscious state.

As cerebral oedema develops intracranial pressure rises. This can disrupt blood supply to cause irreversible brain damage. It is important to keep the intracranial pressure low. If the patient is being ventilated, give morphine 0.01 mg/kg. Initially use hyperventilation to acutely reduce intracranial pressure Start an infusion of 1 g/kg of 20% mannitol over 10 minutes, and notify the neurosurgeon. Steroids are useless to control intracrannial pressure after head injuries. A late sign of raised intracranial pressure is dilation of one or both pupils. Unfortunately, by the time this has occurred, the brain will be damaged.

Cerebral aneurysm clipping

Vasospasm is a problem after surgical clipping of intracranial aneurysms. Vasospasm slows intracerebral blood flow, and predisposes to strokes. Aim to keep the PaO_2 greater than 150 mmHg (19.7 kPa) and the mean blood pressure greater than 100 mmHg. Give at least 35% oxygen by mask. You may need a dopamine, or a noradrenaline infusion to maintain the blood pressure. To dilate the cerebral arteries, and override vasospasm a nomedopine infusion is often used.

Stereotactic surgery

Postoperative bleeding after stereotactic needle biopsy can be devastating. Even if these patients are fully conscious monitor them in recovery room for at least two hours after surgery.

Hypophysectomy

Surgical ablation of the pituitary gland is performed through the nose. This presents the problems of a patient who has had both a nasal, and an intracranial operation. Monitor them as for a patient who has had a craniotomy. Occasionally bleeding occurs around the base of the brain triggering excessive sympathetic nerve activity. This will cause hypertension, and cardiac arrhythmias, and aggravate further bleeding.

If massive polyuria occurs and persists for more than an hour commence fluids with 0.45% saline (1/2 N saline), and 5 mmol potassium per litre to replace urinary losses. Measure urinary electrolytes, and replace deficits accordingly. Give desmopressin (DDAVP®) 2 micrograms as a slow intravenous infusion to control the polyuria. The syndrome usually resolves in 2–3 days.

Brainstem surgery

Occasionally patients who have had brainstem surgery get lower cranial nerve dysfunction, with vocal cord paralysis, difficulty in swallowing, and partial airway obstruction. Make sure they fulfil the criteria on page 21 before extubating them. Watch them closely for obstruction on loss of gag reflex. If this happens then reintubate the patient.

Spinal cord surgery

Spinal cord surgery is painful if the cord is intact. If the surgeon agrees to place the catheter during the procedure, then a thoracic epidural is the best way to control the pain. Otherwise use high doses of morphine, but watch for respiratory depression. High spinal cord injury can cause *Ondine's Curse* where the patient appear to forget to breathe. It may be necessary to re-intubate, and ventilate these patients. The problem usually resolves after 2–3 days. High spinal cord injury (or surgery) can disrupt sympathetic outflow tracts causing hypotension and bradycardia. Vasopressors may be needed to support the blood pressure. Tracheal suction gives these patients a bradycardia. Use atropine 0.6 mg intravenously to prevent this.

NEWBORN (See also page 62)

After delivery, or caesarean section, neonates sometimes come to the recovery room with their mothers. Likely problems are:
• hypothermia;
• hypoglycaemia due to stress;
• cardiorespiratory problems that arise at birth.

Make sure the baby has been dried, and is well wrapped to prevent hypothermia. (See also page 165.)

Hypoglycaemia is possible if the birth has been stressful, or the mother is diabetic, or has received a large glucose load within a few hours of delivery.

Neonatal respiratory problems arise from the aspiration of meconium, or amniotic fluid. Sometimes mild respiratory distress or transient tachypnoea of the newborn (TTN), occurs. The signs are nasal flaring, grunting respiration, indrawing of the sternum, and cyanosis. If any of these signs occur, arrange for the baby to be assessed by a paediatrician, and consider transferring the baby to a neonatal intensive care unit.

OBSTETRIC PATIENTS

Obstetric patients are most often young, and healthy. More than half have had regional anaesthesia for the delivery of their baby. Both the mothers and their babies undergo massive physiological changes in the first few hours following delivery. For this reason they require high nurse–patient ratios. In many hospitals the obstetric operating theatre is in a different part of the hospital to the main operating suite. If this is the case in your hospital, the obstetric recovery room needs to be scrupulously maintained, equipped, and staffed, with the same standards as the main operating suite. Resist the temptation to relegate older equipment to this area.

Let the mother have her baby as soon as she is fully conscious. Lie her on the left side with her baby beside her. Apart from routine admission procedures, and monitoring, check frequently for vaginal blood loss. Check that the fundus is firm and well contracted. Make sure the intravenous drip is running freely, and check the rate of any oxytocic infusion.

Many women will have had their operation, or delivery under epidural, or spinal anaesthetic. Make sure clear instructions have been written for continuing epidural infusions, and the lines are clean and well secured, with no uncovered injection ports.

Air emboli

Air emboli occur surprisingly often during caesarean sections. They seldom seem to do much harm, but may account for the feelings of alarm, and restlessness that occur sometimes after delivery of the baby. Occasionally they are severe enough to cause hypotension, breathlessness and chest pain which persists into the recovery room[7].

Missed abortions

Patients who have had dilation, and curettage for missed abortions should not be separated from other obstetric cases, and recovered in an area isolated from the recovery room. Treat them as normal patients, and admit them routinely to the recovery room. If they are upset and miserable; allow them to grieve appropriately.

Premature Delivery

Cervical sutures are used to prevent premature delivery. In the recovery room patients are sometimes kept in a head down position for several hours, while being monitored for spontaneous uterine contractions. If contractions occur the obstetrician may start *tocolytic therapy*.

β_2-adrenoceptor agonists relax uterine muscle, and are used in selected patients in an attempt to inhibit premature delivery. Their main purpose is to postpone the delivery until corticosteroids are given, or other measures are instituted to improve perinatal survival. They are indicated for the inhibition of uncomplicated premature labour between 24 and 33 weeks of gestation. Three agents are used: ritodrine, salbutamol, and occasionally terbutaline. Ritodrine is the only drug passed by the Federal Drug Authority in the USA. Elsewhere salbutamol is widely used.

TOCOLYTIC AGENTS

Because of the complexity of dosage regimes in obstetrics, in every case consult the detailed specialist literature that comes with the drugs.

Ritodrine is given by infusion initially at 50 microgram per minute, gradually increasing to 150–350 microgram per minute, and continued for 12–48 hours after the contractions have ceased.

Salbutamol is started at 10 micrograms per minute, and gradually increased to a maximum of 45 micrograms per minute until the contractions have ceased, then gradually reduced.

Both these drugs cause tachycardia, hypertension, hypokalaemia (especially if potassium depleting diuretics have been used), aggravate tachyarrhythmias, and cause hyperglycaemia. Use them with utmost caution in pre-eclampsia. You will need to monitor the pulse rate (which should not exceed 135–140 beats per minute), and the blood pressure. Fatal pulmonary oedema has been reported with ritodrine, and although the cause is multifactorial, fluid overload is probably the most important factor. Tocolytic therapy can cause post-partum haemorrhage; counteract this with β-blockers.

Take care—do not guess doses.

Postpartum haemorrhage

If more than normal bleeding has occurred during the delivery, or caesarean section, monitor the patient closely. Use an automated blood pressure machine, and a pulse oximeter. Record the blood pressure every five minutes for the first 30 minutes, and then every 10 minutes. Watch the amount, and character of the vaginal bleeding. If unexplained tachycardia, or hypotension occurs, initially assume the cause to be haemorrhage and treat it as described on page 349.

Ergometrine, or oxytocin (Syntocinon®, Syntometrine®) are used to reverse uterine atony. Atony is the commonest cause of the bleeding. The two drugs, oxytocin and ergometrine, used together are more effective in early pregnancy. Initially repeat the oxytocin given in theatre (5–10 units intravenously), and start an infusion of 10–30 units in 500 ml of normal saline, run at 250 ml/hour. Be careful if the patient is hypotensive, or hypovolaemic, because oxytocin will cause a dose dependent drop in peripheral vascular resistance, causing the blood pressure to fall sharply. This can occur at doses as low as 200 milliunits. Ergometrine is very effective at reversing uterine atony, but it frequently stimulates nausea and vomiting, and hypertension.

A prostaglandin F_2 α called carboprost, (Hemabate®) is used for severe postpartum haemorrhage that does not respond to ergometrine or oxytocin. The dose is prostaglandin F_2 α 250 micrograms, and it is injected by deep intramuscular injection. It has nasty side effects including: bronchospasm, nausea, vomiting, diarrhoea, and flushing. Excessive doses can cause the uterus to rupture. Check the dose, and administration with another member of staff before giving it.

If bleeding persists the patient will have to go back to the operating theatre for an examination to find out whether the bleeding is coming from the cervix, or the uterus.

Aspiration pneumonitis[8]

Patients are at high risk from aspiration pneumonitis. Aspiration pneumonitis (*Mendelson's syndrome*) in obstetric patients is particularly fulminant and often fatal. The anaesthetist will not remove the protective endotracheal tube until he is absolutely certain the patient can manage her own airway, and her pharyngeal, and laryngeal reflexes are intact. The patient is normally awake with all her reflexes intact before reaching the recovery room. If she is drowsy, or comatose, lie her in the recovery position. The anaesthetist should personally supervise her care.

If aspiration has occurred on induction the patient will remain intubated, and should be transferred to intensive care unit for further management. If it occurs on extubation, the patient would probably be re-intubated, sedated and ventilated; but if not she will require high oxygen flows. Nurse the patient on her left side if she will tolerate it. It is generally accepted that steroids, bronchial lavage, and prophylactic antibiotics are not warranted in the early stages of aspiration pneumonitis. If lumps of food have been vomited up then consider a bronchoscopy to eliminate blockage of a major airway. Chest X-ray changes will not show up for 2–3 hours.

Toxaemia of pregnancy

About 5 per cent of obstetric patients have toxaemia of pregnancy. The term *toxaemia of pregnancy* includes pre-eclampsia and eclampsia. Pre-eclamptic patients behave as if they are severely volume deplete, with excessive adrenergic drive pushing their blood pressure up. They respond well to colloid fluid loads. Pre-eclamptic patients run the risk of convulsions for up to 48 hours after delivery. Patients who fit, or lose consciousness have progressed from pre-eclampsia to eclampsia. Women who already show signs of toxaemia such as hypertension, proteinuria, oedema, hyperreflexia, and muscle twitching, headache, confusion, or thrombocytopaenia may get worse in the recovery room. Pre-eclamptic patients may arrive in the recovery room with an intravenous infusion of magnesium sulphate running. The infusion rate is about 0.5 mg/kg/hour. Magnesium will reduce the probability of convulsions, control hypertension and improve cardiac stability and renal function. Other drugs used to reduce the chance of convulsions are phenytoin, or occasionally a benzodiazepine such as diazepam or clonazepam. You must be certain about how to care for these infusions. You will need written protocols about them, the expected progression of the disease, and when to notify the obstetrician. These patients need close monitoring for a minimum 24 hours, and usually longer.

Severe hypertension, that is, a diastolic blood pressure greater than 110 mmHg, needs immediate treatment. Hydralazine, nifedipine, labetalol, or even nitroprusside may be required (see page 244). Use an arterial line to guide your therapy.

Pulmonary oedema is a risk, and is usually due to fluid overload, or less commonly, cardiac failure. Monitor oxygenation with a pulse oximeter, check the lungs for creptitations, listen to the heart for added heart sounds. The best signs that pulmonary oedema may be developing are increasing respiratory rate, and the progressive onset of shortness of breath. A chest X-ray will confirm your diagnosis. (See page 283 for management.)

Amniotic fluid embolism[9]

This is an uncommon complication (1:50 000), and is characterized by sudden collapse at the time of delivery, with cyanosis, haemorrhage, and disseminated intravascular coagulation. There is no consistent specific test to confirm the clinical diagnosis, even though fetal cells can sometimes be isolated from the maternal circulation. The patient will require ventilation in the intensive care unit, with ionotrope support, antibiotics, and management of their coagulopathy. The outcome is poor, with a mortality of 80 per cent.

OESOPHAGECTOMY[10]

Oesophagectomy is a traumatic operation performed for cancer of the oesophagus. Bowel is pulled up through the mediastinum, and a piece with its blood supply intact is used to replace the oesophagus. This operation is a major physiological insult, that predisposes the patient to cardiac arrhythmias, especially atrial fibrillation, and major respiratory complications. Be prepared to digitalize the patient. These patients are frequently hypomagnesaemic which contributes to the cardiac arrhythmias sometimes seen in recovery room. The patient will often remain intubated on admission to the recovery room, and will have all the problems associated with a long operation. If the carcinoma has involved the larynx, he will have a tracheostomy, and be unable to speak.

A nasogastric tube is needed to prevent the stomach distending, Make sure the nasogastric tube is well secured, because it crosses the anastomosis. and moving it puts stress on the stitches holding the anastomosis together. If the nasogastric tube comes out it can be a disaster, because it cannot be easily replaced, and the distending gut may tear the anastomosis apart.

ORTHOPAEDICS

Operations on bones are painful. Young patients especially, need more than the average amount of opioid to control their pain. It is best to start pain relief before they leave the operating theatre so that they already have had a loading dose on reaching the recovery room. Many orthopaedic operations are now being performed with epidural anaesthesia, and regional blockade, so pain relief can be continued in the ward.

Athroscopy

Arthroscopy is a painful procedure. Many surgeons instil a long-acting local anaesthetic such as bupivacaine into the joint to help control the pain. Addition of morphine to this solution improves the duration of analgesia. Following knee operations the legs are often elevated on pillows.

Tourniquets

Operations performed under tourniquet, such as total knee replacements, may bleed vigorously in the recovery room, so watch the drain bottles for losses. It is not unusual for a knee replacement to lose a litre of blood in the first few hours after surgery. Check that blood is cross-matched, and available.

Hip surgery

During hip replacements and femoral neck fractures, several litres of blood can be lost. Blood spilled on the floor, and drapes makes it difficult to estimate the blood loss during surgery, and the patient may come to the recovery room either hypovolaemic, or having had too much fluid. Often patients continue to bleed after coming to the recovery room, and if this is not detected the patient may become shocked later after returning to the ward. Up to a litre of blood can be lost into the thigh before it starts to swell noticeably. Occasionally a patient will neglect to tell the medical staff he has been taking aspirin in one of its many guises, which may explain excessive postoperative ooze.

It is usually the elderly, with all their other medical problems, who have hip surgery. These patients commonly become hypoxic in the recovery room, especially if they have had a general anaesthetic. Periodic hypoxaemia occurs for up to five days after surgery[12]. If a patient has fractured her neck of femur, she will probably be already hypoxic before coming to the operating theatre; and the hypoxia will be worse postoperatively[13]. Hypoxia, (together with fat emboli) are the main reasons for postoperative confusion that is so common in these patients[14]. The problem is aggravated if opioids are used for postoperative pain control, and severe hypoxia occurs when the patient is asleep[15]. If the patient has been taking antidepressants the postoperative confusion is even worse.

Hypoxia is a constant threat
to elderly patients
having orthopaedic operations.

Abduction pillow

After hip replacement an *abduction pillow* (or Charnley pillow) is used to keep the legs apart, and strapped in the extended position. This pillow is often put on by staff in recovery room. Before you put on the pillow check the skin on the legs thoroughly for signs of break down or abnormality, and the perfusion of the limbs. Put the wide end between the ankles. Apply the straps in such a way that you can easily slip your finger between the strap and the skin. Be careful not to compress the peroneal nerve with the straps. Check the pedal pulses, and the perfusion of the feet before the patient leaves recovery room.

Routine orthopaedic checks
- Check drain bottles every 30 minutes; and record their patency, the amount of drainage, its colour, and its character.
- Check neurovascular status every 30 minutes. This includes; peripheral pulses, limb colour, limb temperature, capillary refilling, presence of numbness, or tingling, swelling, and if possible movement.
- Check the position. Keep the limb in the correct position, set by the surgeon. Initially the bed should be flat. While the patient is lying flat have a sucker ready, because they are at risk of aspirating if they vomit.
- Check for signs of fat emboli (see below).

Plaster checks
- warmth, colour, and capillary refilling;
- movement of fingers or toes;
- sensation and presence of pain, numbness or tingling;
- pulses;
- state of plaster.

To help prevent a plastered limb from swelling elevate it on a pillow. Do a plaster check every half hour, and record your findings. The main danger is that the limb will swell inside the tight plaster, and cut off the distal circulation. If this occurs the patient will complain of 'pins-and-needles', followed by pain and then numbness. These important symptoms may be absent if a local, or regional anaesthetic has been used. Feel the character of the pulse, and compare it with the pulse in the unplastered limb; they should be the same. Look carefully to see that the extremity is not changing colour, and that the skin capillaries are not congested and blue. Check capillary return by pressing on a nail bed, and note how fast the capillary fills when you let it go. This should be about one second, but if the limb is congested it will be faster. If the limb is ischaemic, the capillary will fail to fill. It will be necessary to split the plaster if the limb perfusion is impaired.

Check that blood is not seeping through the plaster. If it is, then mark out the boundaries with felt tipped pen so its progress can be followed. The surgeon should review the plaster before the patient returns to the ward.

Fat emboli

Orthopaedic, and trauma cases are at risk from fat emboli, (sometimes called fat emboli syndrome, or FES). It occurs in up to 10 per cent of bone trauma, and in the past has been a major cause of death. It is thought that fat from the bone marrow is released into the circulation. In the blood stream enzymes change some of it to free fatty acids. These are toxic to alveolar cells in the lungs, resulting in pulmonary oedema and disturbance in oxygen diffusion into the body. The fat may also trigger disseminated intravascular coagulation (DIC). The syndrome usually occurs 12–72 hours after injury; but more acutely, may appear in the recovery room, especially in cases of trauma admitted the day before.

Signs of fat emboli seen in the recovery room may include:

- a respiratory rate increasing to more than 20 breaths per minute, with a developing respiratory alkalosis;
- fine moist sounds especially in lung's bases;
- hypoxia;
- headaches;
- disorientation, confusion, and deteriorating conscious state;
- possibly fitting;
- fever;
- scattered petechiae may be seen on the chest wall;
- retinal petechiae.

Prevention of fat emboli includes early immobilization, and stabilization of fractures. Treatment may include ventilation for a few days in intensive care unit.

Deep vein thrombosis (DVT)[16]

Hip fractures and pelvic fractures are at risk of deep vein thrombosis. Up to 50 per cent of these patients have evidence of deep vein thrombosis. Up to 2 per cent die from pulmonary embolism with elective surgery and up to 7 per cent from emergency surgery. Epidural and spinal anaesthesia decrease the risk slightly; probably by increasing blood flow to the limbs during the operation. How to prevent deep vein thrombosis, and pulmonary embolism remains a controversial issue[17].

Risk factors include:

- emergency surgery;
- increasing age;
- previous history of thrombosis, or embolism;
- obesity;
- malignancy;
- prolonged immobilization;

- oral contraceptives containing oestrogen;
- cardiac failure.
    Prophylaxis in the recovery room include:
- encouraging active leg, and foot exercises;
- low dose heparin, or low molecular weight heparins used preoperatively, and sometimes given again in the recovery room. Low molecular weight heparins are more effective than standard heparin
- less effectively, intra- and postoperative infusions of dextran 70; use 10 ml/kg;
- graduated compressive pressure stockings;
- where possible raise the patient's legs to prevent pressure on the calf muscles.

Pulmonary embolism (PE)

Pulmonary embolism uncommonly occurs in the recovery room, and is more likely to occur in the ward 2–14 days postoperatively. Consider pulmonary embolism if a patient becomes abruptly short of breath, has pleuritic chest pain, or collapses. Patients with an acute pulmonary embolis are apprehensive, fearful and panicky. A chest x-ray, or ECG in recovery room usually reveals nothing at this early stage. A wheeze can be sometimes heard over the affected lung. Treatment is difficult in the first few days after an operation, because thrombolysis with streptokinase will dissolve all clots, precipitating postoperative bleeding. Heparin can be commenced cautiously.

PERINEAL OPERATIONS

Operations on the perineum are painful. The anaesthetist sometimes puts in a caudal block to control the pain. Warn the patient he may have a numb bottom for some hours, but as soon as the anaesthetic starts to wear off to ask the ward staff for pain relief. Caudal anaesthesia tends to wear off abruptly.

PLASTIC SURGERY

Do not let patients become restless after plastic surgery operations. If patients thrash about they are likely to disrupt the surgery. This applies especially to skin grafts, vascular flaps, and nerve and tendon repairs. Diazamul, or diazepam, 1–5 mg intravenously is suitable sedation. Give it slowly in 1 mg increments, and supplement it with oxygen by mask.

Check the perfusion of pedicle grafts. Signs of poor perfusion are pallor, coolness, blue discoloration, and poor capillary return.

Plastic surgery is frequently performed under deep anaesthesia. To avoid emergence delirium let the patients wake up slowly, and quietly.

Epidural analgesia will provide continuing regional anaesthesia for operations on the abdomen, or lower limbs; and additionally will keep the operation site well perfused.

Tissue grafts

Following microsurgery for free vascularized tissue grafts, put patients on supplemental oxygen, and keep the surgical site warm. A good blood supply is essential for a successful graft. Good analgesia will help prevent cutaneous vasoconstriction that might jeopardize the graft. Do not let the patient become hypotensive or hypovolaemic. Monitor his oxygenation with a pulse oximeter. If the grafted tissue appears pale, or white suspect problems with its arterial blood supply. If it appears dark, or blue the venous drainage is impaired. In either case, inform the surgeon.

Hypotensive anaesthesia

Some plastic procedure operations are performed under hypotensive anaesthesia to reduce bleeding, and make it easier for the surgeon to see what he is doing. When the blood pressure is returned to normal the surgical site may bleed. Be prepared for this. Do not discharge the patient to the ward until his blood pressure has been stable at preoperative levels for an hour.

If a patient is confused, restless, slow to awaken, or complains of a headache after hypotensive anaesthesia inform the anaesthetist. This may be a sign of intraoperative cerebral hypoxia.

THORACOTOMY

Analgesia is best achieved with either a thoracic epidural, or intercostal blocks. (Some surgeons use a cryoprobe on the intercostal nerves as they are closing up. It takes some weeks for the nerves to regain function.) In the recovery room the patients are nursed in the sitting position. Check the underwater drains to ensure they are draining and swinging. The drain tubes must never be tied to the bed linen, or the cot side. As the patient moves the drains can be accidentally pulled out. Under some circumstances it is dangerous to clamp thoracic drain tubes, particularly if the drain tubes are bubbling into the bottle. Clamping a bubbling drain will cause a pneumothorax, because the air cannot escape from the chest. Never clamp drain tubes if the patient is receiving positive pressure ventilation (see page 28).

THYMECTOMY

This operation is performed to relieve the symptoms of myasthenia gravis. The patient will normally be taking neostigmine, or physotigmine to counteract muscle weakness. These drugs are usually omitted on the morning of surgery, and recommenced in the recovery room. Their side effects are bradycardia, weakness, and excessive oral and bronchial secretions.

The Tensilon® test

The Tensilon® test is used to find the optimal postoperative dose of neostigmine. Edrophonium (Tensilon®)is a short acting anticholinesterase. If a dose of edrophonium causes an increase in muscle power then increase the dose of neostigmine.

Do not extubate the patient until he has achieved maximum strength. Following extubation the patient must be watched for weakness in the facial, and neck muscles, and for any difficult in swallowing secretions.

As after any mediastinal operation, watch for the signs of concealed haemorrhage, respiratory distress; or subcutaneous emphysema, indicating the patient has developed a pneumothorax.

THYROIDECTOMY AND PARATHYROIDECTOMY

Sit these patients up as soon as they regain consciousness. Their bandages will need to be checked and resecured. The patients are usually nauseated, because of surgical traction on, and around the vagus nerve. Give metoclopramide (Maxolon®) 5–10 mg intramuscularly. If nausea persists give prochlorperazine (Stemetil®) 6.25 mg intramuscularly.

Stridor

Concealed bleeding from below the deep fascia in the neck can cause airway obstruction. If the patient develops noisy breathing, or stridor in the recovery room immediately notify the anaesthetist, or the surgeon. Do not attempt to reintubate these patients unless you are skilled; because the laryngeal opening, and even the pharynx, will be obscured by oedema. Intubation requires an inhalational induction.

If you cannot find someone to help, relieve the obstruction yourself.

Stridor is a medical emergency.

MANAGEMENT OF STRIDOR AFTER THYROID OPERATIONS

Step 1. Put the patient on high inspired oxygen, and sit him up.

Step 2. Take out the skin clips or sutures. The wound will fall open.

Step 3. Using sterile instruments take out the sutures running transversely in a straight line in the bottom of the wound. The tissues will fall open, and allow the blood to drain out. No harm can be done by this procedure, and it may save the patient's life.

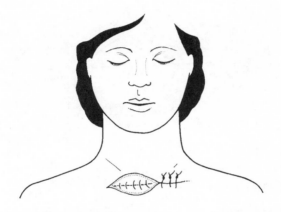

Fig 9.4 Removal of sutures after a thyroidectomy

TONSILLECTOMY

Following tonsillectomy concealed bleeding into the pharynx is a danger. Recover these patients in the coma position without a pillow until they are fully conscious. For patients under 50 kg, put a pillow under their hips, and drape them head down; this lets blood drain from their mouth. For larger patients use the recovery position (see page 11).

Tonsillectomy is painful, but there are problems if the patient is deeply sedated after this operation, so check with the surgeon, and anaesthetist before giving further opioids. This precaution applies especially to patients who have a history of sleep apnoea. These patients are at risk of obstructing their airways, and with an opioid depressing their respiratory centre, silently become apnoeic. Have a working sucker under their pillows. Do not use metal suckers, but rather soft plastic suction catheters that will not damage the friable surgical site. Tonsillectomy patients need a intravenous infusion for 24 hours after surgery. Give adults metoclopramide (Maxolon®) before they return to the ward, because they tend to swallow blood and feel nauseated.

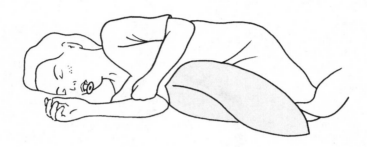

Fig 9.5 Tonsillectomy posture

TRACHEOSTOMY

This may be performed as part of a laryngectomy, or on patients who have been intubated for a period in the intensive care unit.

Keep the airway clear. Use soft plastic Y-catheters to suck out blood and secretions. Thoroughly pre-oxygenate the patient before carrying out this procedure. While suctioning the patient hold your breath and mentally count to 10. Never suck longer than this without stopping to give the patient a rest, and some more oxygen. Suctioning is a sterile procedure; use sterile gloves, and a non-touch technique. (See page 19.)

Change the dressings before the patient returns to the ward. Check to make sure the tracheostomy tube has been formally and firmly stitched in place, rather than just tied in with tape. Warn the ward staff if it has just been tied in place. If the tracheostomy tube falls out in the next 3–4 days it is almost impossible to replace, because a clear tract will not yet have formed through the oedematous tissue. Send sterile dressing scissors, tracheostomy dilators, and a spare tracheostomy tube back to the ward with the patient. These instruments will be needed urgently, if the tracheostomy falls out. Keep them in a sterile plastic bag on the head of the bed until the stoma hardens in 4–6 days.

Humidification

Start humidification with a heated humidifier as soon as possible. Spontaneously breathing patients can be humidified, and oxygenated using a T-piece (see page 408). Do not use a condenser humidifier unless it has been specially designed for tracheostomies. Jamming a normal condenser humidifier (eg. Humidi Vent™) on to the tracheostomy tube can suffocate the patient if he coughs up a glob of phlegm which blocks the paper filter.

UROLOGICAL SURGERY

Most of the recovery room problems follow transurethral resection of the prostate.

Hypotension

Nausea is a sign of hypotension in patients after spinal, or epidural anaesthesia. Sometimes frusemide (Lasix®) is given to patients to encourage a urine output, and flush away clots. The combination of a spinal anaesthetic, a diuretic, and an elderly patient with poor cardiac function is a potent recipe for hypotension. Use an infusion of colloid to restore the blood pressure. Give in 100 ml aliquots until either the blood pressure or the jugular venous pressure (JVP) rises. Heart failure may be a problem. If the JVP rises, and the blood pressure remains low, suspect heart failure. Give ephedrine in 5 mg doses slowly intravenously repeated at 5 minute intervals up to a limit of 1 mg/kg. If the problem persists use a dopamine infusion to support the blood pressure (see page 460).

After a spinal anaesthetic, if the patient sits up abruptly the blood pressure will fall. Sit him up slowly, and measure his blood pressure frequently. If he becomes hypotensive, lie him flat.

Beware of hypotension in the urological patient
Measure the blood pressure frequently.

Hypothermia

A falling core temperature is a problem in elderly urological patients, who may have received many litres of cool bladder irrigation fluid. (See hypothermia, page 165.)

Catheters - see page 33
Drains - see page 27

A confused urological patient?
Consider hypoxia, and water intoxication.

Spinal headaches

The larger the needle used for the spinal anaesthetic, and the younger the patient, the more likely he is to get a headache. Although customary to lie patients flat for some hours after spinal anaesthesia, this is not necessary, and will not reduce the incidence of post-spinal headache. Good hydration helps prevent spinal headache. Even if the patient is eating, keep his drip running for the first 24 hours.

Danger of damage to a numb limb

The patient will normally be fully conscious but unable to feel the lower half of their body. This total analgesia persists for 1–4 hours depending on type of the local anaesthetic agent used. The patient may be injured if a numb leg falls off the trolley, or the patient is knocked while being transferred from the trolley to his bed.

Water intoxication

Water intoxication occurs when the serum sodium falls to less than 130 mmol/litre. It is more serious if the onset is sudden, for instance, after urological surgery, than if it occurs slowly over a number of days. Water intoxication may first present in the recovery room with an obtunded patient who is slow to rouse, or who has muscle twitches. Water intoxication is almost always a result of medical therapy.

The causes are:
- Irrigation of the bladder during transurethral resection of the prostate (TURP) allows water to enter the open prostatic veins—even if glycine 1.5% is used instead of water it may still occur;
- endoscopic endometrial cautery, where water was used as the irrigating solution;
- excessive use of 5% dextrose solutions;
- rarely, inappropriate antidiuretic hormone secretion.

In the recovery room the patient complains of:
- dizziness;
- headache;
- nausea;
- a tight feeling in the chest;
- shortness of breath;

- sometimes abdominal pain.
  He may become
- restless;
- confused, and disoriented;
- start retching;
- develop muscle twitching;
- start wheezing from acute left ventricular failure
  Then
- the blood pressure rises;
- the urine may turn brown due to haemolysis;
- pulse slows to a bradycardia;
- ECG shows a widening QRS complex, and T wave inversion.

If not quickly treated, the patient will become cyanotic, hypotensive, and have a cardiac arrest.

Measure the serum sodium if you suspect acute water overload. A serum sodium of less than 130 mmol/litre is diagnostic. In adults each decrement of 3 mmol/litre of sodium ion indicates approximately a one litre water overload.

Acute water overload is particularly dangerous in children especially if the serum sodium drops below 125 mmol/litre. The mortality is high, and survivors are often brain damaged.

Pathology tests will reveal haemolysis, haemoglobinuria, hyponatraemia, and haemoglobinuria.

Management.

1. Initially give 100%, oxygen measure the vital signs, and stop any infusions containing dextrose.
2. If the patient is stable, and the serum sodium is greater 120 mmol it can be managed conservatively by simply giving neither water nor 5% dextrose for the next few days.
3. If the patient's clinical state is deteriorating acutely you may need to give up to 100 ml of 5% sodium chloride with 100 ml of 20% mannitol intravenously. This should be run in slowly over 30 minutes.
4. Give frusemide 40–120 mg if the patient is developing cardiac failure.
5. A dopamine infusion may be needed cardiac failure develops.
6. Transfer to a high dependency unit where the patient can be monitored for the next few days.

Transient blindness

Transient blindness occurs, rarely, after transurethral resection of the prostate (TURP). It may be due to glycine toxicity. The patient complains of blurred or foggy vision. The fully dilated pupils are alarmingly unreactive. Vision usually returns to normal after 4–6 hours. The cause is unknown.

Septicaemia and toxaemia

The prostate harbours a variety of bacteria. If the prostatic venous sinuses are opened during surgery, irrigation can push bacteria into the blood stream. On occasions these patients develop a short episode of hypotension, severe chills, fever, and capillary dilatation. These symptoms only last a few hours, and then the patient recovers spontaneously. These events are probably due to bacterial endotoxins entering the circulation. Gentamicin is used as the antibiotic of choice. Use an initial loading dose of gentamicin 2 mg/kg intravenously.

Glycine toxicity

When glycine enters the circulation in large amounts it is toxic to the heart and the retina. This effect can be counteracted by adding the amino acid, arginine, to the irrigating glycine solution. The signs of glycine toxicity are nausea, vomiting, convulsions, slow respiratory rate, spells of apnoea, hypotension, cyanosis, and anuria. Transfer the patient to ICU for supportive treatment.

Ammonia is a by product of glycine metabolism. Ammonia toxicity occurs within one hour of surgery, with signs of nausea, vomiting and then deteriorating conscious state which quickly becomes a coma. Blood levels of ammonia may exceed 500 micromol/litre (normal level, 10–35 micromol/litre). The patient will remain in coma for 10–12 hours to emerge from his coma when the blood ammonia level falls below 150 micromol/litre. Ammonia toxicity may be due to arginine deficiency. Transfer the patient to ICU for supportive treatment.

Confusion

Postoperative confusion occurs in about 6–10 per cent of patients undergoing transurethral resection of the prostate. If a patient remains confused or aggressive after prostatic surgery, transfer him to a high dependency nursing area for further management. These patients can be a disturbing problem on a normal ward. Confused patients pull on their catheters causing trauma to the raw urethral surface. Dilutional thrombocytopaenia occasionally occurs, so check their platelet count if bleeding persists. Sometimes particles of prostate gland, rich in tissue thromboplastin, enter the circulation and trigger disseminated intravascular coagulopathy (see page 362).

Deafness (See page 151)

VASCULAR SURGERY

Angiographic procedures

Problems presenting in the recovery room include intimal dissection at the puncture site, haematoma, embolism of debris or clot to the limb causing ischaemia or infarction, and hypersensitivity to the contrast dye. The radiocontrast dye can induce an osmotic diuresis that may present with urinary retention, or hypotension, secondary to an osmotic diuresis.

Perfusion

It is most important to be alert to the risk of the graft blocking in the first few hours postoperatively. The risk is higher in the recovery room, because of the coagulation and blood flow changes that occur during emergence. The graft is more likely to block after general anaesthesia than regional anaesthesia[19]. Check the perfusion of the limbs below the surgery. Record the warmth, colour, pulses and perfusion of the limb on the recovery room chart.

Myocardial ischaemia

About 60 per cent of patients with peripheral vascular disease have ischaemic heart disease. Many of these patients will have no signs of heart disease, but still suffer from silent ischaemia. They have a high risk of myocardial infarction in the first postoperative week. Frequently the first signs of ischaemia develop in the recovery room, and the staff should be alert to detect this complication. If the patient returns to the ward with unrecognized ischaemia there is a high risk that he will have a myocardial infarct, or cardiac arrhythmia and die. The risks rise to a maximum on the first and second postoperative day. Monitor all vascular patients with an ECG, and pulse oximeter in the recovery room. Watch for signs of myocardial ischaemia (see page 276). Many anaesthetists will prescribe prophylactic beta blockers with the premedication for vascular patients. Nitroglycerine paste is also frequently used.

Hypertension, and tachycardia
may precipitate cardiac ischaemia.

Analgesia

Vascular patients need good analgesia. Ideally this should be provided with an epidural infusion, but if not, opioids will help reduce the added stress of postoperative pain.

Hypothermia

Patients undergoing aortic surgery frequently become hypothermic. Do not attempt to extubate vascular patients until their temperature is at least 36.5°C. Hypothermia delays metabolism, and excretion of drugs, and there is a danger of persistent residual effects of opioids, and muscle relaxants. To overcome this risk, the patient may need ventilating, monitoring, and ionotropic support in recovery room for a few hours. After prolonged vascular surgery patients are often acidotic, but providing the cardiovascular system remains stable, and is responding to ionotropes, this does not need correction, and will rapidly resolve as the patient warms.

Renal function

Up to 25 per cent of aortic surgery patients develop deterioration in renal function postoperatively[20]. A renal dose of dopamine (an infusion of 3–5 micrograms/kg per minute) will help improve renal blood flow, urine output, drug excretion and renal function. This is usually started in theatre, transferred to recovery room, and continued in the ward for at least 24 hours. Aim to maintain a urine output of greater than 60 ml/hour. Resist the urge to use frusemide to maintain a urine output unless it is less than 20 ml/hour in which case before giving frusemide 40 mg IV, check that the patient:

• is not volume deplete;
• has warm hands and feet;
• and a CVP of between + 2 cm and + 9 cm of water above the mid-axillary line;
• has a urinary catheter that is not blocked.

The commonest cause of low urine output
after vascular surgery is hypovolaemia.

Major aortic surgery

These patients appear haemodynamically stable on the operating table at the end of the procedure, but as soon as they are moved on to their bed to trolley for transport, they may drop their blood pressure and central venous pressure. If the patient arrives in the recovery room hypotensive, then raise his legs on pillows. Tipping a patient head down will achieve no more than raising his legs, and may have the disadvantage of altering blood flow through the lungs worsening his oxygenation. Check the surgical blood loss. Has it been replaced? Check his jugular venous pressure (or central venous pressure). If it is not elevated, rapidly infuse 5 ml/kg boluses of blood, polygeline (Haemaccel®), hetastarch or plasma. Repeat these boluses until the jugular (or central) venous pressure rises, the pulse slows and the urine output increases. In an adult you may need to infuse a litre or more. After each bolus, listen to the chest for fine rales indicating cardiac failure. Check respiratory rate, and monitor the oxygen saturation with a pulse oximeter. If the respiration rate is rising and rales are heard, or the oxygen saturation falls, then overload may be the problem. X-ray the chest to check for pulmonary oedema. If the jugular venous pressure (JVP) rises and no urine appears, consider starting a dopamine infusion of 3–5 micrograms/kg per minute through a central venous catheter.

(See page 288 for treatment of shock.)

Carotid endarterecomy[21]

Patients undergoing carotid endarterectomy have a high incidence of coronary artery disease, so watch carefully for postoperative arrhythmias. The patient should have intra-arterial blood pressure monitoring.

The operation removes the thick plaque lining the artery to improve cerebral blood flow. In the first few postoperative hours haemorrhage into the neck, may not present with external swelling, but distend into the pharyngeal mucosa causing airway obstruction. This can occur suddenly, but is usually preceded by difficulty in swallowing saliva, noisy breathing, and then stridor. If this occurs notify the anaesthetist and the surgeon. Look for this complication if blood does not come out of the drain tube.

A major problem is a blood clot forming on the raw lining of the carotid artery. This occurs in 1–7 per cent of patients, usually in the first 2 hours after operation, and will cause a stroke. If the artery is surgically unblocked within 30 minutes the stroke may resolve. Watch for changes in conscious state, and diminished power in the limbs. Check that the patient can lift each leg off the bed, and has a firm hand grip. Check his co-ordination by asking him to touch the tip of his nose with each forefinger. Watch for any slurring of speech, difficulty in swallowing, facial drooping, or changes in the size, or reactivity of the pupils. Report to the surgeon immediately if any of these signs occur.

Hypertension is defined as a systolic blood pressure greater than 180 mmHg, or 40 mmHg above preoperative levels, or a diastolic greater than 100 mmHg. Hypertension may be the first sign of impending deterioration of neurological function[21]. Up to 65 per cent of patients get reflex hypertension, particularly if the patient has been previously hypertensive.

This is probably due to the surgery disturbing the baroreceptors located at the bifurcation of the common carotid, and internal carotid arteries. Usually there are no symptoms, but cardiac ischaemia may be revealed by the ECG monitor. You will need good minute-to-minute control of the blood pressure to reduce the risk of clots and strokes. Treat the hypertension with a nitroglycerine infusion 0.3–2 micrograms/kg per minute. Avoid giving hypotensive agents such as hydralazine, in an uncontrolled manner intramuscularly, and avoid long acting drugs.

Up to 45 per cent of patients will become hypotensive in the recovery room, or within 2–3 hours of returning to the ward. The patient may show evidence of cerebral hypoxia, such as confusion, agitation, or disorientation. Hypotension often leads to cardiac ischaemia. Watch for nausea and vomiting as a sign of developing hypotension. Initially treat it with ephedrine, or phenylephrine, while restoring the patients vascular volume. Once an adequate vascular volume is achieved, treat persistent hypotension with a dopamine infusion.

Hyperperfusion syndrome, with loss of autoregulation of cerebral blood flow, sometimes causes unilateral migraines.

1. Jakobsen C. J., Alburg P., et al. (1991). Acta Anaesthesia Scandinavia, 35: 238–41
2. Shiozaki T., Kishikawa M., et al. (1993). American Journal of Surgery, 165: 326–30
3. Lanigan C. J. (1992). British Journal of Anaesthesia, 68: 142–5
4. Magos A. L., Bauman R., et al. (1989). Lancet, 2: 925–6
5. Wheatley S. A., Miller J. M. (1994). British Journal of Obstetrics and Gynaecology, 101: 443–6
6. Benevenuti D. (1993). Plastic Reconstructive Surgery, 92: 1423
7. Fong J., Gadalla F., et al. (1990). Canadian Journal of Anaesthesia, 37: 262–4
8. Sage D. J. (1993). Current Opinion in Anesthesiology, 6: 471–5
9. Clark S. L. (1991). Critical Care Clinics, 7: 877–82
10. Blyth P. L., Mullens A. J. (1991). Australian Clinical Review, 11: 45–50
11. Nagawa H., Kobori O., et al. (1994). British Journal of Surgery, 81: 860–2
12. Dyson A., Henderson A. M., et al. (1988). Anaesthesia and Intensive Care, 16: 405–10
13. Fugere F., Owen H., et al. (1994). Anaesthesia and Intensive Care, 22: 724–8
14. Gustafson Y., Berggren D. (1988). Journal of the American Geriatric Society, 36: 525–30
15. Catley D. M., Thornton C., et al. (1985). Anesthesiology, 63: 30–28
16. Dehring D. J., Areus J. F. (1990). Anesthesiology, 73: 146–64
17. Gooucke C. R. (1989). Anaesthesia and Intensive Care, 17: 458–65
18. Warner L. O., Rogers G. L., et al. (1988). Anesthesiology, 68: 618–21
19. Rosenfeld B. A., Beattie C., et al. (1993). Anesthesiology, 79: 435–43
20. Martin L. F., Atnip P. A. (1994). American Journal of Surgery, 60: 163–8
21. Garrorich M. A., Fitch W. (1993). British Journal of Anaesthesia, 71: 569–79

10. PRE-EXISTING DISEASE

This chapter does not cover every condition you encounter, but it does include many diseases that directly affect the care of the postoperative patient. Cardiac and respiratory problems are dealt with in Chapter 14 and Chapter 16.

Surgery is frequently performed on unfit patients. Their illness may be a result of their life style of smoking, drinking or overeating, or due to an acquired or inherited disease. In the 1940s the American Society of Anesthesiologists issued a scale of fitness of patients presenting for anaesthetics. This scale is known as the ASA grading. Despite its deficiencies it is still widely used for describing patients' fitness.

ASA GRADINGS	
ASA I	Patient is fit for age
ASA II	Patient has mild systemic disease which does not interfere with day to day activity.
ASA III	Patient has severe disease which does limit day-to-day activity
ASA IV	Patient has severe disease which is a constant threat to life
ASA V	Patient is not expected to live 24 hours with or without surgery
An E is added if the surgical procedure is an emergency; for example ASA IV E	

ADULT RESPIRATORY DISTRESS SYNDROME (ARDS)

ARDS is a form of respiratory failure resulting from a variety of direct and indirect insults on the lung, all of which present with similar pathophysiological changes. It is characterized by respiratory distress, progressive refractory hypoxaemia, diffuse pulmonary infiltrates and increased stiffness of the lungs (reduced pulmonary compliance).

About one-third of the patients who die following successful resuscitation after major trauma succumb to progressive respiratory failure. ARDS may occur in any age group, but is particularly obvious in a previously fit young person with no pre-existing heart or lung disease.

The lung (unlike the skin for instance), has only limited ways to respond to injury, by becoming permeable to fluid from the circulation. The outcome is the same no matter what the insult is, in other words when injured the basement membrane between the circulation and the alveolae is damaged, and the lungs leak.

Predisposing factors include:
- aspiration of gastric contents;
- sepsis;
- fluid overload;
- multiple transfusions;
- prolonged hypotension;
- massive adrenergic discharge, such as after head injury;
- fat emboli;
- uraemia;
- burns;
- pancreatitis;
- lung contusion;
- cardiopulmonary bypass.

Less than 5 per cent in each of the above risk factor groups develops ARDS, and there appears to be no one factor that is dominant. If more than three factors are present there is more than a 70 per cent chance of the patient developing ARDS. Shock combined with any of the above factors increases the incidence many fold.

Regardless of the cause, ARDS is always associated with an increase in the amount of fluid outside the circulation and within the lung tissue. It is sometimes called *low pressure pulmonary oedema*. This is unlike cardiogenic pulmonary oedema, where fluid leaks into the lung tissue because of increased back pressure in the capillaries, (*high pressure pulmonary oedema*).

At first the patient is free of respiratory symptoms and signs. Some 12 hours after the injury his respiratory rate rises, followed by dyspnoea and a falling PaO_2 and oxygen saturation, despite a low $PaCO_2$. Oxygen improves the PaO_2 initially. Examination of the chest reveals little, apart from scattered noises in supine zones. About 24–36 hours after the triggering event the chest x-ray shows patches of interstitial oedema. The lungs become stiff and the work of breathing increases. Other features include increased pulmonary secretions, and a decreased functional residual capacity, followed by hypoxaemia, tissue hypoxia and lactic acidosis.

Management includes
1. Careful fluid administration.
2. Controlled oxygen therapy.
3. Diuretics.
4. Turning the patient, because the dependent lung is the worst affected.

5. Using a pulmonary flotation (Swan Ganz®) catheter to keep pulmonary vascular pressures as low as possible.
6. As a last resort, assisted ventilation, with positive end expiratory pressures (PEEP) to improve oxygenation.

AIDS[1]

Groups at high risks of HIV/AIDS include homosexual and bisexual men and their partners, haemophiliacs, intravenous drug users, and children of affected mothers. The main problem is the danger of *needlestick injury*. Seroconversion is uncommon, and estimated to be about 1:300–400[2] needlestick injuries. Recapping needles is the commonest cause of needlestick injuries.

Never, never recap needles.

Dispose of syringes into a proper sharps disposal unit. Do not leave used syringes lying around on benches. Do not use sharp needles for drawing up drugs. Read Chapter 4 on infection control and take *universal precautions* at all times, and not just when you have a patient with HIV/AIDS in the recovery room. Patients with AIDS syndrome are highly susceptible to acquired infections. The HIV carrier rate in Australasia now is thought to be about 1:330 people. Many more carry either Hepatitis B or C, and this is a much greater risk to recovery room staff than HIV.

ALCOHOLICS

Patients who drink alcohol every day are tolerant to some of the sedative drugs. As they emerge from anaesthesia they tend to be restless, often moving about in a semipurposeful manner before they wake properly. They may try to sit up, and open their eyes before spitting out their airway. During this time they appear dazed, will not respond when you talk to them, and occasionally become violent. Do not remove the airway, let them take it out themselves.

Alcoholics are susceptible to spontaneous hypoglycaemia, especially when stressed after operations. If they remain obtunded, or become sweaty or restless check their blood sugar. It should be greater than 4 mmol/litre. If it is less than 3 mmol/litre give 25 ml of 50% glucose slowly through a freely running drip.

Thin alcoholics are often hypothermic in the recovery room. Do not discharge them until their temperature is greater than 36.5°C.

ANAEMIA

Anaemic patients are pale, particularly on the mucosa of the cheeks and lips. In coloured patients check their fingernail beds which should be pink. White nail beds may indicate anaemia. Anaemia disguises the warning signs of cyanosis, and the pallor associated with shock. Hypoxia develops rapidly in an anaemic patient, and will be made worse by bradycardia, reduced cardiac output, respiratory depression, or hypotension (see page 307). In the tropics hookworm, malnutrition, malaria, and chronic tuberculosis cause severe anaemia.

A subtle cause of *relative anaemia* occurs in patients who have had a large blood transfusion in the operating theatre. Although the measured haemoglobin may be acceptable, the donated red cells are reluctant to release oxygen to the tissues. Transfused red cells take 18–24 hours to regain their normal function.

Management:
1. Monitor the patient with a pulse oximeter and an ECG. Watch particularly for signs of cardiac ischaemia, or cerebral hypoxia.
2. Give high inspired oxygen concentration by mask. This needs to be continued in the ward for at least 24 hours, until the red cells are functioning properly again.
3. Replace blood loss early and adequately. Transfuse a susceptible patient to a haemoglobin 20 per cent above his preoperative level.
4. Do not allow the patient to become hypotensive, or allow his perfusion to fall. He may require dopamine to maintain his renal perfusion and cardiac output.
5. Initially assume confusion or disorientation is due to hypoxia. Treat it, and then look for other causes for the confusion.

ASTHMA (See page 335)

CHRONIC OBSTRUCTIVE AIRWAYS DISEASE
(See page 338)

DIABETICS

The recovery room needs some means of measuring blood glucose, such as a portable glucometer. All diabetics must have their blood glucose checked on admission to the recovery room.

Hypoglycaemia

Hypoglycaemia is more commonly seen if the patient has had a reduced dose of their morning insulin, and then been fasted for an afternoon operation. The most disastrous thing for a diabetic to suffer is unrecognized hypoglycaemia. Like hypoxia, hypoglycaemia is rapidly fatal. The clinical signs of hypoglycaemia, sweating, confusion, tachycardia, pallor and anxiety are difficult to detect in the postoperative patient.

Alcoholics and neonates are also susceptible to hypoglycaemia, and need to have their blood glucose checked in the recovery room.

Beta blocking agents, such as metoprolol, or propanolol, mask the warning signs of hypoglycaemia by preventing the sympathetic discharge that accompanies a low blood glucose. They prevent the patient sweating, getting a tachycardia, or becoming anxious.

Hyperglycaemia

Postoperatively, uncontrolled pain can cause hyperglycaemia and ketosis. A carefully given anaesthetic, minimizing sympathetic stimulation, and a well planned recovery is unlikely to unbalance the diabetic.

HYPEROSMOLAR CRISIS

A nonketotic hyperosmolar crisis can lead to coma in the postoperative diabetic patient as a complication of poor metabolic control. It presents as severe hyperglycaemia without ketoacidosis, and usually occurs in middle aged or elderly patients. As the blood sugar rises, serum osmolarity increases. The patient develops a high urine output, and becomes confused, and obtunded. Signs appear when the blood glucose exceeds 25 mmol/litre. This is likely to occur in a poorly controlled diabetic. You can check on the stability of the patient's diabetes by the glycolysated haemoglobin level (HbA$_{1C}$). The HbA$_{1C}$ indicates the average glucose level over the past 2–3 months. The normal value is 5–7.5%; and a level of greater than 10% indicates poor control.

Management of abnormal blood sugars

Try to keep the blood glucose in the range of 5.5–11 mmol/litre while the patient is in the recovery room.

A simple practical approach is:
1. If the blood glucose is less than 5.5 mmol/litre withhold insulin.

2. Treat a blood glucose of less than 3.5 mmol/litre with 25 ml of 50% dextrose.
3. If the blood glucose is greater than 11 mmol/litre then give short acting soluble insulin 5 units intravenously with 60 minutes between boluses. Check the blood glucose every 30 minutes.
4. Maintain a background infusion of 125 ml/hour of 5% dextrose (that is 6.25 grams/hour of glucose).

There are many other regimes. Check which regime the patient's physician prefers.

Significant problems are:
• renal vascular disease;
• autonomic neuropathy causing postural hypotension, bradycardia and urinary retention;
• peripheral neuropathy may affect the pharynx and sleep apnoea is a particular hazard. Neither diabetics, nor any one else should be allowed to snore in the recovery room.

METABOLIC EFFECTS OF SURGERY IN A DIABETIC PATIENT.

During and after surgery, a patient releases catecholamines including adrenaline in response to the stress. Adrenaline does four main things:

1. It breaks down glycogen in the liver and converts it to glucose, (glycolysis).
2. It accelerates the breakdown of fat tissue into free fatty acids, (lipolysis).
3. It increases the conversion of amino-acids to form glucose, (gluconeogenesis).
4. It inhibits the release of insulin from the cells in the pancreas.

Stress also causes the release of cortisol, growth hormone and glucagon; these hormones suppress the secretion of insulin. The overall effect is that glucose is released into the blood stream, while insulin secretion is being suppressed. As the stress subsides, a normal patient will secrete insulin. Insulin facilitates the transport of glucose into muscle cells. Diabetics cannot do this, and without insulin the blood glucose continues to rise; meanwhile the glucose starved muscle tissue breaks down to make more glucose.

Autonomic neuropathy

Diabetics are at great risk from coronary artery disease, hypertension, and autonomic neuropathy. Preoperative postural hypotension is a reliable sign that the patient has coronary autonomic neuropathy (CAN). Autonomic neuropathy is a problem, because the patient does not experience chest pain when his myocardium becomes ischaemic or infarcts. Watch the ECG monitor for developing ST depression while he is in the recovery room. This may be the only sign of myocardial ischaemia. Postural hypotension can be severe, so sit him up slowly, and watch his blood pressure. If he becomes hypotensive lie him down and check his perfusion status. He may require a colloid fluid load to restore his vascular volume.

HINTS

- Dextrose is another name for glucose.
- Although insulin is adsorbed by glass, and some plastics, it is not significant enough to affect treatment when insulin is given in a intravenous infusion, or with a plastic syringe. It is not necessary to prime the IV tubing with glucose and insulin.
- One unit of regular insulin in a 70–80 kg stable diabetic lowers the blood glucose by about 1.5 mmol/litre.
- 10 grams of glucose raises the blood sugar in a 70–80 kg patient by about 1.5–2 mmol/litre.
- To convert mmol/litre of glucose to mg/100 ml multiply by 18.
- The effects of subcutaneous soluble insulin starts in 30 minutes, reaches a peak in 2–4 hours and wears off in about 6–8 hours.
- Given intravenously soluble insulin has a half life of only about 5 minutes, and its effects disappears within about 30 minutes.

DOWN'S SYNDROME[3]

Patients with Down's syndrome have airways that easily obstruct. They have large tongues, small mouths, stiff necks and they are difficult to intubate. They are at risk of extubation stridor, especially after long procedures. Give warmed humidified oxygen, and keep them in recovery room until you are sure this is not going to be a problem. They tend to dribble so nurse them in the recovery position until they are conscious. They sometimes have unstable atlanto-occipital joints, so be careful when you extend their necks, you could dislocated their cervical spine and render them quadraplegic. They are resistant to sedative drugs, but quite sensitive to opioids, a small dose can cause sedation. Start analgesia with a small dose of opioid intravenously.

DRUG ADDICTS

Street addicts and intravenous drug abusers often have malnutrition and are in poor physical health. They have a high risk of carrying Hepatitis and HIV. Universal precautions are your best protection against acquiring these diseases (see page 35).

Drug addicts often have thrombosed veins, and it is difficult to find sites to insert drips or take blood. Ask the patient where his best veins are, he will know.

Amphetamine and cocaine

Amphetamine (*Speed*) and cocaine addicts are depleted of endogenous noradrenaline, and can become alarmingly hypotensive in the recovery room. They may require a noradrenaline infusion to restore and maintain their blood pressure. Use phenylepherine or methoxamine as an interim measure if noradrenaline is not readily available.

Hypotension may also be due to suppressed adrenal cortical function. If an addict becomes hypotensive, consider giving a dose of hydrocortisone to cover the stress of the postoperative period. Make sure the patient is volume replete, then give hydrocortisone succinate 100 mg intravenously. If the blood pressure responds within 5–20 minutes, maintenance hydro-cortisone (about 100 mg 6 hourly) will be needed; refer the patient to a physician.

Opioid addicts

Pain relief is best achieved with regional local anaesthetic techniques, but do not withold opioids if pain relief is required. Recovering addicts may refuse an opioid, so use a regional technique where possible. Active heroin addicts need higher than normal doses of opioid to achieve adequate pain relief. Be careful though, active addicts tend to overstate how much heroin they take. The street drugs are usually diluted with glucose or worse. Titrate morphine intravenously until the desired level of analgesia is achieved. Do not use partial opioid agonists such as pentazocine or nalbuphine which can precipitate acute withdrawal symptoms. Withdrawal may occur for the first time in recovery room with sweating pallor and abdominal cramps. These signs can cause diagnostic confusion. Some addicts are being treated with methadone. Check the methadone dose; and be prepared to substitute morphine if necessary. Initially give a quarter of their methadone dose, as morphine, slowly intravenously and watch for drowsiness, and respiratory depression. For instance if a patient is taking 32 mg of methadone a day, start with 8 mg of morphine intravenously given over 10 minutes.

Opioid addicts may be slow to breathe postoperatively because their respiratory drive has been suppressed. This insensitivity to carbon dioxide persists for several months after their last *fix*.

EPILEPSY

Epileptics may fit in the recovery room. This is more likely if they have not had their routine daily medication.

Propofol is a cause of convulsions in the recovery room. The latency of onset may vary from minutes to hours. Of concern is a report of a day case patient who fitted after discharge and sustained a mild head injury[4]. In view of the current uncertainty about the association of propofol with convulsions it would be wise to be cautious about early discharge if any abnormal muscle movement occurs, and if in doubt, to consider admission.

Other drugs that can cause fitting are enflurane, methohexitone, and pethidine. There have been a number of reports of patients developing fits within 48 hours of commencing pethidine infusions. This is due to the toxicity of norpethidine which is excreted only by the kidney. The total dose should not be more than 24 mg/kg/24 hours[5], and less if the patient has renal impairment. It is unwise to use pethidine in patients with renal failure.

Initial management of fitting:

1. Turn the patient into recovery position.
2. If possible clear the airway with a sucker.
3. Administer 100% oxygen with a mask.
4. Support breathing if necessary.
5   Get help.
6. Bring the resuscitation trolley to patient.
7. Do not try to force anything into patient's mouth to try to stop him biting his tongue.
8. Restrain him, so that he does not damage himself.
9. Record the blood pressure, pulse and respiratory rate.
10. Attach pulse oximeter, ECG and automated blood pressure machine.
11. Secure intravenous access.
12. It may be necessary to intubate him to maintain his airway and ensure proper oxygenation.

Further management:

Fitting can be acutely controlled with intravenous thiopentone 2–5 mg/kg or diazepam 0.15 mg/kg. While this is being given it will be necessary to support the patient's airway and breathing. Phenytoin may be needed if the patient has not received his morning dose. Give the replacement maintenance dose of 1.3 mg/kg slowly intravenously. If he has not had phenytoin before, a loading dose of 12–15 mg/kg will be needed. Consider the possibility that the patient may have aspirated during the fit. If he remaina in a coma intubate him to protect his airway and to ensure adequate cerebral oxygenation.

HAEMOPHILIA

Haemophiliacs have generally been treated with cryoprecipitate (antihaemophilic globulin) before coming to the operating theatre. Fresh frozen plasma can be used as a substitute. They usually do not bleed immediately postoperatively, but may do so in the ward some hours later. Bleeding from superficial wounds although staunched by pressure, will resume when the pressure is released.

HYPOTHYROIDISM

Occasionally unsuspected hypothyroid patients undergo anaesthesia. They are usually obese and elderly with dry, coarse hair, podgy features and a large tongue. They come to recovery room cold and comatose, and are difficult to wake up. They may be hypotensive and have a bradycardia. Muscle relaxants are difficult to reverse and the patients may have to go to the intensive care unit for further management.

LIVER DISEASE

Hypoxia or acidosis is poorly tolerated in patients with liver disease, particularly if the patient is hypoglycaemic. Keep him well oxygenated, and maintain tissue perfusion if necessary with the support of an inotrope.

To avoid renal failure in jaundiced patients (*hepato-renal syndrome*) try to keep their urine output above 1 ml/kg/hour. Start with mannitol 1.5 g/kg, and if needed add dopamine 3–5 micrograms/kg per minute. Insert a urinary catheter to monitor the urine output.

Patients with liver disease metabolize most drugs slowly and their recovery may be prolonged. Use opioids with care as respiratory depression will aggravate their liver disease.

Morphine and papaveretum can precipitate biliary pain in patients who have had a cholecystectomy. Use pethidine instead.

Spontaneous hypoglycaemia occurs without warning in patients with liver disease so check the patient's blood glucose on their admission to the recovery room. Suspect coagulation disorders in all patients with liver disease especially if they have prolonged bleeding from venous or arterial puncture sites.

Keep patients with liver disease warm. Shivering can rapidly deplete reduce muscle glycogen stores and predispose to hypoglycaemia.

LUNG DISEASE (See Chapter 16)

MUSCULAR DYSTROPHY[6]

Patients with muscular dystrophy are weak. They require smaller amounts of all anaesthetic agents than normal patients and are especially vulnerable to muscle relaxants. Make sure they can sustain a head lift from the pillow for a minimum of five seconds, and that they have the capacity to deep breathe and cough before the anaesthetist leaves the recovery room. Where possible use regional blockade for pain relief. If opioids are needed use increments of about one-fifth of the estimated dose and watch for respiratory depression before repeating. These patients are at risk of malignant hyperthermia.

MULTIPLE MYELMATOSIS

Patients with multiple myeloma often have fragile vertebra and ribs. Be careful how you position and move them. The excessive protein they excrete can damage their kidneys, so keep their blood volume up, and do not allow them to become hypotensive or dehydrated. These patients have syrupy, protein laden plasma and are at risk from deep vein thrombosis. Prophylaxis depends mostly on adequate fluid replacement, and moving their legs around to prevent venous stasis. A low molecular weight heparin can be given, and the use compression stockings is recommended.

MUSCULO-SKELETAL DISEASE

Patients with musculo-skeletal disease and myopathies are susceptible to malignant hyperthermia. This will present in the recovery room so monitor their temperature and watch for the signs of sweating, rising respiratory rate and tachycardia.

Patients with low muscle mass are very sensitive to muscle relaxant drugs. Keep a watch for signs of inadequate reversal of these drugs (see page 172) especially as neostigmine wears off after about 45 minutes. You may need to give a second dose cautiously.

Thin atrophic skin and pressure sores or injuries are common. Be careful when moving these patients, not to drag them across the bed sheet, because of the risk of tearing their fragile skin.

NEUROFIBROMATOSIS (Von Recklinhausen's disease)

Patients with neurofibromatosis may have neurofibroma in their airway that causes stridor or upper airway sounds. They occasionally have undiagnosed phaeochromocytomas causing alarming hypertension postoperatively.

NEUROLOGICAL DISEASE

Strokes

Patients with a history of strokes present a variety of problems in the recovery room. Depending on the type of dysfunction they may have:

• difficulty in coughing and deep breathing;
• problems in adjusting their position;
• inability to tell you if they are in pain, or have a full bladder.

It is helpful to make up a chart on a piece of white cardboard so that dysphasic patients can point to a symbol, or a picture which tells you they are in pain, want to empty their bladder, wish to move their position, would like to write something down, are too hot or too cold, and so forth.

Multiple sclerosis

The weakness of multiple sclerosis may be aggravated by regional anaesthesia[7]. These patients are predisposed to deep vein thrombosis and pulmonary embolism. Encourage stir-up exercises and leg movements in recovery room, as most thrombi start to form here. Compression stockings should be fitted before their operation.

Myaesthenia gravis[8]

Patients with myaesthenia gravis are at risk of respiratory difficulties in recovery room for two reasons. Firstly, they have intrinsic muscle weakness and are not able to cough adequately to clear their mucus. Sputum will then block bronchi causing collapse of the lung. Secondly, neostigmine is often used to improve their muscle power, and this can cause salivation, bronchorrhoea and bradycardia (the so-called *cholinergic crisis*). Treat these unpleasant side effects with atropine 0.6–1.2 mg intramuscularly.

Quadraplegics

Pain and hypoxia may trigger autonomic hyperreflexia with fulminating hypertension and cardiac arrhythmias. Once the hypertension is treated the arrhythmias usually resolve spontaneously.

Eaton–Lambert syndrome

Patients with carcinoma of the lung sometimes have Eaton–Lambert syndrome with muscular weakness causing respiratory distress. They will need to be re-intubated, supported on a ventilator and transferred to the intensive care unit. Other patients with dystrophica myotonia and familial periodic paralysis occasionally develop similar problems.

DIABETIC NEUROPATHY (See page 122)

OBESITY[9]

Obesity is a common health hazard, sufferers die early, and have many life threatening chronic diseases such as:
- peripheral vascular disease;
- heart disease;
- breathing problems;
- pulmonary disease;
- liver disease;
- diabetes mellitus;
- diaphragmatic hernias;
- hyperlipidaemias;
- polycythaemia.

OBESITY

Obesity is said to occur when a persons body weight is 10% over their ideal weight. The term morbid obesity applies to people more than twice their ideal body weight. Ideal height weight tables vary from place to place, so it is easier to calculate body mass index (BMI).

$$BMI = \frac{\text{weight (kg)}}{\text{height (m)}^2}$$

Normal	BMI < 25 kg/m^2
Overweight	BMI 25–30 kg/m^2
Obese	BMI > 30 kg/m^2

Monitoring problems

Monitor the patient with an ECG, pulse oximeter. Blood pressure cuffs rarely fit properly, consequently you cannot rely on the readings. An arterial line is useful if the patient has had major surgery. Oxygen consumption is increased, so maintain supplemental oxygen. Fat obscures the surface landmarks so ECG dots are hard to place accurately. Intravenous lines are difficult to insert. Secure them well. Sometimes a central venous line will have been inserted in theatre. Make sure it too is well secured, and consider stitching the cannula to the skin.

Respiratory problems[10]

Large intrapulmonary blood shunts, poor compliance, and co-existing lung disease substantially increase the risk of hypoxia. Furthermore the muscular effort of just breathing is hard work, and uses lots of oxygen. These patients breathe with rapid short shallow breaths, characteristic of a restrictive respiratory disorder. Getting them to cough effectively is difficult. Incentive spirometery is a good way to help them expand their lungs.

Airway management is difficult in fat patients with bulky necks. There is a risk in using laryngeal masks in obese people, because they usually have hiatus hernias with oesophageal reflux, and may regurgitate and inhale (aspirate) their stomach contents. Many anaesthetists give these patients prophylactic antacids and oral ranitidine 150 mg about 2 hours before the anaesthetic to lessen the risk of acid aspiration pneumonitis. If they start to vomit, or regurgitate it is difficult to turn them on their sides. You will need strong and capable help. Ideally, obese patients should not be extubated until they are fully awake. If they come to the recovery room lying on their backs (and often there is no alternative), and still intubated or with laryngeal masks, turn them into the coma position if possible. Do not extubate them until they are awake and then sit them up at 45°. When they can lift their head from the pillow, and touch the tip of their nose with a finger on command, they can then be extubated.

Do not tilt obese patients head down because nearly all obese patients have hiatus hernias. If they regurgitate or vomit while lying on their back in a head down position they will almost certainly aspirate, because you will not be able to move them on to their sides quickly enough.

Nearly all obese patients have sleep apnoea syndrome. They get a bradycardia when they stop breathing and a tachycardia when they start again. These patients need constant attention to maintain an unobstructed airway. A nasopharyngeal airway often helps overcome obstruction due to a floppy soft palate.

Morbidly obese patients may develop the *Pickwickian syndrome* with hypoxia and chronically raised carbon dioxide levels leading to pulmonary hypertension. Opioids further depress their respiration so take special care if you give them.

Administration of drugs

Do not prescribe drugs on the basis of their weight, because you will overdose the patient. Consider obese patients as just thin people inside a fat body. Attempt to assess their lean body mass. A practical way is to feel your wrist and compare it with the patient's wrist to gauge their normal build. Big boned people have more muscle mass than those with fine bones. Then estimate what a person of that body build, and height would approximately weigh if they were of normal build.

Avoid intramuscular injections, because the needles may not be long enough to reach well perfused muscle, and the dose may be deposited in fat from where it will be poorly absorbed. Give analgesics intravenously. Pain relief is best achieved with regional blockade, but that is not always possible. Patient controlled analgesia with pethidine may be useful in these patients, but it is safer to avoid continuous opioid infusions.

Deep vein thrombosis

Obese patients are at risk from deep vein thrombosis and pulmonary emboli. Polycythaemia, immobility, heart failure, and increased intra-abdominal pressures which compress the vena cava make this risk worse. These patients should put on compression stockings before going to the theatre and be encouraged to move their legs in the recovery room. Low dose heparin by subcutaneous injection is widely advocated to prevent deep vein thrombosis in obese patients. It does not require laboratory monitoring. The low molecular weight heparins such as dalteparin (Fragmin®) and enoxaparin (Clexane®) are as effective and safe as unfractionated heparin. In orthopaedic practice they are probably more effective.

Core hyperthermia

Obese patients can become alarmingly hyperthermic because their hot core is insulated by surrounding fat. This may not be immediately obvious, because the patient has cool or cold skin, and poor peripheral perfusion (see page 162 for treatment). If his skin feels cold, but he is sweating slightly, suspect this problem.

Transport

Obese patients are best transported on their beds in a semi-sitting position (30–45°). This saves moving them on and off patient trolleys.

PAGET'S DISEASE

Paget's disease may be missed on preoperative assessment. Classically the patients have a prominent forehead, and a prominent tibial ridge. The patients have a high cardiac output, which if depressed with β-blockers, or other cardiac depressants jeopardises their tissue oxygen supply. Blood loss can be quite overwhelming after orthopaedic surgery, so be prepared for this. Their oxygen requirements are high, because they shunt blood from their arteries to their veins through sinuses in their bones, bypassing the tissues. Continue supplemental oxygen in the ward.

PARKINSON'S DISEASE

These patients are often treated with L-dopa. They may develop arrhythmias or hypertension in recovery room because their adrenergic nerve endings are overloaded with noradrenaline that can be released by a trivial stimulus. Monitor them with an ECG and be prepared to use a β blocker, such as metoprolol, to control tachyarrhythmias. Phentolamine in 1 mg increments can be used to control a rapid rise in blood pressure. This drug acts quickly and lasts about 4–7 minutes. It will give time for either a nitroprusside or labetalol infusion to be set up.

PEPTIC ULCERATION

Peptic ulceration may be exacerbated by surgery. Over the perioperative period, cover this probability with one or more of the following: prophylactic H_2 antagonists (for example ranitidine), a prostaglandin mediator (misoprostol), a surface covering agent (sucraflate) or a proton pump inhibitor (omeprazole). Avoid non-steroidal anti-inflammatory drugs (NSAIDs) because they exacerbate ulcers.

PORPHYRIA

These are a family of diseases of inborn errors in the synthesis of haem, the porphyrin unit of haemoglobin. ALA synthetase is an enzyme which manufactures the precursors of haem. These precursors can cause disturbances in many organs with: acute abdominal pain, vomiting, neuropathies, epilepsy, psychiatric disturbance and even coma. There are three acute hepatic porphyrias, all of which can be triggered by drugs that increase ALA synthetase. Barbiturates are absolutely contraindicated.

Other drugs which can cause problems include anticonvulsants and alcohol.

PSYCHIATRIC DISORDERS

Some psychiatric patients will become acutely disturbed in recovery room. If necessary sedate them with haloperidol 5–10 mg intravenously. Avoid haloperidol in patients taking lithium because it may precipitate neuroleptic malignant syndrome (see page 164). Always exclude hypoxia and hypoglycaemia as a cause of agitation in these patients. For retarded or mentally handicapped patients it is helpful to have someone the patient trusts available to be with them when they awaken from their anaesthetic.

PULMONARY DISEASES (See Chapter 16)

Position affects ventilation and perfusion of the lung[11]. If the patient is on a ventilator, the non-dependent areas of the lung are better ventilated; but if the patient is breathing spontaneously, the dependent areas are better ventilated. Dependent areas of the lung are better perfused, and this increases gas exchange. In the recovery room the patient will have better gas exchange and oxygenation with his good lung down.

RENAL DISEASE

The main problems are delayed excretion of drugs, hypertension and compromised tissue oxygen delivery because of anaemia.

Drugs

Drug excretion is increasingly delayed as the glomerular filtration rate falls below 30 ml per minute. With the exception of atracurium, the action of all the long acting muscle relaxants is prolonged in renal failure. If partial curarization returns (neostigmine has a shorter half life than the relaxant drugs), it is better to sedate and re-intubate the patient; and ventilate him until the effects have worn off, than to try other pharmacological measure to reverse the muscle relaxants.

Intraoperative fentanyl is well tolerated, and rarely lingers to cause a problem in recovery room. Morphine is partly metabolized in the kidneys. It is well tolerated in small doses administered at longer intervals between each dose. Pethidine is poorly tolerated by patients with renal failure as one of the metabolites, norpethidine, is toxic and is excreted only by the kidneys. Norpethidine rapidly accumulates causing irritability, confusion, and eventually convulsions and coma.

*Small doses of morphine given at frequent intervals
is the analgesic of choice for patients with renal disease.*

Oxygen delivery

Oxygen delivery is compromised by anaemia and heart failure if present. Confusion, restlessness or agitation should be regarded as hypoxic in origin and treated with oxygen.

Bleeding

If the creatinine is above 600 mmol/litre the patient is likely to bleed. Avoid major regional nerve blockades because of the risk of haemorrhage into a neurovascular bundle.

Veins are precious. Avoid damaging them because they may be needed for future haemodialysis. Use small cannulae. Insert drips using strictly sterile techniques. Check to ensure intravenous access is no longer needed before removing it.

Thrombophlebitis must never occur. Remove drips at the first sign of tenderness along a vein and reinsert them at another site. These patients are immunocompromised and very susceptible to infection. All dressings should be done as a strictly sterile procedure.

Avoid using the radial artery punctures for blood gases, because this site may be needed for future access for haemodialysis and any stenosis or damage to the artery will preclude it use.

Fluids

Take care not to overload these patients with fluids. Up to one litre of intravenous saline is usually safe. If the patient comes to the recovery room with a second litre running, slow it to a 12 hourly rate unless you receive authoritative instructions and reasons for an alternative regime. Renal patients have no way of excreting fluid. All drips should be attached to burettes or infusion pumps to limit the rate of administration.

If there is any doubt about the management
of renal patients. Consult the renal physician.

Be wary of reducing the cardiac output in an anaemic renal patient, because he needs his high output to deliver oxygen to his tissues. Use vasodilators rather than β blockers for management of hypertension.

RHEUMATOID ARTHRITIS

Rheumatoid arthritis affects 2 per cent of men, and 5 per cent of women over the age of 65. Patients with rheumatoid arthritis are more susceptible to opioid induced respiratory depression than normal people[12]. They are more prone to respiratory obstruction in the recovery room, in particular, to sleep apnoea. They have stiff necks and brittle bones, so be careful when turning them or transferring them from the trolley to the bed. They often have thin, atrophic skin which tears easily, and can rip of when you remove adhesive dressings. Similarly their veins are fragile; so make sure drip cannulas cannot move up and down in the veins. They often have temporomandibular joint destruction, so be careful, when inserting or removing airways, not to over extend their lower jaw. Hypothermia may become a problem.

Pulmonary fibrosis inflicts a restrictive lung disorder on these patients, so they tend to have a higher resting respiratory rate than normal people, and find it difficult to cough or deep breathe effectively. Chronic anaemia can contribute to tissue hypoxia. Patients may be taking steroids (see page 136).

SICKLE CELL SYNDROMES[13]

Suspect sickle cell trait in African negroid people. *Sickle cell trait* (HbAS) occurs in 25 per cent of negroid patients and those from the malaria belt of Africa, Central America and around the Mediterranean Sea. *Sickle cell disease* (HbSS) occurs in 4 per cent of negroid people. At oxygen tensions below 60–70 mmHg (8–9.3 kPa) haemoglobin molecules deform and destroy the red cell. Multiple organ and tissue infarcts occur as the deformed red cells clog the microcirculation. Susceptible patients characteristically have large livers and spleens, but minimal jaundice. A *sickle cell crisis* can be triggered by a tourniquet. A *haemolytic crisis* can precipitate renal failure, particularly in the presence of sepsis.

Patients with the full disease (HbSS) usually undergo a series of preoperative exchange transfusions to reduce the number of abnormal circulating red cells. Never let these patient become hypoxic or acidotic. Keep their inspired oxygen high, keep them warm and ensure their perfusion status is good. Beware if they show signs of poor peripheral perfusion. They require early replacement of blood loss and maintenance of a good cardiac output. Monitor them with a pulse oximeter while they are in the recovery room. To guarantee red cell oxygenation they should return to the ward and remain on oxygen for at least 8 hours, in the case of the sickle cell trait (HbAS), and for at least 48 hours in the case of the full disease (HbSS).

SMOKERS

Elderly smokers are usually arteriopaths with ischaemic heart, and peripheral vascular disease.

Adverse effects of smoking include:
• increased airways resistance makes them wheeze;

- excessive sputum production;
- tracheobronchial ciliary paralysis delays the clearance of sputum predisposing to pneumonia;
- polycythaemia with increased blood viscosity increases the work of the heart and predisposes to myocardial ischaemia;
- increased incidence of coronary heart disease predisposing to postoperative myocardial ischaemia;
- elevated carbon monoxide levels reduce the oxygen carried by haemoglobin predisposing patients to occult hypoxia. The effect lasts many hours after their last cigarette[14];
- nicotine increases heart rate, systolic and diastolic blood pressure and causes peripheral vasoconstriction predisposing to cardiac ischaemia[15]. The vasoconstriction can persist for up to 24 hours after the last cigarette.
- enzyme induction increases analgesic requirements.

Smokers often cause problems in the recovery room. Monitor them closely. They often cough uncontrollably especially after bronchoscopy. The anaesthetist may have sprayed the throat during the procedure. Persistent cough can often be controlled by lignocaine 1–1.5 mg/kg intravenously as a bolus[16].

On the other hand some older smokers will make no effort to cough postoperatively. They seem oblivious of the sputum rattling in their airways, or are unable to muster the lung reserve to cough it free. These patients are likely to suffer partial lung collapse and pneumonia. Encourage them to deep breathe and cough. Use a laryngoscope to clear the sputum from the upper airway. If possible use intercostal blocks or regional blockade for pain relief. Morphine will depress the desire to cough, and pethidine dries out the sputum making it thick, tenacious and difficult to cough up.

STEROIDS

Patients on long term systemic or oral steroids will require extra hydrocortisone support during the stress phase of their injury. Adrenal suppression caused by systemic steroids lasts for many months, and possibly years after the last dose of a long course of steroids. It is important to check if the patient has had systemic steroids in the last year.

Postoperative patients with adrenal suppression may need up to 500 mg hydrocortisone a day for the first 4 or 5 days after surgery, or as long as the stress phase of injury goes on. Use hydrocortisone 100 mg I/M, 6 hourly.

Adrenocortical reserves are diminished in:
- Addison's disease either treated or untreated;
- after bilateral adrenalectomy;
- following steroid therapy in the past year or so;
- pituitary ablation.

No patient should be allowed to die
of refractory hypotension,
without a big dose of hydrocortisone.

THYROID DISEASE

The diagnosis of myxoedema is often overlooked during the pre-anaesthetic work up since the patient is a slow thinker and often a poor historian. All drugs are metabolized slowly. Patients with myxoedema are particularly sensitive to the opioids. Normal doses may have profound effects.

TRAUMA

Patients are at risk from a full stomach and alcohol intoxication. The stomach may take 36 hours or more to empty. Vomiting frequently occurs in the recovery phase so nurse them in the recovery position, and have someone to help, and a big sucker near by.

Patients who have a large amount of tissue trauma need careful control of their fluid balance to minimize the effects of adult respiratory distress syndrome (ARDS). This usually appears about 36 hours after the trauma and presents with a rising respiratory rate, and decreasing PaO_2 on blood gases.

It is unwise to extubate patients with large segments of flail chests. They should be ventilated for some days postoperatively until the flailing segment has stabilized. Tension pneumothorax may present with sudden collapse of the patient while in the recovery room.

Keep in mind the patient may have unsuspected concealed haemorrhage compromising his circulation. This presents in the recovery room with a persistent tachycardia and a tendency for the blood pressure and urine output to fall.

Occult head injury may cause diagnostic confusion if the patient does not fully recover consciousness after the anaesthetic.

Multisystem organ failure (MSOF) is a hazard in major trauma. In particular, renal function can easily deteriorate during the first few postoperative hours. If the patient develops acute renal failure, the prognosis is not good. Record the patient's urine output half hourly. Ideally try to maintain urine output above 1 ml/kg per hour. If it falls below 0.5 ml/kg per hour act quickly to prevent acute renal failure. The threatened kidney does not tolerate hypoxia or hypotension well.

Most patients with severe trauma are transferred on their beds straight from the operating theatre to the intensive care unit. If you do keep them in the recovery room, make a list of all their problems on a board where it they can be seen by all the staff.

ARDS (See page 117)

Fat emboli (See page 103)

Hypothermia (See page 165)

Bleeding patient (See page 349)

Acute renal failure (See page 342)

VON WILLEBRAND'S DISEASE (PSEUDO HAEMOPHILIA)

Patients with von Willebrand's disease have defective platelet adhesiveness and a factor VIII deficiency. Excessive bleeding may be helped by tranexamic acid which inhibits plasminogen activation and fibrinolysis. Desmopressin (DDVAP®) is often given before surgery. This can make the patient pale and nauseated. Cryoprecipitate can be used to help control bleeding if necessary, but it may carry the risk transmission of hepatitis or HIV. Patients with von Willebrand's disease who are surgically stressed often have other changes in their blood that make them clot more readily than they normally would. If they are going to bleed postoperatively it usually reveals itself in the recovery room, whereas other clotting deficiencies bleed some hours later. Superficial bleeding can usually be controlled by pressure. Be careful when taking their blood pressure not to leave the cuff inflated, because they will develop a shower of purpura all over their arm.

WEGNER'S GRANULOMATOSIS

These patients sometimes have friable granulomas in their mouths that can bleed if damaged by a sucker or an airway.

1. Jones M. E. (1989). *Anaesthesia and Intensive Care,* 17: 113–17
2. Rogers P. L., Lane H. C., *et al.* (1989). *Critical Care Medicine,* 17: 113–17
3. Powell J. F. (1990). *Anaesthesia,* 45: 1049–51
4. Reported to the Victorian Consultative Council on Anaesthetic Mortality and Morbidity. Information Bulletin No. 3 February (1994).
5. Stone, McIntyre, *et al.* (1993). *British Journal of Anaesthesia,* 71: 738–40
6. Smith C. L., Bush G. H. (1985). *British Journal of Anaesthesia,* 57: 1113–8
7. Alderson J. D. (1991). *Anaesthesia,* 45: 1084
8. Baraka A. (1992). *Canadian Journal of Anaesthesia,* 39: 1002–3
9. Shankman Z., Shir Y. (1993) *British Journal of Anaesthesia,* 70: 349–59
10. Pasulka P. S., Bistrian B. R., *et al.* (1986). *Annals of Internal Medicine,* 104: 540–6
11. Gillespie D., Rehder K. (1987). *Chest,* 9: 25–9
12. Gardner D. L., Holmes F. (1961). *British Journal of Anaesthesia,* 33: 258–64
13. Galloway S. J., Harwood-Nuss A. L. (1988) *Journal of Emergency Medicine,* 6: 213–16
14. Tait A. R. Kyff J. V. *et al.* (1990). *Canadian Journal of Anaesthesia,* 37: 423–8
15. Egan T. D., Wong K. C. (1992). *Journal of Clinical Anesthesiology,* 4: 63–72
16. Gefke K., Andersen L. W. (1983). *Acta Anaesthesia Scandinavia,* 27: 111–12

11. Difficulties and Disasters

Occasionally an emergency occurs in the recovery room. Stay calm, give instructions in a slow clear voice. Never shout, or alarm more junior staff, or other patients. Regularly practise what to do in various emergencies. Design a resuscitation protocol, and fix it to the wall. (See page 146.) It is better to design one specifically for your recovery room, than to rely on commercially made ones.

AGITATION (See delirium page 153)

AIR EMBOLISM
(SOMETIMES CALLED GAS EMBOLISM)

Air embolism is a cause of sudden collapse. It usually occurs during the insertion, or after disconnection, of a central venous line. With a 5 cm of water gradient, 100 ml of air can be sucked in through a 14 G needle in one second. Despite this alarming fact most episodes of air embolism are minor, and over almost as soon as they are diagnosed.

*Suspect air embolism if a patient collapses
while a central venous line is being handled.*

A bolus of gas in the right ventricle makes the blood froth. The froth blocks the flow of blood to the lungs, and the patient rapidly becomes hypoxic and hypotensive.

Reports of gas embolism are becoming more frequent because of the increasing use of carbon dioxide to inflate the abdomen during laparoscopic procedures. Fortunately carbon dioxide is more soluble than air, and therefore less likely to cause stable emboli.

Eleven per cent of caesarean section patients have detectable air emboli[1] during the procedure, but most are clinically insignificant. They present with breathlessness, hypotension, and arterial desaturation, and the patient is often fearful. These effects may continue when the patient returns to the recovery room.

Other procedures associated with air embolism include laminectomy, head and neck surgery, total hip replacement, hysterectomy, and epidural catheterization.

Signs

Not all of the following need be present to suspect air embolism. Less severe cases may present in the recovery room with a brassy dry cough, wheeze, chest pain and dyspnoea.

Severe cases present with:

- Cyanosis with rapid oxygen desaturation, as measured on a pulse oximeter.
- hypotension and a feeble pulse;
- tachycardia;
- engorged neck veins;
- the characteristic *mill-wheel murmur* over the anterior chest is a late sign. It sounds like water squelching about inside a gum (Wellington) boot;
- tachypnoea progressing to irregular gasping respirations;
- pulmonary oedema;
- sudden collapse;
- cardiac arrest.

MANAGEMENT

Immediate management:

- Stop further air getting into the circulation;
- put your finger over the hole where the air entered;
- call for help;
- give high flow, 100% oxygen;
- tip the patient head down, and turn him on to his left side so that the froth in the right ventricle is carried away from the entry to the pulmonary artery (*Durrant's manoeuvre*);

    If the patient has no carotid pulse, treat as a cardiac arrest.

- External cardiac massage may help break up the froth.
- If he has a central line *in situ*, try aspirating air. This manoeuvre is only worthwhile in the first couple of minutes.
- If the patient becomes moribund, the surgeon could try direct needle aspiration of air from the right ventricle.

    Continuing management:

- patients should stay on high oxygen concentrations for at least 6 hours, to help remove any nitrogen gas bubbles;
- where available, further treatment with hyperbaric oxygen is an option.

Occasionally bubbles of gas will pass through a patent foramen ovale, or through a ventricular septal defect to embolize some other region. If the gas bubble occludes part of the cerebral circulation the patient will have a stroke.

AIRWAY OBSTRUCTION (See page 330)

ANAPHLAXIS

Anaphylaxis is an acute allergic reaction. It occurs in sensitive individuals when foreign compounds (such as penicillin or incompatible blood) are injected into the body.

Anaphylactic reactions

Anaphylactic reactions are an immune mediated response involving the antibody immunoglobulin E (IgE). When the foreign substance (*antigen*) combines with IgE on a mast cell or basophil, large amounts of histamine and other inflammatory mediators are released. Only a tiny amount of antigen is necessary to trigger a huge response. The sudden vasodilation, and catastrophic fall in blood pressure can cause a cardiac arrest. If the patient survives this first insult, capillary beds all over the body leak large amounts of fluid into the tissues. This causes facial, airway and pulmonary oedema. Histamine release may cause an urticarial rash.

Anaphylactoid responses

Anaphylactoid responses occur when some drug or chemical, causes histamine release, either locally, or throughout the whole body. The reaction is not immune mediated, does not involve IgE and is related to the dose and the speed of injection.

Therapeutic principles

1. Any unexpected reaction to a drug or blood products should be suspected as anaphylactic.
2. The patient frequently deteriorates rapidly.
3. The mainstay of treatment is adrenaline since the effect of steroids and antihistamines take some hours to work.
4. Use adrenaline at the first suspicion of anaphylaxis.
5. Adrenaline is safe and effective, but you may need more than one dose.
6. Additional vasopressors are rarely needed. The combination of adrenaline and plasma volume expansion will return the blood pressure and cardiac output to acceptable levels.

Signs

Signs and symptoms include:
Early:
- sensation of warmth or itching especially in the groin and the axillae;
- acute anxiety, restlessness, panic;

- nausea and vomiting.
    Later:
- erythematous or urticarial rash;
- oedema of face, neck, eyelids, and soft tissue.
    Progressing to:
- bronchospasm, cough and wheeze;
- laryngeal oedema with dyspnoea, stridor, drooling, aphonia;
- hypotension sometimes severe enough to cause coma;
- tissue hypoxia with cyanosis;
- arrhythmias and cardiac arrest.

MANAGEMENT
    Immediate management:
1. Stop the administration of the agent causing the reaction.
2. Give high flow oxygen by mask.
3. Assist ventilation if necessary.
4. Lay the patient flat.
5. Call for help.
6. Attach ECG, pulse oximeter and automated blood pressure monitor.
7. Stay with the patient and ensure the airway is patent.
8. Get the emergency trolley and prepare for a rapid infusion of fluids.
    Further management
1. Lay the patient flat and raise his legs.
2. If unconscious clear the airway, intubate and assist ventilation; give high flow oxygen.
3. First give adrenaline. For adults give intramuscular adrenaline 0.3–0.5 ml of 1:1000 (1 mg/ml). For children give intramuscular adrenaline 0.01 ml/kg of 1:1000 (1 mg/ml). If necessary repeat at 5 minute intervals.
4. Now start a wide bore peripheral drip with either colloid or normal saline.
5. Give intravenous adrenaline if there is no response to intramuscular adrenaline, or if no blood pressure or pulse is detectable. For adults give adrenaline 5 ml of 1:10 000 (0.1 mg/ml) slowly over 5 minutes. For children give adrenaline 0.1 ml/kg of 1:10 000 (0.1 mg/ml) slowly over 5 minutes.
    Additional measures once the patient's blood pressure is restored
1. Give a stat dose of hydrocortisone 5 mg/kg inravenously.
2. Give intravenous promethazine (Phenergan®) 0.5 mg/kg.
3. Treat bronchospasm with 2 ml nebulized 0.5% salbutamol through face mask.

4. If necessary give salbutamol 1.5 micrograms/kg intravenously.
5. If wheeze persists, treat it with aminophylline 6 mg/kg intravenously over 10 minutes, followed by an infusion of 0.6 mg/kg/hour.
6. If wheeze still persists, suspect aspirated foreign material (see page 336).

Laryngeal oedema is life threatening. The onset of stridor warns total airway obstruction is only moments away. Consider immediate tracheostomy or cricothyroid puncture. Intubation will be difficult because swollen laryngeal tissue will obscure the vocal cords, and the opening to the trachea. (See also page 333.)

Penicillin allergy

Many patients state that they 'allergic to penicillin'. Often this statement is accepted without question by the medical and nursing staff. Once labelled as 'allergic to penicillin', they can be denied this life saving group of drugs in an emergency. Closer questioning often reveals that they do not have a true allergy, but that they felt 'sick after the tablet', or 'it upset their stomach', or 'the injection hurt' , or some other non-allergic response. True *allergy* is marked by urticarial rash, wheeze and tissue oedema.

ANGINA (See page 276)

ARTERIAL INJECTION (ACCIDENTAL)

Accidental intra-arterial injection of catecholamines, or other toxic compounds, can cause the loss of a limb. It can be treated by diluting phentolamine 10 mg in 10 ml of saline. Injecting it in 1 ml increments directly into the artery. If necessary continue this as a slow continuous infusion to maintain arterial patency. Watch the blood pressure, because phentolamine causes vasodilation and hypotension. Continuous brachial plexus block has sometimes been used, but the results are not encouraging.

Keep careful notes about what has been done because of the medico-legal consequences.

ASTHMA (See page 335)

see also Wheezing, page 180

ASPIRATION (See page 336)

AWARENESS

Estimates of the incidence of awareness vary from 0.2 per cent to 0.9 per cent[2]. Emergency caesarean section under general anaesthesia, is the commonest operation associated with awareness. Patients who have been aware, or partially aware during their general anaesthetic are often distressed, fearful and crying in the recovery room. They may appear confused, and are often unable to say why they are so upset. If a patient tells you she has been aware during the anaesthetic, do not dismiss her claim, it may be true. If you suspect this complication reassure her and attempt to allay her anxiety. Notify the anaesthetist because there may be medicolegal consequences. Carefully record in the history only what you see, and measure, and not your opinions. The anaesthetist and an experienced colleague should consult the patient, take an accurate, witnessed, written record of the patients claims, and organize a series of consultations. The patient may need treatment for *post traumatic stress disorder* (PTSD)[3].

Patients who remember their stay in recovery room sometimes complain about this afterwards. The commonest complaint is 'Something must have gone wrong, because I woke up in pain, and I had to be given oxygen'. This *pseudo-awareness* can be avoided if anaesthetists warn their patients preoperatively they will wake up in the recovery room with an oxygen mask on.

BLEEDING (See page 347)

BREAST FEEDING MOTHERS[4]

Breast feeding women produce between 500–1000 ml of milk daily. If more than 6 hours elapse between feeds the mother becomes very uncomfortable. Allow the mother to express the milk. A well timed anaesthetic avoids most of the problems.

Following a minor operation, the mother may safely breast feed within a few hours of surgery. After major surgery the mother should express the first postoperative feed and discard it.

Avoid drugs with high lipid solubility, such as diazepam, and morphine, because they readily enter breast milk and sedate the baby. A single dose of pethidine is less likely to do this[5]. Avoid non-steroidal anti-inflammatory (NSAID) drugs, because they enter the breast milk. Indomethacin has been reported to cause neonatal convulsions, and aspirin carries the theoretical risk of Reye's syndrome (see page 206). Paracetamol causes no problems in full term babies, but avoid it if the mother is breast feeding a premature baby. All antiemetics are contraindicated because they may cause dystonia, and sedation in the infant.

Stress and fluid restriction depress breast milk production. To help a breast feeding mother keep up her milk supply, make sure she is well hydrated. Even after minor surgery, consider a saline infusion, especially if she has been fasting overnight.

BRUISING

If you do not apply firm pressure to a puncture wound after you withdraw the needle, the patient will get a bruise. Venipunctures stop bleeding after about one minute of firm pressure. Do not just tape a piece of cotton wool over the puncture site, and assume the job is done. Underneath that cotton wool a hidden, painful haematoma will develop. Arterial punctures must receive firm pressure for at least 5 minutes, timed by the clock.

CARDIAC TAMPONADE (See page 287)

CHEST PAIN

Causes of chest pain include:
- angina (see page 276);
- pneumothorax (see page 339);
- air emboli (see page 140);
- pulmonary emboli (see page 339);
- trauma during surgery (in one case it was the assistant's elbow resting on the chest while holding a retractor).

COLLAPSE

Start with the Three Cs.
Call for help, emergency trolley, and defibrillator
Check, pulse, colour, oximeter, and ECG.
Check the clock.

A = Airway
Is the patient cyanosed?
Is the patient's airway patent?
Is he receiving adequate oxygen?

Consider:
- laryngospasm (see page 331);
- foreign body (see page 332);
- fluid in the pharynx.

B = Breathing

Is the patient breathing?
Check air is moving in and out of the chest with a stethoscope, and by feeling the expired air with your hand.
Consider:
- bronchospasm (see page 180);
- pulmonary oedema (see page 283);
- pneumo- or haemothorax (see page 339);
- lobar collapse.

C = Circulation

Check the pulse rate, rhythm and blood pressure. Do an ECG.
Consider:
- cardiac arrest (see page 289);
- hypotension (see page 237);
- arrhythmias (see page 245);
- cardiac tamponade (see page 287);
- tension pneumothorax (see page 339);
- air embolism (see page 140).

D = Drugs, drips and infusions

Are they all running properly?
Consider:
- wrong drug;
- wrong dose;
- air embolism (see page 140).

E = Endocrine status, check for hypoglycaemia

Expose the patient for a complete examination.

F = Fitting

Is the patient fitting?—see below
Eliminate the killers:
- hypoxia (see page 323);
- hypoglycaemia (see page 164).

CONFUSION (See delirium page 153)

CONVULSIONS

If the patient begins to fit, do not try to force his mouth open, or put a gag between his teeth unless he is biting his tongue. You can easily damage teeth if you use force.

Causes include;
- hypoxia;
- hypoglycaemia;
- propofol[6];
- local anaesthetic toxicity;
- epileptics, especially if he has not received his daily medication;
- hypocarbia;
- pyrexia;
- hypocalcaemia;
- water intoxication;
- eclampsia;
- malignant hypertension.

A fitting patient?
Always exclude hypoxia and hypoglycaemia.

MANAGEMENT
Immediate management:
Check the carotid pulse, if it is not present then treat for cardiac arrest.
1. Call for help.
2. Clear the airway.
3. Support breathing.
4. Give high-flow oxygen by mask.
5. Lay the patient on to his side.
6. Attach ECG, pulse oximeter, and automated blood pressure machine.
7. Stay with the patient and ensure the airway is patent.
8. Bring the emergency trolley.
9. Check the blood sugar level.
Further management:
Fitting is usually controlled with:
1. Thiopentone (Pentothal®), 2–5 mg/kg intravenously.
2. Diazepam (Valium®), 0.15 mg/kg intravenously (up to 20 mg in an adult).
3. Phenytoin (Dilantin®, Epinutin®), 250 mg intravenously. And if patient has not already been receiving phenytoin, then up to 1 gram can be safely given over 30 minutes.

4. If the patient remain comatose, consider re-intubation to guard the airway against aspiration of gastric contents.

COUGHING

Coughing is a sign of an irritation in the larynx or lower airway. Causes include:

- laryngoscopy, bronchoscopy or abrasion of the airway during intubation;
- aspiration of foreign material, blood or mucus into the larynx or lower airway;
- oedema or inflammation of the bronchi and bronchioles, as in asthma and pulmonary oedema.

With excessive coughing the patient is unable to get his breath, becomes distressed, and turns purple in the face from vascular engorgement. He may become cyanosed and hypoxic. Coughing can tear stitches especially following plastic facial surgery, middle ear surgery, or repair of a retinal detachment. It might also break ribs (*cough fractures*) in the elderly, contribute to cardiac arrhythmias, and disrupt abdominal sutures.

MANAGEMENT

If coughing becomes a problem, or is threatening oxygenation:

1. Sit the patient up.
2. Give high flow oxygen by mask.
3. Attach a pulse oximeter and ECG.
4. Ask the anaesthetist to examine the airway with a laryngoscope to check for foreign material.
5. If the coughing is due to simple irritation of the mucosa, give a bolus dose of lignocaine 1.5 mg/kg intravenously[7] over 30 seconds, this quickly solves the problem.
6. If the patient becomes hypoxic or develops cardiac arrhythmias, it may be necessary to sedate, and re-intubate him and re-assess the situation.

Morphine is a good cough suppressant, but pethidine is not. If a patient is producing excessive sputum, then it is unwise to suppress his cough reflex. The accumulating secretions may block airways causing lower lobe collapse, and pneumonia. Coughing can sometimes develop into stridor with laryngeal spasm, a life threatening situation (see page 330).

CRYING PATIENTS

Occasionally patients sob when emerging from anaesthesia. Often they do not know why they are crying. It does not necessarily mean they are in pain. It is sometimes a sign that the patient has been aware during the operation. Unpremedicated patients, and those who have been anaesthetized with propofol for a short procedure are more likely to cry on waking. Patients suffering from anxiety or depression sometimes cry too.

CYANOSIS

Cyanosis is a bluish discoloration of the mucous membranes or skin. If in doubt, compare the patient's tongue with the colour of a staff member's tongue.

Treat cyanosis as life-threatening hypoxia until you are sure of the cause. (See Collapse, page 147.)

Causes include:
- Hypoventilation caused by residual anaesthetic agents, muscle relaxants, opioids, or benzodiazepines.
- Airway obstruction, such as laryngospasm, asthma or inhaled vomitus.
- Lung disease, such as pneumonia, lung collapse, or pulmonary oedema.
- Mechanical problems, such as haemo- or pneumothorax.
- Cardiac failure, air emboli, or fat emboli.
- Abnormal haemoglobin, such as incompatible transfusion with massive haemolysis, methaemoglobin, sulphaemoglobin, or carboxyhaemoglobin

There are two types of cyanosis, central cyanosis and peripheral cyanosis.

Central cyanosis

Central cyanosis is seen as blue lips, tongue and mucous membranes. It is a sign of severe hypoxia (see Chapter 15).

Peripheral cyanosis

Peripheral cyanosis causes blue hands, feet and fingernail beds. If the patient has central cyanosis he will have peripheral cyanosis too; but peripheral cyanosis with no central cyanosis, indicates the patient is cold, has venous congestion, or is shocked. Cyanosis is difficult to detect in a dark-skinned person. Check his nail beds, the insides of his mouth or the inner part of his lower eyelid; even so you cannot always tell. A pulse oximeter is not influenced by skin colour and gives an accurate reading.

DEAFNESS

To help your deaf patient orient themselves, put their hearing aids back before they recover consciousness. If you are wearing a mask, take it off so your patient can read your lips. Don't shout. Warn staff not to use a painful stimulus when the patient does not respond to a verbal stimulus.

If nitrous oxide was used during the anaesthetic, patients with previous reconstructive middle ear surgery may suffer from pressure changes in their middle ear, causing a transient loss in hearing.

Deafness has occurred after spinal anaesthesia. A loss of 10 decibels, or more has been recorded in 3.7 per 1000 cases[9].

CYANOSIS

Cyanosis is not seen until the patient has at least 3 grams of deoxyhaemoglobin in their blood. This corresponds approximately to a PaO_2 less than 50 mmHg (6.6 kPa), and a pulse oximeter reading less than 85%. Occasionally central cyanosis is caused by drugs, such as methylene blue, or prilocaine; or an incompatible blood transfusion.

Anaemic patients may not become cyanosed even when dangerously hypoxic. Patients with polycythaemia, such as chronic bronchitis can look blue in the face (plethoric) without being hypoxic.

Good lighting is needed to detect cyanosis properly. Daylight is preferable, but special fluorescent tubes can be used. Ordinary fluorescent tubes cast a blue light on the patient. The yellow light from a normal incandescent light bulb also makes cyanosis difficult to detect.

Methaemoglobinaemia may present as cyanosis. The drugs prilocaine, benzocaine, and nitroglycerine are the usual causes. The arterial blood looks dark, almost brown, when a sample is taken. Methaemoglobin forms when a chemical agent oxidizes the haemoglobin, changing the iron from a ferrous (Fe^{+2}) to a ferric (Fe^{+3}) form. Methaemoglobin cannot carry oxygen and tissues become hypoxic. The pulse oximeter misleading gives a an oxygen saturation reading of about 80%, irrespective of the true saturation[8]. Take blood for methaemoglobin levels if you suspect this condition, repeat at 2 and 8 hours. A level greater than 15% will cause hypoxia, greater than 60% in dangerous and greater than 70% is fatal. Treatment is with methylene blue 1 mg/kg over 10 minutes. Methylene blue, itself, makes the patient cyanosed. Excess methylene blue can cause more (Fe^{+3}) to form. Measure blood gases, the PaO_2 may well be normal, but if the patient is hypoxic then an acidosis will develop.

DEATH IN THE RECOVERY ROOM

From time to time a patient will die in the recovery room. For medico-legal reasons carefully document the events leading up to the death, and the resuscitation attempts. As these notes could be required in court, it is essential they should record fact only, and not opinion. They should be detailed enough to give a record, that does not rely on memory, even years later.

Staff involved may be upset, especially if the patient was young, or the death perceived as avoidable. Counselling may be needed for staff members.

Have suitable protocols already set up to cope with this event. You need guidelines about how to inform relatives, who should be present at this interview and where the interview should be held. It is important for senior medical staff, not junior or nursing staff, to initially tell the relatives. Telephone the relatives to ask them to come to the hospital. It is possibly unwise to tell them over the phone of the death, simply inform them there has been a problem. Suggest they bring someone with them. Many medico-legal and litigatory problems can be avoided if this difficult task is done in a humane, honest and sensible manner by the senior staff responsible for the patient. Litigation usually arises when relatives believe they are being deceived.

DELAYED EMERGENCE

Sometimes patients take a long time to emerge from their anaesthetic. The reasons for this (in order of incidence) are:
1. Prolonged action of anaesthetic drugs.
2. Metabolic causes.
3. Brain damage.

1. Prolonged action of the anaesthetic drugs

Sometimes patients take more than 90 minutes to excrete or metabolize the drugs given during the anaesthetic. This is a process that cannot be hurried. Do not use painful stimuli in an attempt to hurry the process. Droperidol, scopamine, and diazepam can often have a more sedating effect than anticipated.

Naloxone will reverse opioids; but you should consider the metabolic and physiological consequences of catapulting the patient into agonizing pain. (See page 198 for dose and precautions.)

Flumazenil will reverse the actions of the benzodiazepines, but it only works for about 35 minutes. The dose is 3 micrograms/kg intravenously over 15 seconds. It can be repeated at 60 second intervals to a maximum of 15 micrograms/kg.

Drug interactions. Occasionally drug interactions can be responsible; for instance, erythromycin and ketoconazole prolong the action of midazolam by many hours [10].

2. Metabolic causes

Hypothermia, hypoventilation hepatic, and renal dysfunction delay the metabolism and excretion of drugs.

3. Neurological damage

A serious complication is brain damage caused by hypoxia, stroke, fat embolism, air embolism, intraoperative hypotension. Water overload after prostate surgery, or uterine endoscopic procedures, can cause coma or hemiparesis. Consider occult head injury or alcohol intoxication in trauma patients who are slow to wake up.

Treatable causes

Exclude hypoglycaemia with a blood glucose reagent stick in all diabetic and alcoholic patients as soon as they are admitted to the recovery room. The blood glucose should be above 3.5 mmol/litre (see page 121). Check for and treat water overload (see page 110). A stroke after carotid artery surgery needs immediate re-operation. Air embolism may respond to hyperbaric oxygen therapy.

DELIRIUM[11]

Delirium is sometimes called an *acute brain syndrome*. Some patients become agitated, or belligerent, and need restraint on emerging from anaesthesia. The patient appears to have perceptual difficulties, not knowing where he is, or what is going on. Incoherent speech, disorientation and a clouded consciousness are other features. He may well know his name, and even respond to it, but remains confused.

The commonest causes of delirium are:
- hypoxia, this can maim or kill, so exclude it first;
- pain;
- a full bladder in the presence of sedative drugs;
- hypoglycaemia;
- ketamine;
- scopolamine (hyoscine) used as a premedication.

Even transient hypoxia at some time in the perioperative period will later cause a prolonged period of postoperative confusion, especially in the elderly. Proving a patient is not hypoxic, or has not had a period of hypoxia, is very difficult. Blood gases and pulse oximetry, although reassuring, may not be sufficient to provide this proof (for the subtle causes of hypoxia see Chapter 15).

The confused restless, and agitated patient
is hypoxic until proven otherwise.

The cause of delirium may not be clear; but psychological factors as occur with operations threatening body image aggravate the problem.

Factors predisposing to delirium include:

• younger age;
• drug or alcohol abuse;
• amputation;
• mastectomy;
• heart surgery;
• inadequate psychological preparation;
• intraoperative hypoxia, hypotension,
• intraoperative cholinergic drugs;
• intraoperative awareness;
• tricyclic antidepressants.

Pre-existing causes include head injury, hepatic or renal failure, electrolyte abnormalities, mental retardation, dementia, and severe infection. Most of these are obvious preoperatively.

MANAGEMENT

1. Give 100% oxygen and attach a pulse oximeter.
2. Restrain the patient if necessary.
3. If possible, avoid sedation.
4. If you suspect scopolamine, droperidol, phenothiazines, ketamine or tricyclic antidepressants to be the cause, cautiously give physostigmine 0.02–0.03 mg/kg intravenously. It may slow the pulse and cause salivation. Be careful, it may cause convulsions. It has a short action and you may need to give another dose.

THE VIOLENT PATIENT

Occasionally a patient will warn you that they have been violent on emerging from a previous anaesthetic. Take this warning seriously, because you could be confronted with a violent patient who is a danger to himself, or the staff. If you have no intravenous access give ketamine 1.5 mg/kg I/M. It is rapidly absorbed from most sites. This will rapidly bring the patient under control, making him comatose. Then support his airway, and treat him as a comatose patient. Allow him to emerge after giving him haloperidol 5–10 mg I/M.

DRY MOUTH

Some patients will complain of a dry mouth and lips. There are commercial preparations that will help, or ask your pharmacy to make up a lemon flavoured ointment to smear on their lips. Avoid glycerine based ointments, because they dry the lips even further. Dry mouths make some patients restless. Give them small sips of water, or let them suck on wet gauze or ice. In many recovery rooms after minor surgery it is now permissible for patients to have a small drink. Check with the surgeon and anaesthetist before offering fluids.

DYSPNOEA
(see also Chapter 16)

Dyspnoea is an uncomfortable feeling of shortness of breath. Dyspnoea occurs when the patient has to work harder to breathe than he would normally need to. The extra work is detected by stretch receptors in the lung tissue (*J receptors*) and special muscle spindles in the intercostal muscles and diaphragm.

Causes of dyspnoea in the recovery room include:
- Inadequate reversal of muscle relaxants.
- Airway obstruction, such as laryngospasm, laryngeal oedema, asthma, bronchiol inflammation due to aspiration.
- Mechanical causes, such as haemo- or pneumothorax.
- Stiff lungs (meaning low lung compliance) that occur in pneumonia, pulmonary oedema, and ARDS.
- Hypoxaemia with a PaO_2 less than 55 mmHg (7.24 kPa), or hypoxia the tissue have switched to anaerobic metabolism causing a lactic acidosis.
- Sepsis, water overload, or saline overload, where fluid accumulates in the lung tissue.
- Post-thoracotomy.
- Cardiac failure.
- Shock or malignant hyperthermia with lactic acidosis.
- Rarely in recovery room, diabetic ketoacidosis.

Dyspnoeic patients do not tolerate an oxygen mask; they pull it off their face in effort to 'catch their breath'. It takes tact and persistence to keep the mask on. A hypoxic dyspnoeic patient can be aggressive.

EXTRAVASATION

Some drugs are tissue toxic, and if they extravasate during an intravenous infusion they cause tissue death. If there is any pain at the site of an infusion, take it out and re-site it elsewhere.

Extravasated adrenergic drugs, such as the adrenaline, dopamine, noradrenaline and isoprenaline cause intense vasoconstriction.

Surrounding muscle and skin become ischaemic and die. The results can be horrific, with muscle, skin, and tendon necrosis requiring disfiguring, and destructive debridement. Dilute phentolamine 10 mg to 10 ml in saline. Inject the dilute phentolamine in 1 ml boluses around, and into the area of the extravasation. Watch the blood pressure because phentolamine causes hypotension.

Extravasation of drugs such sodium bicarbonate, potassium containing solutions, calcium chloride and some antibiotics cause similar problems. Keep the needle in and inject saline into the area to dilute the drug. Apply warm 40°C compresses to dilate the vessels serving the area. Block the nerves to the region with local anaesthetic to provide analgesia and improve tissue perfusion.

EYES

Red eyes

Unconscious patients do not blink. It only takes a few minutes for ulcers to form once the cornea dries out. Keep unconscious patient's eyelids closed. Use a lubricating ointment, such as methyl cellulose (Lacrilube®) to protect the eyes of a comatose patient. Do not use chloramphenicol ointment because of the slight risk of bone marrow suppression.

Sore, dry or gritty eyes occur if they have been open during the operation. If the patient complains of this, make a note about whether his eyes were taped shut during the operation, and which ointment, if any, was used. If you are concerned then stain the affected eye with fluorescein to reveal corneal or scleral damage. Irrigate the eye with saline, tape it shut and refer the patient to an ophthalmologist.

Foreign bodies

When used to splint fractured noses, plaster of Paris can get into the eye. Wash out the grit with normal saline.

Trauma

Surgical instruments have been known to rest, or even be dropped on the eye during surgery. If this occurs notify an ophthalmologist, even if there appears to be minimal or no damage. He will examine the fundus with an ophthalmoscope. There may be medico-legal consequences.

Pressure on the eye from an anaesthetic mask can cause retinal haemorrhages and detachment. Diabetic patients are especially at risk. Hypotensive anaesthesia has also caused vitreous haemorrhages.

Drugs

In susceptible patients atropine, glycopyrrolate, ketamine, and trimetephan, can precipitate acute closed-angle glaucoma. It presents with agonisingly painful red eye, corneal clouding, and a dilated pupil. The vision goes fuzzy, and the patient may become nauseated and vomit. This event is an emergency, and if not treated promptly the patient will go blind. If you suspect acute glaucoma start acetazolamide 10 mg/kg intravenously, and an infusion of 3 ml/kg of 20% mannitol. Call an ophthalmologist for help.

Blindness

Rarely, transient blindness occurs after transurethral resection of the prostate (TURP) (see page 111).

Retinal haemorrhage can be caused by pressure from a face mask, especially if it has been held tightly in place by an elastic harness. The patient will complain of blotchy vision. Retinal haemorrhages can also occur after epidural injection[12].

Retrobulbar haemorrhage sometimes occurs after retrobulbar injections for cataract surgery, or even after cosmetic blepharoplasty[13]. Unless rapidly decompressed this calamity will cause blindness. Report visual disturbances to the surgeon without delay.

FEVER (See hyperthermia page 159)

Fever is uncommon in the recovery room
do not ignore it.

FINGERNAILS

If a patient has long fingernails, and her hand is allowed to lie on her chest, the pressure from the nails may ulcerate the skin. This can happen surprisingly quickly in comatose patients.

HAEMORRHAGE (See page 347)

HAIR

Coagulated dry blood occasionally remains in the hair after head and neck surgery. Dried blood is hard to get out, and putrefies if it is left. Wash and comb the hair with aqueous cetrimide being careful not to get it in the eyes, and then rinse with ample water.

HEADACHE

Headache occurs in 10–30 per cent of patients particularly after minor surgery. Those people who suffer from frequent tension headaches are more prone to get them postoperatively. Place a cool wet towel on the forehead. Start with simple analgesics, such as paracetamol 500–1000 mg. If the patient cannot take oral medication, use paracetamol suppositories. Pethidine 0.5–1 mg/kg is a stronger alternative, but avoid morphine because it can aggravate headaches.

Other causes include:
• intraoperative tension on neck muscles or cervical spine joints;
• spinal anaesthesia;
• accidental dural tap during epidural anaesthesia;
• underventilation;
• opioids;
• intraoperative hypotension or hypoxia;
• caffeine withdrawal;
• severe hypertension;
• water intoxication.

HICCUPS

Hiccups frequently occur after laparoscopy, or more rarely after abdominal procedures when the operation has been close to the diaphragm. Usually they respond to gently sucking out the pharynx. If hiccups persist, metoclopramide 5–10 mg intravenously, or ephedrine 5 mg intravenously may help. Sometimes hiccups resist treatment. In the past chlorpromazine has been used, it never seems to work, and causes hypotension and prolonged sedation.

HOARSE VOICE

A hoarse or croaky voice is more likely in patients who have been intubated for some hours. The endotracheal tube forcibly abducts the vocal cords, and may actually dent them. The hoarse voice usually resolves in a few hours. Recurrent laryngeal nerve damage can occur during a thyroidectomy or operation on the neck. This will paralyse one or both of the vocal cords. Characteristically the patient is unable to say 'Eeeee' in a higher pitched voice. Inform the surgeon if you suspect this complication.

Infants and children with a hoarse voice following intubation may go on to get airway obstruction some hours later. Children with stridor or a hoarse voice should be admitted and closely observed. (See page 62 for management of stridor.)

HYPERCOAGUABILITY

Postoperative hypercoaguability is a complex disorder involved in a wide range of thrombotic complications. You may notice it because blood samples clot on the way to the laboratory, or intravenous infusions stop running. Haemostatic mechanisms are normally finely adjusted to produce a clot at the site of vascular injury, and to avoid clot formation in areas where the endothelium is intact. Hypercoaguability predisposes to deep venous thrombosis, stroke, myocardial infarction and occlusion of vascular grafts. Epidural blockade, by producing sympathetic blockade, increases blood flow through the operative site. It also, in some obscure ways, affects platelets, and some blood factors to decrease blood coagulability, and reduce the incidence of thrombotic complications[14]. If you suspect hypercoaguability consider using compressive stockings, nitroglycerine transdermal patches, or low molecular weight heparins.

HYPERVENTILATION (See page 322)

HYPERGLYCAEMIA (See page 121)

HYPERTHERMIA[15]

Fever (pyrexia) usually refers to a temperature of 37.8–40°C
Hyperthermia usually means a temperature greater than 40°C
It is rare for a patient to become febrile in recovery room, but when it does happen it is always significant.

Fever

Fever occurs because the patient's heat production is faster than his heat loss. Normally the body produces about as much heat as a 100 watt light globe to keep the body at about 37°C. At about 42°C brain enzymes are damaged, and muscle tissue breaks down (rhabdomyolysis) releasing myoglobin into the blood stream.

Oxygen consumption increases by about 15 per cent for each degree Celsius rise in body temperature. The heart needs to increase its stroke volume and heart rate to meet the tissue oxygen demands; to compensate for vasodilation, and the increased work of breathing. Arrhythmias and cardiac failure occur if the heart is unable to increase its output.

A rise in body temperature can be generated by:

1. Rise in general metabolic activity as occurs in:
   • sepsis due to aspiration pneumonia, following urinary surgery, or drainage of abcess;
   • thyroid storm;
   • phaeochromocytoma;
   • reactions to blood or blood products (see page 353);
2. Increased muscle activity, such as
   • shivering and shaking (see page 174);
   • malignant hyperthermia (see below).
3. Very obese patients may fail to lose heat and suffer from core hyperthermia (see page 162).
4. Drug reactions.
   • Atropine or scopolamine can cause delirium, dry mucous membranes, dilated pupils flushed skin, and tachycardias. This is best treated with cooling, sedation, and only if necessary, physotigmine.
   • Allergic response.
   • LSD, amphetamines, but particularly cocaine can cause an adrenergic storm.
5. Central nervous system catastrophes, following events such as, intracranial haemorrhage are associated with an adrenergic storm.
6. Occasionally the patient may have been covered with drapes, or plastic sheeting in the operating theatre and therefore unable to lose heat.

Malignant Hyperthermia (MH)[16]

Also known as malignant hyperpyrexia.

This rare condition occurs in about 1:15 000 children, and perhaps in 1:50 000 of the adult population. It tends to run in families as an autosomal dominant gene. It is triggered by many drugs including halothane, isoflurane, ketamine, and especially suxamethonium.

The prognosis is not good. With treatment the mortality is about 21 per cent, and without treatment it is more than 70 per cent[17]. If you are to save the patient's life the disease must be recognized quickly.

Prepare written protocols so even if the situation arises at 3.00 am everyone will know what to do. Regular practice is the key to success.

The first sign is an unexplained tachycardia, and an increase in respiratory rate (reflecting a rise in CO_2 production) shortly followed by a fulminating rise in body temperature. The temperature rises rapidly to above 40°C, the patient is hot and flushed (almost beetroot coloured). He then becomes rapidly acidotic and blue with a mottled skin. His muscles are twitching or tightly and stiffly contracted.

Laboratory findings show marked metabolic acidosis, hyperkalaemia with myoglobinaemia, and myglobinuria.

Use dantrolene for treatment. It is an expensive drug, and groups of hospitals find it cheaper to pool their resources instead of each hospital having a full stock. Keep dantrolene refrigerated. Keep full instructions on how to use it and a MH protocol with the drug. Do not lock the dantrolene away in a pharmacy. It must be immediately available should you need it. Dantrolene is an orange powder, which is hard to dissolve, and requires a special solvent (containing mannitol and sodium hydroxide). Make sure you have enough. You will need up to 18 vials as a starting dose to treat one case.

MANAGEMENT

Immediate management.

1. Give 100% oxygen and continue it in an attempt to keep up with the enormous rise in oxygen consumption.
2. Attach an ECG and pulse oximeter, insert a rectal temperature probe; attach an end tidal PCO_2 monitor.
3. Summon help.
4. Prepare to insert an arterial line, a central venous line, and consider a pulmonary artery flotation catheter.
5. Prepare for rapid intravenous infusion.
6. Assemble cooling equipment and at least 12 litres of ice cold saline.
7. Monitor blood gases frequently to check pH and oxygenation.

Further management.

At this stage it is better to move the patient to an intensive care unit.

1. Measure blood gases early and prepare to support ventilation if necessary. Take serial blood gases every 20 minutes.
2. If the patient is still intubated hyperventilate him vigorously. Start with a minute volume of 12–14 litres per minute. Use the blood gases and an end tidal CO_2 monitor as a guide. The arterial PCO_2 is roughly inversely proportional to the patient's minute volume. Should you need to paralyse your patient use vecuronium as the preferred relaxant and sedate the patient with morphine.
3. Commence a dantrolene infusion starting at 2 mg/kg which should be repeated every 7 minutes until muscle rigidity resolves. Give at least 6 mg/kg[18]. Do not exceed 10 mg/kg.
4. Cool the patient with ice packs in the axillae and groin. Supplement the ice with a wind tunnel cooled with water. Peritoneal lavage with cool (but not iced) fluids may help.

5. Infuse cold (but not iced) solutions. The usually rate is 1000 ml given every 10 minutes for the first 30 minutes. A central venous line, urinary catheter and possibly pulmonary artery flotation catheter will guide the fluid replacement therapy because cardiac and renal failure are constant threats.

6. If the pH is less than 7.10 correct the acidosis with sodium bicarbonate 0.5–1.0 mmol/kg, and then recheck the blood gases and pH. It may be necessary to repeat the sodium bicarbonate. Keep the arterial $PaCO_2$ between 35–45 mmHg (4.6–5.9 kPa) by hyperventilating the patient.

7. Correct electrolyte disturbances. Hyperkalaemia and hypoglycaemia are hazards.

8. To prevent myoglobin and haemoglobin sludging up the kidneys, maintain the urine output over 1.5 ml/kg/hour. Give 0.3 g/kg of mannitol over 15 minutes and if necessary supplement with frusemide 0.06–1.5 mg/kg.

9. Give hydrocortisone 100 mg intravenously each hour.

10. Treat tachyarrhythmias prophylactically with procaine amide 15 mg/kg intravenously over the first 60 minutes. Do not use lignocaine, because it is a known trigger agent.

11. Complications include coagulopathies, renal failure, pulmonary oedema and hypothermia from over enthusiastic cooling.

Core hyperthermia

Obese people sometimes generate heat faster than it can escape through the fat. They shut down their cutaneous circulation if they are in pain, or become fluid deplete. Although their skin feels cold, their core temperature may rise to more than 40°C. Adequate analgesia and fluid replacement will prevent the cutaneous shut down. If necessary, start with a tiny dose of chlorpromazine, 0.015 mg/kg intravenously, to vasodilate them, and allow them to dissipate heat. Larger doses of chlorpromazine will drop the blood pressure dramatically.

Thyroid Storm

Many of the features of thyroid storm are similar to malignant hyperthermia: hot flushed skin, sweating, tachycardia, atrial arrhythmias, hypotension, pulmonary oedema, nausea, vomiting and perhaps diarrhoea. As the temperature rises convulsions and coma will occur. The temperature will probably be in the region of 38–41°C. Females in their late 30s or 40s are the most susceptible. Thyroid storm is a result of, either undiagnosed, or poorly treated thyrotoxicosis. It usually occurs 8–16 hours after severe stress or an operation, and is not often seen in recovery room. Preoperative stress, such as anxiety, apprehension, iodine withdrawal, pain, trauma, prior surgery, or infection may cause it to occur in recovery room.

Treatment includes:

1. Supporting oxygen and fluid requirements along with reducing the patient's temperature as outlined in the treatment of malignant hyperthermia.
2. Control arrhythmias with propanolol 0.015–0.03 mg/kg intravenously every 10 minutes until tachycardia drops below 100 per minute.
3. Propylthiouracil 12.5 mg/kg loading dose down a nasogastric tube; followed by 0.5 mg/kg every 8 hours.
4. Sodium iodide 30 mg/kg intravenously. Theoretically this should not be given until the propylthiouracil had time to reduce the iodine uptake by the thyroid gland.
5. Hydrocortisone 3–5 mg/kg intravenously will help inhibit further thyroxine release. Adrenal insufficiency is a feature of thyroid and adrenergic storms.

Phaeochromocytoma[19]

This is a catecholamine secreting tumour, usually in, or near the adrenal gland. It is said to occur in 0.5–1 per cent of hypertensive patients, usually in the 30–50 year age group. In patients with unsuspected phaeochromocytomas 50 per cent of deaths occur either in association with anaesthesia, or in the recovery room.

Often the stress of intubation or the onset of pain postoperatively is the trigger for the tumour to release its catecholamines. However drugs, such as the dopamine antagonists, metoclopramide, and droperidol; or any drug with the potential to cause histamine release, such as the opioids, may trigger an attack.

This disease is a great mimic. It usually creates a hypertensive crises, and may be followed by hypotension, but it may also imitate renal colic, syncope, shock, sepsis, ischaemic heart disease or cardiac failure. Other features are hyperglycaemia, nausea, vomiting, postural hypotension, and sweating but not flushing.

MANAGEMENT

1. Give oxygen, attach an ECG, pulse oximeter, and non-invasive blood pressure monitor, and establish an intravenous line. Prepare to insert an arterial pressure monitor.
2. Use an α-adrenoreceptor blocking agent. Preferably give phentolamine 0.015–0.03 mg/kg intravenously and repeat it every 30 seconds until blood pressure starts to fall. Set up an infusion of phentolamine 10 micrograms/kg per minute. Treat the reflex tachycardia with β blockers

intravenously, and repeat as necessary to bring the pulse rate below 100 per minute to a total of 0.1 mg/kg. Only use after using the phentolamine otherwise the blood pressure will rise. This paradox occurs, because beta blockers cause peripheral vasoconstriction.

3. Prazocin and phenoxybenzamine may be started after the initial crises is over.
4. Esmolol 1–10 micrograms/kg bolus intravenously could be used to control the heart rate for about 20 minutes.
5. Direct vasodilators, such as nitroprusside infusion are useful to control the blood pressure.
6. Lignocaine is a useful adjunct to the propanolol in the control of any ventricular arrhythmias. As a rule once the blood pressure is controlled the arrhythmias tend to resolve.
7. Use cooling measures as outlined in the management of malignant hyperthermia if needed.

HYPERTENSION (See page 239)

THE NEUROLEPTIC MALIGNANT SYNDROME[20]

The neuroleptic malignant syndrome (NMS) is an uncommon, but life threatening condition. Most cases occur in patients receiving therapeutic doses of neuroleptic drugs, but it also occurs with other agents that interact with the dopaminergic systems in the brain. The features are hyperthermia, muscle rigidity; and signs of autonomic dysfunction tachycardia, pallor, labile blood pressure, sweating, and urinary incontinence. Drugs triggering this syndrome include the butyrephenones, phenothiazines, and the tricyclic antidepressants. Do not give patients with a history of this disease any of these drugs.

HYPOGLYCAEMIA

Healthy adults experience symptoms when the blood glucose concentration falls below 2.5 mmol/litre (30–45 mg/100 ml).

If you suspect hypoglycaemia
do not wait for the results
treat it!

May occur in:
- diabetics (see page121);
- alcoholics (see page 119);
- neonates (see page 168);
- infants (see page 68).

Most symptoms and signs are those of excessive sympathetic discharge, these include:
- sweating;
- tachycardia;
- hypertension;
- confusion;
- restlessness;
- slurred voice, aggressive behaviour;
- obtunded mental state, progressing to coma and convulsions;
- brain damage and death.

Hypoglycaemic patients are
sometimes aggressive and abusive.

MANAGEMENT
1. Measure blood sugar with test strips or glucometer. To get accurate results, follow the maker's instructions exactly. Send blood for a formal laboratory measurement.
2. Treat hypoglycaemia if the blood glucose is less than 3 mmol/litre. Give 0.5–1 ml/kg of glucose 50 per cent intravenously into a large vein, and the patient should improve within minutes. (Dextrose is another name for glucose.)

HYPOTENSION (See page 237)

HYPOTHERMIA

Hypothermia becomes a problem when the core body temperature falls below 36°C. About 60 per cent of patients arrive in the recovery room with temperatures less than 36.5°C[21]. Elderly people, small children, infants and neonates are particularly susceptible to hypothermia. Other patients likely to be hypothermic are burn victims, those unable to shiver; and those who have had major vascular, abdominal surgery or trauma surgery. Two units of blood transfused at 4°C can lower the core temperature of a patient by 0.5°C[22].

Shivering

The normal patient will shiver in response to hypothermia, shutting down his skin blood flow so that heat production will exceed heat loss. Shivering muscle produces large amounts of heat, by increasing the metabolic rate and oxygen consumption five- to seven-fold. To deliver oxygen to the highly active muscle tissue, the heart must increase its cardiac output proportionately. Hypothermia causes peripheral vasoconstriction, so the heart has to work even harder to pump blood through the constricted vessels. This can result in myocardial ischaemia, tissue hypoxia, and a lactic acidosis.

Once the temperature falls below 33°C, the patient ceases to shiver, and his conscious state becomes increasingly obtunded.

Epidural opioids depress shivering and increase heat loss particularly after caesarean section[23]. The rate of heat loss is greater under epidural anaesthesia than local anaesthesia, and furthermore patients are slower to re-warm than after general anaesthesia.

Infants and neonates

Neonates and infants do not shiver. Neonates increase their heat production by metabolizing specialized *brown fat* tissue. At best this stratergy only works for a few hours. Brown fat metabolism increases oxygen consumption, uses glucose stores, and can cause hypoglycaemia. Hypothermia in infants causes hypoventilation, acidosis, and a falling cardiac output. The drowsy neonate, or infant who becomes less responsive may be becoming hypothermic. Check his temperature frequently.

An increasingly drowsy infant
may be hypothermic.

Pathophysiology

An anaesthetized patient loses the ability to maintain their body temperature at, or above, the normal of 36.8°C. They lose heat by radiation, conduction, convection and evaporation. The loss is made worse, because operating theatres are cooled to 18–20°C to suit those in gown and gloves, rather than to maintain the patient's temperature.

Hypothermia delays the metabolism and excretion of drugs, prolonging the actions of sedative drugs and opioids, so patients often arrive in the recovery room still deeply anaesthetized. The kidneys fail to concentrate urine, and urine output increases. Coagulopathies occur because, platelets are sequestrated in the liver, and the actions of all the clotting enzymes slow down. Hypothermic patients are slow to regain consciousness, and do not guard their airways well. Hypothermic patients may cool further, before beginning to warm. This phenomenon is called *after fall* and is caused by cold blood coming back from muscle beds and skin as circulation in these areas is restored.

> *It is better to prevent hypothermia in the operating theatre,*
> *than to treat it in the recovery room.*

Diagnosis

   If you suspect hypothermia feel the skin temperature on the patient's chest with the palm, (not the back) of your hand. Confirm your suspicion with a tympanic membrane sensor, or an oesophageal or rectal thermistor probe. Do not use a normal clinical thermometer, because these do not measure low temperatures. Never put a glass thermometer into the mouth of an unconscious or semiconscious patient.

MANAGEMENT[24]

   Many patients remember being freezing cold when they wake up. They are comforted by a warm blanket. Unless myxoedemic or hypoglycaemic, most postoperative hypothermic patients will warm themselves up if they are protected from further heat loss.

   It can take 12 hours or more to rewarm a severely hypothermic patient. Proceed slowly. Active warming, beyond the use of a forced air convection heater or a heated humidifier can cause complications. You may need to transfer the patient to ICU for continuing treatment.

1. A patient should remain intubated, paralysed and ventilated until his core temperature has risen to at least 35.8°C. In the elderly, or sick patient; or after major surgery, do not attempt extubation until the patient is fully re-warmed. Re-warm no faster than 0.8°C per hour.
2. Give high concentrations of oxygen, because shivering will greatly increase oxygen consumption, and can make the patient hypoxic.
3. Monitor the patient with an ECG. At temperatures of about 33°C, the ECG will show prolongation of the PR and QT interval, and J waves.

   Moderate hypothermia, (less than 33°C) progressively depresses the heart, resulting in hypotension and bradycardia. With severe hypothermia, (temperatures lower than 28°C) ventricular fibrillation can occur, and is more likely with rewarming. Arrhythmias due to hypothermia are difficult to treat.

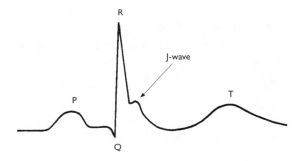

Fig 10.1 J wave seen on ECG in hypothermia

4. Use a forced convection warming device, such as Bair Hugger™ (see page 416).
5. If you do not have a forced convection warming device, cocoon the patient in a metallic (Mylar®) space blanket. These do not actively warm the patient, but prevent heat loss by radiation and convection. Separate the space blanket from the patient's skin by at least a cotton sheet. Place the reflective side towards the patient, and cover it with warm blankets. Domestic electric blankets, and hot water bottles, have no place in the recovery room, and can easily burn a comatose patient.
6. Check the recovery room temperature is at least 25°C with a relative humidity of 50 per cent.
7. Warm intravenous fluids with an in-line blood warmer. As the patient rewarms in the recovery room he will vasodilate as shivering increases blood supply to muscles. Be prepared to give fluids during the rewarming phase to prevent worrying hypotension.
8. Use a heated humidifier if the patient is still intubated.
9. Neonates and infants need incubators, or overhead heaters.
10. For interpretation of blood gases in the hypothermic patient (see page 375).

HYPOXIA (See Chapter 15)

Causes seen in the recovery room include:
• Hypoventilation caused by residual anaesthetic agents, muscle relaxants, opioids, or benzodiazepines.
• Airway obstruction, such as laryngospasm, laryngeal oedema, asthma, bronchial inflammation due to inhaled material.
• Mechanical causes, such as haemo- or pneumothorax.

- Lung disease, such as pneumonia, lung collapse, pulmonary oedema, and ARDS.
- Anaemia.
- Abnormal haemoglobins including incompatible blood transfusion causing haemolysis, and methaemoglobinaemia.
- Sepsis, water overload, or saline overload, where fluid accumulates in the lung tissue.
- Post-thoracotomy.
- Cardiac failure.
- Shock.
- Malignant hyperthermia.
- Rarely, cyanide toxicity from sodium nitroprusside.

It cannot be said too often, that hypoxia is the most frequent, dangerous, and insidious cause of damage to patients that occurs in the recovery room. And it is preventable!

ITCH

Itch is a sign of histamine release. If itch starts straight after giving a drug or blood transfusion suspect an anaphylactoid response.

Opioids can cause a red flare along the vein when injected intravenously. This sometimes itches, but resolves spontaneously within 10–15 minutes and leaves no residual effects.

Opioids, such as fentanyl, make patients' noses itch. Patients can often be see rubbing their nose vigorously in the recovery room. This is a problem if the patient has had reconstructive surgery on their nose. To prevent the itch, use promethazine (Phenergan®) 12.5 mg intramuscularly. Naloxone will resolve the itch, but reverse the relief of pain.

Use a cream, such as Lanosil® (heparinoid 5000 units and hyaluronidase 15 000 units) on the skin over injection sites if a drug extravasates from a cannula, causing local histamine release.

LARYNGOSPASM
(See page 331)

MUSCLE WEAKNESS

See postoperative residual curarization, page 172.
See neuromuscular diseases, page 128.

NUMBNESS AND TINGLING[25]

Numbness (*anaesthesia*) or pins-and-needles (*paraesthesia*) occurs when a nerve is damaged. Regional neural blockade sometimes damages nerves, but the diagnosis is not normally made in the recovery room. Patients who have had a brachial plexus block, or other regional anaesthetic sometimes feel distressed with tingling, and paraesthesia as the blockade wears off. Give analgesia if needed.

On the operating table, poor positioning of a patient can cause peripheral nerve damage. The nerve can be stretched, compressed or made ischaemic (usually with a tourniquet). The incidence is about 1:800 operations. Injury is more common in alcoholics and diabetics; possibly because these patients are already susceptible to peripheral neuropathies. Apart from direct damage during surgery, the commonest injuries are to the brachial plexus where the ulnar nerve is most frequently involved. Brachial plexus palsies also occur when an arm is hyper-extended from the shoulder on an arm board during the anaesthetic. This presents with wrist drop and weakness in the arm.

If an arm is not padded properly on the operating table, there is a risk of injuring the ulnar nerve as it passes through the groove on the medial epicondyle at the elbow. It can also be injured by a direct hit to the 'funny bone', usually on the frame of the patient trolley. Damage presents with numbness and tingling along the ulnar side of the hand to the little finger. The common peroneal nerve in the leg can be damaged if it is compressed against the head of fibula while the patients legs are in stirrups on the operating table. The patient develops foot drop, with numbness and tingling over the lower leg.

During attempts to maintain an airway the facial nerve can be compressed against the mandible. This will cause a facial palsy and drooping mouth, or eyelid, on the affected side.

Extravasation of irritating substances, such as thiopentone, in the medial side of the antecubital fossa, can damage the median nerve. This presents in the recovery room as numbness over the palm and clumsiness of the fingers. The antecubital fossa will be painful and inflamed.

If a patient complains of numbness, or tingling, trace out the area involved carefully with a marking pen, and inform the surgeon. This enables you to determine later whether the injury is resolving. To cover yourself in future litigation make a careful note of what you see, and what the patient tells you in the history. Most injuries are fortunately transient neuropraxias that resolve without treatment.

Numbness and tingling around the face and mouth is one of the signs of lignocaine toxicity.

PACEMAKERS

Patients with heart block have pacemakers to provide the heart with a rhythm that maintains an adequate cardiac output. Patients sometimes come to theatre with one either permanently implanted, or temporarily inserted.

Assess pacemaker function when the patient returns to the recovery room. Do a 12-lead ECG. Note the heart rate and rhythm, compare this with the patient's pulse. Check the ECG for the pacemaker spikes that precede the R wave.

Normal serum potassium levels are necessary for a pacemaker to function well. If arrhythmias occur, or the pacemaker misbehaves; check the serum potassium. Diathermy or electrosurgery will not upset modern pacemakers, but older models can be damaged by current surges. Cardioversion can damage pacemakers. If possible consult a cardiologist before performing cardioversion in a patient with a pacemaker in place.

Do not insert central lines or pulmonary artery flotation (Swan Ganz®) catheters into patients with pacemakers because you may dislodge the pacemaker wire from the right ventricle.

PALLOR

If the patient appears abnormally pale or is sweaty consider:
• hypoxia;
• shock;
• bleeding;
• pain;
• angina;
• nausea;
• anaemia;
• hypoglycaemia;
• drugs particularly pethidine, oxytocin, vasopressin (Por-8®), desmopressin (DDAVP®).
    Initial therapy:
• give high flow oxygen by mask;
• ask the patient if he has chest pain;
• reassure the patient;
• attach an ECG monitor and pulse oximeter;

• perform finger prick test for blood glucose estimation.

    Further management is based on finding the cause.

PNEUMOTHORAX (See page 339)

POSTOPERATIVE RESIDUAL CURARIZATION (PORC)[26]

    Residual effects of muscle relaxants given during the anaesthetic sometime persist to create problems in the recovery room. This is a common complication and up to half of patients receiving muscle relaxants return to recovery room with some degree of residual curarization[27]. The patient may move his arms with jerky, floppy movements. He may have drooping eyelids, and raise his eyebrows in an effort to open the eyes. He will probably have double vision. His ventilatory effort will be poor, and his breathing rapid and shallow. He won't be able to cough effectively, and may panic, because he feels as though he is suffocating. He will be unable sustain a 5 second head lift. To test his grip ask him to squeeze your hand and offer him two (but no more) of your fingers.

    Tracheal tug is seen when the patient does not have enough strength to breathe properly, and uses the strap muscles in his neck to assist the weakened respiratory muscles. You can feel his larynx jerk down every time he breathes in. Postoperative residual curarization increases the risk of aspiration pneumonitis, and contributes to postoperative respiratory failure. It can cause panic and cardiovascular stress, and may give result in hypoxia and hypoventilation.

    Causes of prolonged effects of the muscle relaxants are:
• overdose of muscle relaxant drug;
• delayed metabolism or excretion due to hypothermia, renal or liver impairment;
• abnormal cholinesterase in the blood prolonging the effects of suxamethonium;
• intercurrent disease, such as myasthenia gravis, motor neurone disease or myopathy;
• carcinoma or alcoholism giving rise to abnormally sensitivity to muscle relaxants.

    Diagnosis:
• If the patient is still unconscious, check the return of muscle power with a nerve stimulator (see page 387).
• The most useful test of adequate muscle power is the 5 second sustained

head lift. If a patient can do this he will be able to look after his own airway.

MANAGEMENT

1. Reassure the patient.
2. Give high concentrations of oxygen through a facemask.
3. Assist his breathing with a bag and mask.
4. Attach a pulse oximeter and ECG.
5. Notify the anaesthetist.

Consider the complications, before using a further dose of neostigmine. Neostigmine increases peristalsis, and can disrupt intestinal surgical anastomoses. It can cause bronchorrhoea, bradycardia and excessive salivation. The dose is neostigmine 0.015 mg/kg and atropine 0.03 mg/kg. Do not give more than an overall total of 0.06 mg/kg of neostigmine (4.2 mg in an adult), because it has intrinsic muscle relaxing properties of its own. Do not allow the patient to struggle on. If the patient shows signs of residual curarization, we believe the safest option is to re-induce, intubate, sedate and ventilate the patient until the muscle relaxant has worn off.

PUPILS

The fixed *unilaterally dilated pupil* is a sign of severe brainstem compression. If this develops after neurosurgery immediately notify the neurosurgeon and the anaesthetist. The *oval pupil* is a sign of early brainstem compression.

A unilaterally constricted pupil on the affected side occurs in *Horner's syndrome*. Horner's syndrome is seen when the cervical sympathetic nerves are paralysed after surgery on the neck or thorax, or after spinal, epidural or brachial plexus anaesthetic blocks.

Dilated pupils occur with:
• hypoxia or head injury causing severe damage have a bad prognosis;
• homatropine, used in eye surgery for dilating the pupils;
• trimetaphan.

Pin point pupils occur with:
• pilocarpine eye drops for the treatment of glaucoma;
• narcotic overdose;
• pontine (brainstem) haemorrhage;

Irregular pupils are sometimes seen for a few minutes after anaesthesia with volatile agents. If you test the patient's plantar reflexes at this time, you will find they are upgoing. This phenomenon only lasts about 10 minutes.

These signs can also occur with hypoxic brain damage (low pressure cerebral oedema).

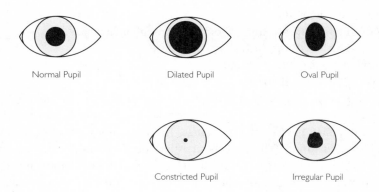

Fig 10.2 Pupils

SHAKING AND SHIVERING[28]

Not all shaking or shivering is due to hypothermia. Many cold patients do not shiver, and furthermore some shaking patients are not cold. The term shivering is best reserved for the cold patient, and shaking for the patient who is not cold.

Between 20 and 50 per cent of patients will shiver or shake after general anaesthesia. It is also occurs after spinal or epidural anaesthesia. Sometimes the shaking is violent, especially in fit teenagers or young adults. Take care to prevent the patient hurting themselves. Once shaking has started it is difficult to insert an airway. Try to keep the airway in until this phase is over.

Patients are more likely to shake if:
• they are teenagers or young adult males;
• the operation is lengthy;
• they have been allowed to breathe spontaneously for more than about 15–20 minutes on a volatile agent;
• an opioid, or an anticholinergic drug, has been used for premedication;
• they have been hyperventilated during the procedure;
• analgesia is inadequate;
• after drainage of abscesses, when it may be a sign of a septic shower of bacteria entering the circulation. Take blood cultures, and consider commencing antibiotics, especially if this is accompanied by

hypotension, or poor oxygenation.

Shivers and shakes are characterized by:

* vasoconstriction;
* pilo-erection (goose bumps);
* clonus;
* spike activity on an EEG;
* increased oxygen consumption;
* increased intraocular pressure.

Shivering and shaking raises the patient's metabolic rate enormously with oxygen requirements rising 5- to 8-fold placing extraordinary demands on the heart's ability to supply the tissues with enough oxygen to prevent hypoxia. In a patient with marginal myocardial reserves, the heart often cannot keep up; resulting in cardiac failure, myocardial ischaemia, lactic acidosis and tissue hypoxia.

MANAGEMENT

Give oxygen by mask. Pethidine has a direct effect on hypothalamic temperature regulating centres to depress shivering and shaking. Use a small dose of pethidine of up to 0.33 mg/kg intravenously. It is even effective if naloxone has already been given, but you will need up to 1

THEORIES ABOUT SHAKING

There are many theories about the causes of shaking seen after general anaesthesia. Suggested causes have been hyperventilation during the anaesthetic, adrenal suppression, pyrogen release, decreased sympathetic activity, and metabolic alkalosis. Electromyographic studies suggest unmodulated spinal cord activity returns before higher centres in the brain have recovered from the anaesthetic agent[29]. In other words the spinal cord wakes up before the brain does.

---

mg/kg or more[30]. About 75 per cent of patients respond to pethidine, but if it fails try doxapram 0.25 mg/kg intravenously[31]. Morphine and fentanyl are not effective against shivering or shaking. Other measures include adequate intraoperative analgesia. (See Hypothermia, page 165.)

To prevent hypoxia in the shivering patient
high flows of oxygen must be given.

Muscle rigidity

Muscle rigidity may occur without shaking. This rigidity wears off after a few minutes, but while it lasts the patient may clamp his jaws so tightly shut they cannot be opened. This is called trismus. Trismus is dangerous because the tongue may be caught between the teeth and injured, or even partially severed, dental caps can be dislodged, or the patient may occlude his airway. Guedal airways have a metal flange to prevent the lumen being crushed. To make the patient open his mouth, pass a soft catheter down his nose until it just touches the posterior pharyngeal wall. This will make him to shake his head from side to side, grimace and gag, and reflexly open his mouth.

Keep the patient's lips, and tongue
out of the way of his teeth until he wakes up.

Muscle rigidity can also be caused by some drugs including the phenothiazines (Prochlorperazine, promethazine and perphenazine), metoclopramide, the butyrephenones (haloperidol, and droperidol). It is more likely to arise with intravenous rather than intramuscular injections. The *Extrapyramidal syndrome* consists of muscle rigidity, and oculogyric crises with nystagmus. Patients can be very frightened by this side effect. To relieve anxiety give midazolam 0.02 mg/kg intravenously, or diazepam 0.1–0.2 mg/kg intravenously. Treat the rigidity with benztropine (Cogentin®) 0.015 mg/kg slowly intravenously.

Persistent muscle rigidity
is a sign of malignant hyperthermia.

SHOCK

Shock occurs when the tissue perfusion is inadequate to maintain the metabolic needs of the cells. This includes inadequate tissue oxygenation, and failure to remove the waste products of merabolism.

There are two types of shock:

Hypovolaemic shock

Where blood volume and extracellular fluid volume are reduced. Causes include:
• burns;
• diabetic ketoacidosis;

- haemorrhage;
- polyuric renal failure;
- prolonged vomiting;
- bowel ileus.

Haemorrhagic shock (see page 349)

Normovolaemic shock

Where the blood volume is normal, but there is a failure of a sufficient head of pressure to perfuse the tissues. Sometimes this is called distributive shock.

Causes include:
- anaphylaxis;
- epidural or spinal anaesthesia;
- cardiac failure;
- myocardial infarction;
- septicaemia;
- tension pneumothorax;
- full bladder;
- hypothyroidism;
- Addisonian crisis.

Cardiogenic shock (see page 288)

Septicaemiac shock

Occasionally reveals itself in the recovery room following:
- bowel resection, where bowel contents have spilled into the peritoneal cavity;
- urological manipulations, such as removal of renal, and ureteric stones;
- drainage of abscess.

The patient presents with signs of low cardiac output, poor perfusion, hypotension, tachypnoea, low urine output, and high jugular venous pressure. Blood gases show a developing metabolic acidosis, and hypoxia. Pulmonary oedema, and acute renal may become a problem. If multisystem organ failure (MSOF) develops the prognosis is poor.

Management includes:
- antibiotics;
- supporting the circulation with dopamine (see page 286);
- transfer to an intensive care unit.

Steroids are contraindicated.

Adrenal failure

A patient who has been receiving long-term steroid therapy may develop refractory hypotension in the recovery room. Supplemental hydrocortisone hemisuccinate 100 mg intravenously will rapidly correct the problem If you suspect this, treat it before confirming the diagnosis.

SNORING

Snoring is a sign of airway obstruction. Never allow your patients to snore; clear and support their airway. (See page 12.)

SORE THROAT

If asked postoperatively almost half the patients complain of sore throats. The causes are:
• atropine, scopolamine or dry gases that desiccate the mucosa;
• damage to the mucous membranes during intubation;
• pharyngeal packs;
• bronchoscopy.

Reassure the patient that sore throats almost always resolve in 24–36 hours.

SPUTUM RETENTION

Sputum retention is especially a problem after upper abdominal operations. When possible use either intercostal blocks, or thoracic epidural anaesthesia, for pain control. In susceptible patients use a heated nebulized humidifier to administer oxygen. It helps to start chest physiotherapy in the recovery room. If sputum blocks a major airway, the patient may need a bronchoscopy to prevent collapse of, or to re-inflate, a lobe of the lung.

SURGICAL EMPHYSEMA

Surgical emphysema occurs when air or gas escapes into the tissues. There is a peculiar crackling feeling to the skin and subcutaneous tissues. The most likely cause is a hole in the lung. It may be caused by accidental breach of the pleura during:
• operations on the neck;
• rib resection;
• kidney operations;

- trauma to the rib cage;
- following external cardiac massage, where ribs are fractured.

If it is associated with a tension pneumothorax, the blood pressure will be low and peripheral pulse barely palpable, and the patient will be gasping for air and panicking. This is an emergency (see pneumothorax, page 339). Subcutaneous emphysema can affect the pharynx and cause respiratory obstruction. If this occurs, the patient will need an urgent transcutaneous tracheostomy.

It is not uncommon to find surgical emphysema in the suprasternal notch. This is caused by air in the mediastinum, and can occur after thymectomy and mediastinoscopy. It is seen as a thin, dark shadow, along the left heart border on the chest x-ray.

SWEATING

Sweating (*diaphoresis*) is a sign something is seriously wrong.
It is associated with:
- nausea;
- hypotension;
- hypoglycaemia;
- hypoxia;
- hypercarbia;
- elevated body temperature;
- cardiac failure;
- opioids, especially pethidine, may cause sweating if given to a patient who is not in pain;
- malignant hyperpyrexia.

MANAGEMENT
Initial management:
1. Give high flow oxygen by mask.
2. Ask the patient whether he has chest pain if so treat for angina.
3. Check for pneumothorax by asking the patient if he can take a deep breath.
4. Reassure the patient.
5. Notify the anaesthetist.
6. Attach an ECG monitor and pulse oximeter.
7. Perform finger prick test for blood glucose estimation.
   Further management depends on the diagnosis.

TEETH

The anaesthetist sometimes damages teeth during intubation. Many patients' teeth are in poor repair, with caries and gum disease. In the recovery room patients emerging from an inhalational anaesthetic often bite down very hard. This masseter spasm (trismus) is probably physiologically similar to that seen during the shivers and shakes. Do not let them bite their tongue. Teeth, and especially crowns and bridges can be damaged if you force open his mouth. A nasopharyngeal airway is useful if the oral airway is obstructed. Choose a size one to two sizes smaller than the appropriate endotracheal tube. Lubricate the nasal airway liberally with 2% lignocaine gel, and pass it straight backwards along the floor of the nose, do not push it upwards.

UNROUSABLE PATIENT (See delayed emegence, page 152)

VOMITING AND REGURGITATION (See Chapter 13)

WATER INTOXICATION (See page 110)

WHEEZE ('bronchospasm')

Bronchospasm is a bad term because it implies muscular constriction of the bronchi, and tempts you to treat this with bronchodilators. It is better to use the term *wheeze* which is what you hear. There are many causes of wheeze.

When airways or their contents vibrate, like the reed in a clarinet, you can hear a wheeze. Generalized wheeze is a sign of turbulent airflow heard especially in smaller airways in asthma, pulmonary oedema, and inflammation of the mucosa. In recovery room consider acute aspiration of gastric contents, or blood. Localized wheeze occurs as air rushes past an inhaled object, or bronchial oedema caused by a pulmonary embolus. Some drugs cause wheezing, such as adenosine, neostigmine and physostigmine.

Anaphylaxis (See page 142)

Aspiration (See page 336)

Asthma (See page 336)

Cardiac failure (See page 281)

Chronic obstructive airways disease (See page 338)

Incompatible blood (See page 353)

Gas emboli (See page 140)

Pulmonary emboli (See page 339)

Fat emboli (See page 103)

1. Karuparthy V. R., Downing J. W., *et al.* (1989). *Anaesthesia and Analgesia,* 69: 620–3
2. Liu W. H., Thorp T. A. (1991). *Anaesthesia,* 46: 435–7
3. MacLeod A. D., Maycock A. E. (1993). *Anaesthesia and Intensive Care,* 21: 653–4
4. Lee J. J., Rubin A. P. (1993). *Anaesthesia,* 48: 616–5
5. Bond G. M., Holloway A. M. (1992). *Anaesthesia and Intensive Care,* 20: 426–430
6. Sutherland M. J., Burt P. (1994). *Anaesthesia and Analgesia,* 22: 733–7
7. Gefke K., Andersen L. W. (1983). *Acta Anaesthesia Scandinavia,* 27: 111–2
8. Rieder H. U., Frei F. J., *et al.* (1989). *Anaesthesia,* 44: 326–7
9. Öncel L., Hasegeli M., *et al.* (1989). *Journal of Laryngology and Oteology,* 106: 783–7
10. Miller A., Olkkola K. T., *et al.* (1990). *British Journal of Anaesthesia,* 65: 826–8
11. Seibert C. P. (1986). *International Anesthesiology Clinics,* 24: 39–58
12. Victory R. A., Hass P., *et al.* (1991). *Anaesthesia,* 46: 940–41
13. Mahaffey P. J., Wallace A. F. (1986). *British Journal of Plastic Surgery,* 39: 213–21
14. Gibbs N. M. (1994). *Australian Anaesthesia 1994,* pp 89–96. Published by Australian and New Zealand College of Anaesthetists, Melbourne.
15. Greenberg C. (1990). *Anesthesiology Clinics of North America.* Vol 8, No. 2, pp 377–97
16. Straziz K. P., Fox A. W. (1993). *Anaesthesia and Analgesia,* 77: 297–304
17. McGuire N., Easy W. R. (1990). *Anaesthesia,* 45: 124–7
18. Cain A. G., Bell A. D. (1989). *Anaesthesia and Intensive Care,* 17: 500–9
19. Crowley W. J., Cunningham A. J., *et al.* (1988). *Anaesthesia,* 43: 1031–2
20. Lev R., Clark R. F. (1994). *Journal of Emergency Medicine,* 12: 49–55
21. Vaughn M. S., Vaughn R. W., *et al.* (1981). *Anaesthesia and Analgesia,* 60: 746–751
22. Morely–Foster P. K. (1986). *Canadian Anaesthetic Society Journal,* 33: 516–27
23. Sevarino F. B., Johnson M. D., *et al.* (1989). *Anesthesia and Analgesia,* 68: 530–3
24. Loning P. E. (1986). *Acta Anaesthesiology Scandinavia,* 30: 601–13
25. Kroll D. A., Caplan, *et al.* (1990). *Anesthesiology,* 73: 202–7
26. Shorten G. D. (1993). *Anaesthesia and Intensive Care,* 21: 782–789
27. Beemer G .H., Rozenthal P. (1986). *Anaesthesia and Intensive Care,* 14: 41–5
28. Crossley A. W. (1993). *British Journal of Hospital Medicine,* 49: 204–8
29. Sessler D. I., Israel D., *et al.* (1988). *Anesthesiology,* 68: 843–850
30. Claybon L. E., Hirsch R. A. (1983). *Anesthesiology,* 59: (3A); S280
31. Crossley A. W. (1993). *British Journal of Hospital Medicine,* 49:204–8

12. PAIN CONTROL IN THE RECOVERY ROOM

Between 30 and 70 per cent of patients experience severe acute pain while in the recovery room[1]. Clinical surveys continue to demonstrate that intramuscular opioids given when needed (PRN) are ineffective in controlling postoperative pain[2]. Acute pain is easy to control, but the planning and management of the analgesic regime is often delegated to an inexperienced member of the surgical team. In the past doctors and nurses did not understand the properties of the analgesic drugs, and had inaccurate prejudices about their use[3]. It was hardly surprising that a ritual of prescribing poorly understood drugs, in inadequate doses, at erratic intervals did little to relieve the patient's pain. The recovery room is the logical place to start postoperative analgesia, and to set up a plan for continuing pain relief in the ward.

Uncontrolled pain is harmful[5] because it:

- causes restlessness, which increases oxygen consumption; this in turn, increases cardiac work, and can result in hypoxia;
- contributes to postoperative nausea and vomiting;
- increases the blood pressure, with the risk of precipitating cardiac ischaemia;
- decreases hepatic and renal blood flow, delaying the metabolism and excretion of drugs, and promoting fluid retention;
- prevents the patient from taking deep breaths and coughing, especially following thoracic, or upper abdominal operations. This increases the risk of postoperative sputum retention and pneumonia;
- discourages the patient from moving his legs, and blood flow through the legs slows. The venous stasis contributes to the formation of deep vein thrombi, and pulmonary embolism;
- increases the postoperative stress response, with greatly increased

Good Reference
The US. Department of Health publishes a comprehensive, detailed, and well referenced, clinical practice guideline titled *Acute Pain Management: Operative or Medical Procedures and Trauma* which is available from the Department of Health and Human Services, Public Health Service, Agency for Health Care Policy and Research, Executive Office Center, 2101 East Jefferson Street, Suite 501, Rockville, MD 20852. Other guidelines have been published by National Health and Medical Research Council [Australia] (1988) *Management of Severe Pain*, Canberra; and The Royal College of Surgeons of England and The College of Anaesthetists (1990); *Report of the Working Party on Pain After Surgery*, London.

cortisol secretion. This delays wound healing, and predisposes to infection[6];

- increases metabolic rate, protein breakdown, and the catabolic effects of injury;
- delays the return of normal bowel function;
- demoralizes the patient, disrupts sleep, and causes distressing anxiety and despair;
- after caesarean section, a mother's pain may impair the bonding with her new born child[7].

FUNCTIONAL COMPONENTS OF PAIN

Pain

Pain has been usefully defined 'as a sensory and emotional experience from actual or potential tissue damage, or described in terms of such damage[4]'.

Hurt

The definition of pain uses the term sensory to describe what we shall call the hurt component of pain. This is the physiological input from peripheral receptors carried to the spinal cord in fine A delta nerve fibres and C fibres. The impulse is then modified by groups of neurones in the dorsal horn of the spinal cord, and carried to centres in the brain. Long lasting uncontrolled severe pain can actually cause cell death of some of the dorsal horn neurones. Once this happens, pain becomes entrenched as chronic pain, and will not respond to analgesics. This tragedy may happen within a couple of days if severe pain is not adequately relieved. The hurt component can be blocked with local anaesthetics, or modified with analgesic drugs such as the opioids, and non-steroidal analgesic drugs.

Fear

The other component of pain in the definition is the emotional component. Anxiety, and fear make pain worse. The fear, (or terror), experienced by patients coming to surgery, activates the sympathetic nervous system's alarm mechanisms. Blood pressure rises, the heart rate increases, and the brain is put on military alert, becoming super-aware of what is happening to the body. Stimuli that previously would have been merely irritating, now become painful and distressing. The fear component can be modified by reassurance and explanation, as well as by drugs that abolish anxiety such as the opioids.

To manage pain effectively you should treat these two components of hurt and fear.

Uncontrolled pain can delay healing,
and increase the risk of infection.

The greatest physiological risk of untreated pain is to frail patients, those with heart or lung disease, those undergoing major procedures such as aortic, abdominal, or major orthopaedic surgery, the very young, and the very old.

The severity of acute pain is determined by the incision, the types of surgery, and patient and staff attitudes to pain.

The incision

Long incisions that cut through muscles, bones and nerves, in thoracic, or abdominal surgery, are more painful than short incisions.

The surgery

Orthopaedic, upper abdominal, thoracic, facio-maxillary, and perineal operations are the most painful. Skin graft donor sites are surprisingly painful.

Patient factors

The experience of acute pain is made up by the stimuli from tissue damage, memory of previous pain, and anxiety. There are often complex psychosocial and environmental factors involved in the perception of pain. Different ethnic groups respond in different ways to pain. Individuals vary in their response to pain, because these factors vary from one person to another. It is probable that most individuals feel pain in a similar way, they just react to it differently. Some patients are more stoic than others. Older people often do not report as much pain as the young, despite being equally affected by it.

People differ in their response to analgesics, and young healthy patients usually require higher doses than older people. Asians seem to recover more slowly from opioids than Caucasians[8].

Pain is likely to be less distressing if the patient:
- expects pain;
- knows it is only temporary;
- feels it is less severe than expected;
- is not anxious about the outcome of the surgery;
- has been taught relaxation techniques before surgery;

Staff attitudes

Pain control is likely to be poor if staff[9]:
- consider pain to be psychological;
- medication is only to be given when patients ask for it;
- are unaware that pain tolerance varies from patient to patient;
- fear respiratory depression or hypotension;

- fear that the patient will become addicted or dependent on opioids;
- do not understand the pharmacology of the drugs they are using.

MANAGEMENT OF PAIN IN THE RECOVERY ROOM

A well planned postoperative analgesic regime starts at the patient's preoperative assessment. Before surgery, discuss with your patients how much pain is to be expected, and the options available to control it. It is too late to do this in the recovery room, because understandably it is difficult to gain the confidence and co-operation of a patient who wakes in unexpected pain. This is especially important, in children, or if the patient is going to take part in his own pain management with a patient controlled analgesia (PCA) pump.

Principles in management of pain are:

1. Pain is easier to prevent than treat, so start analgesia before the pain becomes established. This is the basis of *pre-emptive analgesia*.
2. Attack the pain at more than one point in its pathway. This is the basis of *multimodal analgesia*.
3. In every case, treat both the *hurt* (physiological) component and the *fear* (emotional) component of pain.
4. Do not allow acute pain to remain uncontrolled, because of the risk that it will become uncontrollable chronic pain.

The steps in management are:

1. Establish cause of pain.
2. Assess pain.
3. Reassure patient.
4. Give analgesia.

1. Establish Cause of the Pain

Not all postoperative pain may be due to the surgery, it can be due to something else. Ask the patient, 'Where does it hurt?' Do not give analgesia until you are sure what is causing the patient's pain. Non-surgical causes of pain include:

- myocardial ischaemia or infarction;
- stretched ligaments due to poor positioning of the limbs or spine on the operating table;
- full bladder;
- localized muscle spasm;
- headache.

2. Assess Pain

It is useful to separate the components of pain, and anxiety in your assessment. Subjectively, pain is easy to assess; just ask the patient, and believe what he says. Objectively, pain is difficult to assess. There are a number of pain scores used to quantify pain, explain these to the patient at a preoperative visit.

Unfortunately there are few physical signs of pain. Pain may cause the patient to complain, cry, become agitated or restless. Always exclude hypoxia as a cause of confusion, agitation and restlessness. Agonizing pain can cause bradycardia, hypotension, nausea, vomiting, sweating, dilated pupils and pallor.

Pain is what the patient says 'hurts'.

In adults

The most useful score in an adult is the *visual analogue pain scale* (VAPS). This is a 10 cm long line drawn on a piece of paper. One end of the line is labelled 'the worse possible pain' and the other end 'no pain'. At the preoperative visit ask the patient to mark on this line where he feels his pain (if any) to be at that time. Postoperatively he is asked to re-indicate the degree of pain on the same scale. If necessary his pain can be quantified by measuring his mark in centimetres.

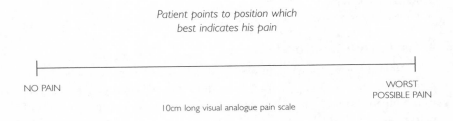

Patient points to position which best indicates his pain

NO PAIN   WORST POSSIBLE PAIN

10cm long visual analogue pain scale

Fig 12.1 Visual Analogue Pain Scale (VAPS)

Other scales use a 1–5; or even a 1–10 point scale. 1 = no pain; 2 = mild pain; 3 = moderate pain; 4 = severe pain; 5 = unbearable pain. Many postoperative patients, especially those with moderate to severe pain, have trouble in quantifying pain in this numerical way. The 1–10 point scale, in particular, is difficult to use. In contrast, the visual analogue scale is easily understood. It is particularly useful just before the patient returns to the ward. Modulate your interpretation of the pain scores with common sense. For analgesia to be effective the dose given must be sufficient to prevent pain when the patient is moving around and deep breathing.

Do not wake up patients
to ask them how much pain they have.

PAIN ASSESSMENT IN CHILDREN

It is difficult to assess pain in children, and no single test works every time. Pain assessment scores are of little use in recovery room. Sometimes a series of five stylized faces showing increments of expressions for the increasing degree of pain are used. At one end the face is smiling and happy and at the other end agonized and crying. In some countries, we have found that children from a village are unable to even recognize these drawings as faces. Furthermore it doesn't take a three-year-old long to realize if he points to a happy face he can avoid a feared injection, because he is unable to link the injection with pain relief.

In neonates and infants[10]

There is ample evidence that pain is felt by (and causes damage to) a neonate. New born infants can mount a neuro-humoral response that is quantitatively greater than adults[11]. Severe stimulus, such as circumcision without anaesthesia, will disturb bonding, disrupt feeding patterns, and cause behavioural changes that persist from days to weeks[12]. Diagnosing pain in infants postoperatively is easy if they cry, but they may be too weak to do so. Look for a furrowed brow, flared nasal openings, and an open mouth.

3. Reassure Patient

Anxiety is a major factor in the perception of pain. Honest, sincere concern and sympathy for the patient and his pain, often relieves it dramatically. Almost all patients, at or beyond middle age, have an understandable fear of cancer. A simple explanation of the cause of their pain, and reassurance 'that everything has gone well' will often take away the anxiety.

4. Administer Analgesia

The two usual ways to control pain in the recovery room are:

- parenteral drugs;
- regional or local anaesthetics. These are dealt with, in detail, later in this chapter.

PHARMACOLOGY OF THE OPIOIDS

The opioids have a number of common properties, but also some important differences.

OPIOID RECEPTORS

Endorphins are a group of naturally occurring opioid peptides synthesized in the central nervous system. They are released in response to pain and latch onto opioid receptors on nerves in the spinal cord and brain, to modify the awareness, and response to pain. The *opioids* are a group of drugs that also interact with the opioid receptors, and mimic the effects of the endorphins. The term *opioids* strictly refers to the naturally occurring opioids such as morphine and codeine, but many of the opioids are synthetic such as pethidine, fentanyl and buprenorphine. There are four main opioid receptors: mu, kappa, delta and chi. It is the mu (μ) receptor or morphine receptor which is the main mediator of pain relief. Unfortunately this is also one of the receptors involved in respiratory depression. The delta receptor in the chemotrigger receptor zone is involved with vomiting. The opioids can be classified in a long series depending on how they act on the opioid receptors.

Peripheral opioid receptors are sited on peripheral nerve terminals. Opioid peptides are found in immune cells that infiltrate inflamed tissue.

Analgesia

Opioids give moderate to good analgesia. They are more effective against constant dull visceral pain, than sharp intermittent pain. Unfortunately the better the pain relief the more severe the respiratory depression. Patients often say that they still feel the pain, but it doesn't hurt any more. Anaesthetists have long known that once pain is established it takes far more opioid to relieve it, than if it was given before the pain begins. This observation is the basis for *pre-emptive analgesia* (see page 193). The effective dose varies greatly from patient to patient; and may be as much as four-fold in any particular age group. This variation can be due, in part, to its euphoric effect, rather than a simple quantitative suppression of pain.

Respiratory depression

Opioids diminish the desire to breathe. Patients may hypoventilate, and slow their breathing to a rate of 8 breaths per minute or less. On arriving in the recovery room many patients, although rousable, seem to forget to breathe; however, they will take a deep breath when asked to. This phenomenon is called *Ondine's Curse*. Encourage the patient to take big breaths, and he will frequently start breathing spontaneously within a few minutes. For a short while you may have to remind him after each breath.

ONDINE'S CURSE

In legend Ondine was a water nymph, who laid a curse on her wayward lover so that he would have to remember to breathe. When he eventually fell asleep, he died.

Respiratory depression is more likely in the following patient groups:
- elderly;
- neonates;
- frail and feeble;
- intercurrent lung disease;
- heart failure;
- diabetics;
- obesity;
- asthmatics;
- liver disease;
- neuromuscular diseases;
- acute drug or alcohol intoxication.

The opioids can kill by causing
respiratory arrest.

With respiratory depression, the arterial $PaCO_2$ rises, and this causes:
- raised intracranial pressure;
- drowsiness;
- excessive secretion of catecholamines causing sweating;
- peripheral vasodilation;
- hyperglycaemia;

• respiratory acidosis.

(For management of opioid induced respiratory depression, see page 198)

EFFECTS OF OPIOIDS ON BREATHING

Opioids reduce the respiratory centres response to a rising carbon dioxide level. They:

- decrease respiratory rate, or,
- decrease tidal volume, or both;
- decrease response to hypoxia;
- alter breathing patterns ranging from periodic breathing through to apnoea.

Cardiovascular effects

Opioids do not alter the patient's blood pressure much. If they do, it is usually because they reduce the sympathetic response to pain. If there is a large fall in blood pressure consider other causes such as: hypovolaemia, hypoxia, cardiac failure, or interaction with other drugs. Pethidine is more likely to cause vasodilation, cardiac suppression, tachycardia and hypotension than the other opioids. The short-acting opioids, fentanyl, (and its son Alfentanil, and daughter Sufentanil) cause bradycardia and profound respiratory depression. Do not use them in the recovery room. Neonates and infants may drop their blood pressure with morphine or pethidine.

Nausea and vomiting

Opioids used during the operation, or in the recovery room cause 20–30 per cent of patients to become nauseated or vomit postoperatively. All opioids seem to be roughly equivalent in their ability to trigger nausea and vomiting. Opioids make patients susceptible to motion sickness, increasing the sensitivity to the input from the vestibular apparatus.

Sedation

Opioids cause drowsiness. Patients lie quietly, and do not move unless prompted. When asked what they are thinking about, they report a non-dreaming, sleep-like state, but are aware of their surroundings. This inability to structure thoughts, anticipate or plan; and the disinclination to move is called *psychomotor retardation*. An interesting phenomenon, is lid lag. The eyelid of a patient who is on opioids blinks down fast, but comes up more slowly than a normal person. The same effect is seen after administration of a benzodiazepine (the so-called *benzo blink*). Do not give any more opioid once the patient becomes sleepy: he has had enough.

Euphoria

Pain has two components; one is hurt, and the other is fear.

Opioids promote an overwhelming feeling of well-being. They abolish anxiety, making it impossible to worry about anything, and fear melts away. As the threatening feelings of alarm and fright dissolve, so does the activity of the sympathetic nervous system. The tachycardia, hypertension, and other metabolic effects resolve. Pain becomes less threatening, and although often still present, does not hurt any more.

Tolerance and addiction

Patients in pain almost never get psychologically dependent (*addicted*) on opioids. It is wrong to withold opioid analgesia from a patient, because of the fear of addiction. A drug addict finds opioids seductive, they enable him to escape from anxiety and feelings he would rather not have. Opioids hijack the addict's judgement, and once tolerance occurs the consequences are well known. Tolerance occurs over days or weeks, with higher and higher doses needed to achieve the same level of analgesia. (Analgesia for opioid addicts is described on page 124.)

A patient with cancer pain and previously receiving oral opioids, who presents for surgery may need up to ten times as much opioid as a normal patient to get control of his pain postoperatively. Consult with the oncology staff about his opioid requirements.

Itch

Opioids are responsible for the itchy noses seen in recovery room. Patients vigorously rub their noses. If this becomes a problem after eye, or plastic surgery on the face or nose, then give a small dose of promethazine (Phenergan®) 0.125 mg/kg. If this fails, naloxone will relieve the itch, but will probably precipitate pain.

Opioids (particularly morphine), used in spinal or epidural anaesthesia commonly cause troublesome itching.

Difficulty with urination

Opioids reduce the desire to pass urine, and cause spasm of the vesical sphincter, and relaxation of the detrusor muscle. Patience, encouragement, privacy, and the sound of running water help overcome the problem. If these methods do not work then pass a catheter.

Amnesia and time compression

Do not tell the patients important information while they are under the influence of opioids. They will almost invariably forget it. Patients must not sign legal documents, such as consent or release forms, while under the influence of opioids. Opioids make it difficult for the patient to judge the passing of time; it appears to pass more quickly.

Other problems

Opioids cause other problems including constipation, constriction of the pupils, biliary spasm, and spasm of the sphincter of Oddi, and bronchoconstriction. Allergic response do occur, but are not common. Histamine release occurs with intravenous morphine, and to a less extent pethidine. In theory morphine should be avoided in asthmatics, but in practice this does not seem to be a problem. Some patients are allergic to opioids, and others have idiosyncratic responses such as blurred vision, dizziness and injected conjunctiva.

Opioids in Common Clinical Use

Morphine and pethidine

Morphine and pethidine are the two most commonly used opioids in the recovery room. Understand their properties thoroughly and you will be able to treat most patient's pain.

Papaveretum

Papaveretum (Omnopon®) is a mixture of morphine and other alkaloids. It is best avoided in women of child bearing age, because the alkaloid noscarpine is thought to interfere with chromosome material.

Morphine
- Good analgesic;
- slower to work than pethidine;
- analgesia lasts for about 3–4 hours;
- unlikely to cause hypotension or tachycardia;
- predisposes to smooth muscle and sphincter spasm, after biliary or ureteric surgery;
- less sedating than pethidine;
- suppresses cough reflex;
- unlikely to interact with other drugs;
- safer in patient with cardiac disease.

If a patient's blood pressure falls after an opioid,
first look for another cause.

Pethidine (meperidine, Demerol®)

- Good analgesic;
- quicker acting than morphine, because it crosses the blood–brain barrier more readily;
- analgesia lasts about 2–3 hours;
- more likely to cause hypotension and tachycardia than morphine;
- useful following biliary and ureteric surgery—it causes less spasm than morphine;
- more sedating than morphine;
- does not suppress the cough reflex;
- may interact with many drugs such as phenothiazines causing excessive sedation or hypotension;
- in renal failure the metabolites accumulate causing disorientation, confusion, and eventually coma and even death.
- Pethidine dangerously interacts with mono-amine oxidase inhibitors used as antidepressants to cause restlessness, hypertension, convulsions, and coma.

Approximately equivalent doses:

Morphine 10 mg = pethidine 100 mg;
= papaveretum 20 mg;
= diamorphine 5 mg;
= fentanyl 100 micrograms;
= phenoperidine 2 mg;
= methadone 10 mg.

PRE-EMPTIVE ANALGESIA[13]

Pre-emptive analgesia

Pain is better prevented than relieved. Clinical anaesthetists have observed that giving an opioid premedication is more effective than giving the same dose to control established pain. Local anaesthetic techniques used during surgery reduce the amount of postoperative opioids needed to control pain.

There is some evidence that the pain of surgery may cause prolonged changes in the way the spinal cord functions, this increases the pain felt postoperatively[14]. Once pain is established it takes high doses of opioid to suppress this hyper-excitable state. Pre-emptive opioids prevent the hyper-excitable state developing in the first place.

Table 12.1

COMPARISON OF MORPHINE AND PETHIDINE		
	Morphine	**Pethidine**
Dose* (intravenous)	0.03 – 0.15 mg/kg	0.5–0.75 mg/kg
Dose* (intramuscular)	0.15 mg/kg	0.75–1.5 mg/kg
Basal infusion rate*	0.03 mg/kg/hr	0.3 mg/kg/hr
Onset (intravenously)	5–10 min	1–2 min
Onset (intramuscularly)	10–20 min	5–10 min
Peak action (intravenously)	45 min	20 min
Duration of action	3–4 hr	2–3 hr
Toxicity in overdose	low	high
Metabolism	conjugated in liver	hydrolysed in liver
Excretion	biliary and renal	renal
Metabolites	active respiratory depressant	toxic (CNS irritability)
Respiratory depression	Equal, but dose dependent	Equal, but dose dependent
Cough suppression	Yes	No
Hypotension after IV injection	Possible	Probable
Interactions with other psycho-active drugs	Possible	Probable
Spasm of sphincters	Big effect	Small effect
Shaking and shivering	Not useful treatment	Most effective treatment

These recommended doses of opioids do not apply to patients with renal or hepatic disease, or other conditions that may increase their effect, or delay their metabolism.

PRACTICAL POINTS IN THE USE OF THE OPIOIDS

Multi-modal analgesia is the term used when several different techniques of analgesia are combined; for example, a patient, after the removal of a renal tumour might have intercostal blocks, an NSAID, and a morphine infusion. The pain control will be much more effective and the doses of drugs needed will be far smaller, than if a single mode of analgesia was used.

OTHER OPIOID ANALGESICS

Diamorphine (Heroin). Its use is illegal in Australia, New Zealand, Canada and the USA. Diamorphine is reputed to have a quicker onset, with less nausea and vomiting than morphine. Dose 0.015 mg/kg intravenously or intramuscularly. It is metabolized in the liver to morphine. Its onset of action is within 5–10 minutes, and it is unlikely to cause hypotension.

Fentanyl (Sublimaze®) is an excellent short-acting analgesic, it is also a profound respiratory depressant (which outlast the analgesia). Given intravenously the patient's respiratory rate drops within a minute or so (the patient may even stop breathing), while the analgesia takes about 5 minutes to peak. Bradycardia may occur. Its analgesic effects last 30–40 minutes. Delayed respiratory depression may occur, especially in the elderly, up to 3–5 hours after the last dose. Because of its respiratory depression, it is difficult to use as an analgesic postoperatively.

Fentanyl is commonly used as an adjuvant to epidural infusions. (see below)

Hydromorphone (Dilaudid®) is a synthetic derivative of morphine. It is 7–10 times more potent than morphine. It is popular in some parts of the USA, because it is believed to be less likely to cause hypotension than morphine.

Methadone (Physeptone®) is a long acting opioid, which is equipotent with morphine, but has a clinical effect for about 20–30 hours.

Papaveretum (Omnopon®) is a purified mixture of opium alkaloids from the opium poppy. (Its slightly pink in colour). Clinically papaveretum 20 mg equals morphine 13 mg. Apart from being more sedating than morphine, its properties are the same. Because it contains noscarpine, which is suspected to cause foetal abnormalities, its use is falling.

Phenoperidine (Operidine®) is a derivative of pethidine, and is similar to fentanyl.

Route

In the recovery room opioids are better given intravenously than intramuscularly. There is up to a 30 minute delay in onset of action when intramuscular injections are used. This delay is unacceptable because the aim is to reduce the stress imposed by pain. In unstable or shocked patients, it is safer to give small increments of well diluted opioids, slowly intravenously, than to risk larger, irretrievable doses into a poorly perfused muscle where absorption will be erratic.

The injection of morphine 1–5 mg into articular spaces, for example, following day case arthroscopies, gives analgesia for up to 48 hours.

Transdermal patches containing fentanyl, which slowly seeps (*iontophoresis*) into the circulation, have been investigated for postoperative analgesia[15]. They are not yet in general use, because of concern about the consistency of the release of the opioid.

Intrathecal and epidural opioids are discussed on page 217.

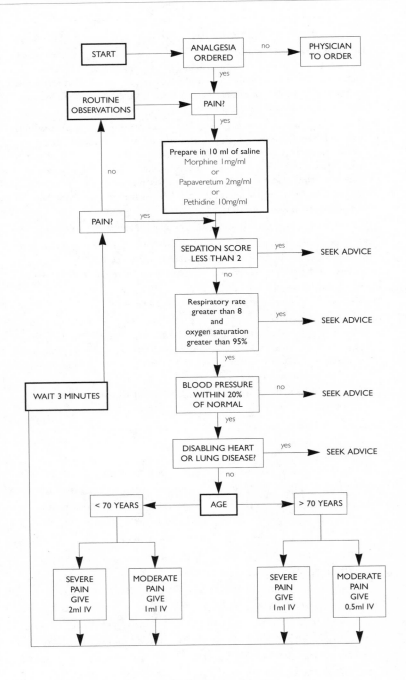

Fig 12.2 Plan for treating pain

Loading dose

To build up adequate blood levels, load the patient with a slow intravenous injection of opioid. Use the pain algorithm set out above to help you. Continue giving the opioid until the pain is relieved or the patient becomes drowsy with drooping eyelids. Stop the titration if the respiratory rate falls below 8 breaths per minute. Some patients will need a lot of opioid, and others will need little. This is to be expected as there is a wide individual variation in the response to these drugs. Young people may need up to 5 times as much opioid as an elderly person of the same weight.

Effective dose

When you have titrated an effective dose the patient should report that his pain is manageable. Other signs that the patient has had enough opioid include:
• drowsiness, with the patient dozing but rousable;
• pupil's less than or equal to 2 mm in diameter;
• a respiratory rate of 8–10 breaths per minute.

Oxygen

Hypoxia can be insidious and dangerous in patients receiving opioids. Give supplemental oxygen to all patients receiving opioids in the recovery room. Send patients back to the ward on at least 35% oxygen.

USING OPIOIDS IN NEONATES AND INFANTS[16]

Neonates, (especially premature babies), or those with neurological abnormalities, or pulmonary disease are likely to become apnoeic, or get respiratory depression with systemic opioids because their blood brain barrier is more permeable. Metabolism and excretion of opioids is at least three times slower than for an older child. The clearance of opioids increases rapidly with age, and approaches adult rates by the age of 3 months (52 post-conceptual weeks). Ideally monitor infants up to the age of 60 post-conceptual weeks, for 12 hours, after an opioid because of the danger of respiratory depression and sedation. If the child has neurological or pulmonary disease and is under the age of one year, monitoring should continue for 24 hours. Apnoea and respiratory depression are dose related. For infants under the age of 3 months the initial opioid dose should be a quarter of the dose recommended for older infants or children. If their pain is not relieved it is easy to give another dose.

Gently massaging their limbs and back, will reduce their pain and calm them. Paracetamol suppositories reduce the amount of opioid required to relieve pain.

Reduce the dose

Either reduce the dose of opioids, use multimodal analgesia, or choose another method of pain control in patients with the following problems:

- hypothermia on admission to the recovery room;
- chronic obstructive airways disease;
- asthma;
- elderly or frail;
- alcohol intoxication;
- liver disease;
- following neurosurgery;
- suspected raised intracranial pressure;
- cor pulmonale;
- known hypersensitivity;
- infants under 3 months;
- patients recovering from nasal or pharyngeal surgery, because of the danger of sleep apnoea.

THE NEWER OPIOIDS

To date the newer opioid drugs seem to have little advantage over older ones, and in many cases are not as good. The overall aim of these new arrivals is good analgesia, without the risks of respiratory depression or addiction. These drugs include buprenorphine, dipipanone, meptazinol, nalbuphine, pentazocine, phenazocine, and tramadol.

Opioid Antagonists

Naloxone

Naloxone (Narcan®) is a potent antagonist to the opioid drugs. It is used to reverse opioid induced respiratory depression, but it completely reverses all the actions of the opioid (and the patient's own endorphins too). This may suddenly plunge the patient into severe pain, causing hypertension, myocardial ischaemia, and even pulmonary oedema[17]. It is a difficult drug to titrate, and seems to work in an all or nothing way. It works for about 35 minutes after an intravenous dose, and may wear off before the opioid, allowing the patient to become re-narcotized. Intramuscular doses last for about an hour. The initial dose is naloxone 0.01 mg intravenously and wait 2 minutes before repeating up to a total of 0.04 mg over 8 minutes. Naloxone is not effective against the respiratory depression caused by buprenorphine, so use doxapram, or if this fails the patient may need ventilation.

Nalorphine

Nalorphine (Lethidrone®) is a partial opioid antagonist. It is most useful, because it is far more easily titrated than naloxone to partly reverse the respiratory depressant effects of the opioids, and is unlikely to abruptly jolt the patient into pain. Start with nalorphine 1 mg intravenously bolus, and repeat at 2 minute intervals up to a total of 10 mg. Its duration of action is about 4 hours.

PATIENT CONTROLLED ANALGESIA (PCA)

Since the patient is the only one who really knows how much pain he is in, it seems reasonable to allow the patient to give themselves enough analgesia to control their pain. Patient controlled analgesia (PCA) is the most effective way to administer opioids. It is safe, effective, and has fewer complications than intermittent intramuscular injections[18].

There are a number of infusion devices that give a bolus dose of opioid when the patient presses a button (see page 409). This is followed by a lock-out time where no further drug is given, no matter how often the button is pressed. If the patient is not in pain, or is drowsy, he will not press the button.

Some devices give a background maintenance infusion. There is no evidence that it is helpful, and in fact may lead to overdose. It is better to have small doses, and a short lock-out time, than to use a background maintenance infusion and longer lock-out times. Basal infusions impose risks of respiratory depression . If you do decide to use them, the hourly basal infusion rate should not exceed the amount of a single bolus dose.

Patient controlled analgesia has the following advantages:
- good safe pain relief;
- readily adapts to changes in the diurnal need for analgesic;
- few sleep disturbances;
- greater spontaneous movement and mobilization;
- decrease in length of hospital stay;
- analgesia is prompt and independent of the availability of nursing staff;
- patients like it initially because they feel in control of their pain;
- lower total doses of narcotics are used;
- can be used in children over the age of about 6 years.

You will need to establish protocols that suit your hospital and its staff. All staff need special training on how to manage the technique.

In many hospitals patient controlled analgesia is started in the recovery room. Here the staff give the first dose of postoperative analgesia, gauge its effect, and then set up a regime that suits the patient. This does increase the work-load on the recovery room staff, but has been shown to be cost effective in terms of patient stay in hospital and reducing demands on busy ward staff.

PCA PROTOCOLS

Protocols should include details of the:

- drug dose and dilution;
- dose increment, which is the dose given when the patient presses the button;
- allowable number of doses per hour;
- lock-out time;
- maximum amount of drug given in a 4 hour period;
- volume remaining in the syringe;
- options to change settings;
- nursing observations and frequency;
- limits of respiratory rate;
- disposal of unused solutions;
- treatment of common side effects;
- details of where to find medical support.

Reducing the Chance of Errors with PCA

There are many different makes of PCA devices on the market, so you must make sure that you are totally familiar with the devices used in your hospital. Check the features on each device before you use it (see page 409). Problems occur with prescription errors, administration errors and patient factors.

Prescription errors include: wrong dose, wrong lock-out time, wrong infusion rates. Make up a standard PCA order form; and set it out so that times and decimal points are clear, and errors difficult to make.

Administration errors include: wrong concentration prepared, wrong interpretation of instructions, equipment wrongly set up, and accidental injection when replacing the syringe. To prevent these errors, two nurses should check the orders at the bedside whenever the syringes are changed. Ideally infusions should have their own separate intravenous line, and

Good Reference **Patient Controlled Analgesia**
Introducing patient-controlled analgesia for postoperative pain control into a district hospital. Norcutt WG, Morgan RJM. (1990). *Anaesthesia*, 45: 401–6

nothing else should run through it. If a line cannot be dedicated to the infusion make sure there is a non-reflux valve correctly fitted into the branch line, so that the opioid will not run backwards up into the other line should the cannula become blocked.

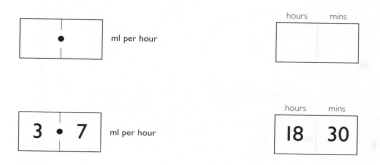

Fig 12.3 Setting time and decimal points on PCA device.

Doses can be either written as milligrams, or millilitres; this is a common source of confusion. The PCA form should be designed to eliminated the chance of error. Orders should be written exactly as they are to be programmed into the machine (see Fig. 12.3).

Patient factors

Confusion or hypoxia make it impossible for the patient to control PCA. Intentional abuse; accidental administration and intercurrent haemorrhage may cause the patient's response to alter. Visitors or staff can, and sometimes do, press the button. If the patient has been given a benzodiazepine, or a phenothiazine, this increases the risk of respiratory depression. Some patients do not like PCA, so respect their wishes.

Doses of Opioids for PCA

The use of background infusions is considered safe and effective in children, but its use is controversial in adults[20]. There is a high risk of respiratory depression in patients receiving background continuous infusions. A background opioid infusion was running in nearly all the reported complications. A constant infusion does not reduce the night time demands for analgesia, nor ensure a better sleep[21].

Table 12.2

ADULT DOSES FOR PCA			
Opioid	Bolus dose	Lock-out time	Infusion (optional)
Morphine	0.5–3.0 mg	5–20 min	0.5–3 mg/hr
Pethidine	5–30 mg	5–15 min	5–30 mg/hr

Table 12.3

CHILDREN'S DOSES FOR PCA			
Opioid	Bolus dose	Lock-out time	Infusion (optional)
Morphine	15–20µg/kg/hr	5 min	15µg/kg/hr
Pethidine	15–20µg/kg/hr	5 min	15µg/kg/hr

Continuous Opioid Infusions

Opioid infusions are still used to give pain relief, but in our experience they are not as safe as PCA. They require constant, skilled supervision to be safe and effective. In a busy surgical ward this may not be possible, in which case, do not use them. The biggest risk is respiratory depression. The danger is that a patient may slip, unnoticed, from sleep into an opioid induced coma; especially at night. Opioid infusions are not suitable for the elderly because their tolerance to opioids is reduced. It is important to have strict and careful protocols for continuous infusions. Despite their popularity we do not encourage their use in adults. They do appear to be safer in children. Unlike adults, oxygen desaturation at night is uncommon in infants and children receiving opioid infusions[22]. The usual doses are: Pethidine: 0.5–1 mg/kg intravenously stat and the 0.25 mg/kg/hour. Or morphine: 0.15–0.3 mg/kg intravenously stat, followed by 30–50 micrograms/kg/hour.

Non-steroidal Anti-Inflammatory Drugs (NSAIDs)

Non-steroidal anti-inflammatory drugs are a group of compounds with anti-inflammatory and analgesic action. They are popular in the management of mild to moderate postoperative pain, because they do not cause respiratory depression, sedation and tolerance[23]. They do have, however, a number of adverse actions limiting their usefulness.

They:
- aggravate asthma;
- jeopardize renal function in hypoxic or hypoperfusion states;
- cause bleeding tendencies;
- cause peptic ulceration;
- cause hypersensitivity phenomena including urticaria, angioedema, and rhinitis.
- interact with, and increase the activity of antihypertensive diuretics (such as the thiazides and frusemide), β-blockers, and angiotensin-converting enzyme inhibitors[24].

NSAIDs

Prostaglandins are a group of compounds involved in the inflammatory response that follows tissue trauma. They are, in part, responsible for the pain associated with injury by stimulating peripheral nerve receptors. NSAIDs interfere with the production of prostaglandins.

NSAIDs are also thought to have a central effect. When tissues are damaged arachanodoic acid is released from the phospholipids in the cell membrane. A group of enzymes called cyclo-oxygenases, oxidize arachanodoic acid into a variety of prostaglandins. The NSAIDs competitively inhibit cyclo-oxygenases, and prevent the formation of the prostaglandins, thus reducing pain. This action is temporary, and is reversible by simply withdrawing the NSAID concerned. For some of the longer acting NSAIDs it can take up to a week for their effects to wear off.

Prostaglandins have many physiological actions in other parts of the body. Inhibition of their action causes a variety of adverse effects including bronchoconstriction and peptic ulceration.

Some clinical points:
- NSAIDs take time to work. They are more effective if they are given before the pain is expected. This allows sufficient time for the drugs to interfere with prostaglandin synthesis. The onset of their analgesic effect occurs after one hour, but they need up to 5 hours to start working. (The analgesia becomes even more pronounced over the next 48 hours.) This time lag is a major disadvantage for their use in the recovery room.
- They are effective orally, or as suppositories. Suppositories are better tolerated, but require larger doses and take longer to work.
- Do not use them in pregnancy or in breast feeding women.
- They appear to be effective in the treatment of ureteric or renal colic[25].
- Bleeding times are prolonged with NSAIDs, but apart from aspirin taken preoperatively, it is rarely a problem.

- When combined with an opioid, NSAIDs reduce the dose of opioid needed, and reduce its side effects. This opioid sparing effect means the dose of opioid can be reduced by 25–50 per cent. This is useful after painful orthopaedic arthroscopic procedures[26].
- Avoid NSAIDs especially ketarolac in patients whom you suspect have poor renal perfusion; eg diabetics, vascular disease, the elderly, or those with heart failure.
- Asthma may be precipitated by any of the NSAIDs, but aspirin, naproxen, indomethacin are particularly bad offenders.
- Try combinations of pain relief (multi-modal therapy). Use NSAIDs and opioids for moderate pain, and add local or regional analgesia for more severe pain.

Paracetamol

Paracetamol (acetaminophen) is the first option for minor pain. It is an effective, safe drug if given in the correct dose. Combined with codeine it enhances the analgesia. The advantages are that it does not aggravate bleeding, cause peptic ulcers or damage the kidney. Use it cautiously in alcoholics, or patients with liver disease because it can cause liver damage. The dose is 0.5–1 gram 4–6 hourly with a maximum of 4 grams daily. This is the ceiling dose, and increasing the dose does not increase its effect. It is hepatotoxic in overdose.

Paracetamol is available in suspensions of 120 mg per 5 ml for children. For analgesia, the oral dose is higher than that recommended for controlling fever. For pain control, the oral dose for children is 20 mg/kg lean body weight 4 hourly. Be careful when you prescribe paracetamol, because a number of different strength formulations are available (24, 48, and 60 mg per millilitre). This may cause confusion, both for staff and parents. The current recommended maximum daily dose is 100 mg/kg. Paracetamol is safe to use for 2–3 days in children. Suppositories give unreliable plasma levels. Use Paracetamol suppositories in doses of 20–30 mg/kg, and give at least 90 minutes before expected pain to be effective. Use the smaller dose range in infants.

Aspirin

Aspirin is used for mild to moderate pain, and often combined with codeine, or paracetamol to increase analgesia. Use a dispersable form. The oral dose is 300–900 mg every 4–6 hours. It will exacerbate asthma, and must not be used in patients who have reported an allergic response to any of the NSAIDs. It is contraindicated in children under the age of 14 years, and in breast feeding mothers because of the presumed risk of Reye's syndrome. Remind families that aspirin is not a drug for children.

ADVERSE EFFECTS OF THE NSAIDs

ASTHMA

Some prostaglandins are bronchodilators. Inhibition of their function in patients with asthma or allergies can precipitate an acute asthma attack. Be particularly careful of aspirin in these patients. Paracetamol, does not cause a problem.

KIDNEY EFFECTS[27]

Prostaglandins have little function in a normal kidney. In a kidney whose blood supply is jeopardised they become important renal vasodilators improving the blood flow and oxygenation of the nephrons. The use of NSAIDs in the elderly, especially if they are dehydrated, hypotensive or hypoxic, impairs renal blood flow and can cause renal failure. It is wise to avoid them in heavy smokers. None of the available NSAIDs is safe in patients with renal dysfunction.

BLEEDING TENDENCY

Platelets are vital for blood clotting. Platelets need prostaglandins called thromboxane A_2 and prostaglandin endoperoxides to function properly. Platelet function should return to normal within three half-lives of the last dose of NSAIDs. Aspirin however, permanently destroys the function of cyclo-oxygenase, and it takes 12–15 days for a new batch of platelets to be produced by the bone marrow. A platelet transfusion is the only way to reverse this if it becomes a problem; fresh frozen plasma will not help.

PEPTIC ULCERATION

All NSAIDs cause chronic mucosal damage, and can trigger peptic ulceration. Even in the short term they can cause upper abdominal discomfort or pain (dyspepsia). This can be minimized if they are taken with milk. Ibuprofen is least likely cause damage. Do not use NSAIDs in any patient who has had a peptic ulcer.

HYPERSENSITIVITY

Urticaria, angioedema, and rhinitis occur in some people. These responses are not true allergic reactions, but due to the pharmacological action of the NSAID. Apart from the synthesis of prostaglandins, arachanodoic acid is also used for synthesis of lipoxygenase compounds, one of which is the slow-reacting substance of anaphylaxis. If the cyclo-oxygenase pathway is blocked there is an overproduction of lipoxygenases which cause the allergic-like response.

DRUG INTERACTIONS

Drug interactions with NSAIDs are a big problem, especially in the elderly on multiple medication. NSAIDs are tightly bound to proteins in the blood, and by displacing other drugs bound to the same proteins, can increase their effect or toxicity. These drugs include: anticoagulants, digoxin, phenytoin, and valproate. NSAIDs reduce the antihypertensive effects of thiazides, loop-diuretics, beta blockers, and angiotensin-converting enzyme inhibitors.

Paracetamol and codeine

Paracetamol and codeine is a good analgesic combination having few side effects. There are many combinations available, a useful one is paracetamol 500 mg with codeine 15–30 mg.

REYE'S SYNDROME

Reye's syndrome is a fulminating encephalopathy associated with liver failure that occurs in children. It occurs after an acute viral illness, and is possibly aggravated by aspirin. The child becomes drowsy, ataxic, starts to vomit and may develop a coagulopathy. It has a high mortality rate.

Ibuprofen

Ibuprofen has the lowest side effects of any of the NSAIDs, but its anti-inflammatory properties are weaker. The oral dose is 200–400 mg 6 hourly. This drug is useful in the management of pain following dental extractions, if given preoperatively.

Diclofenac

The dose of diclofenac is 25–50 mg orally three times daily. Suppositories of 100 mg are available. It is useful for the control of ureteric and renal colic; give diclofenac 75 mg and repeat in 30 minutes if necessary.

Naproxen

The dose is 250–500 mg orally, twice daily. Suppositories of naproxen 500 mg can be given at night.

CLONIDINE

Clonidine[28] has been used in veterinary medicine for 20 years as an adjuvant to other analgesics. In human medicine it has been used for the treatment of hypertension. It is a highly lipid soluble, centrally acting α_2 agonist with analgesic properties. It causes sedation and lessens anxiety in doses of 3μg/kg IV. It potentiates all analgesics, and reduces the incidence of postoperative shivering. It reduces the dose of analgesia required for PCA . It has been used to supplement epidural analgesia in doses of 2 μg/kg. It is potentially a useful drug although the onset of action is slow. It is available in tablets, transdermal patches as well as by injection.

Ketorolac

Ketorolac gives good pain relief. It takes at least 30 minutes to start working. It does not cause a clinically apparent bleeding tendency after one dose of 30 mg, but it is inadvisable to give repeated doses if bleeding could become a complication of the surgery. Aim to use the minimum dose for the shortest period, e.g. ketorolac 0.2–0.5 mg/kg every 6 hours. For patients over the age of 16 start with 10 mg intravenously. It is unnecessary to use a loading dose. Do not use ketorolac if there is any doubt about renal function. Its safety and use in children is controversial and needs further investigation. Avoid its use in patients with coagulopathy, hypovolaemia, renal disease, diabetes, or peptic ulcers. Anaphylaxis can occur with ketorolac. The signs are rash, bronchiole and laryngeal oedema, and acute hypotension. It precipitates asthma, and may cause nausea and vomiting.

REGIONAL ANAESTHESIA

A number of local anaesthetic blocks are used in the recovery room giving pain relief for many hours. This is the best way of controlling postoperative pain.

Thoracic or lumbar epidural blocks (see page 212)

Caudal blocks

Local anaesthetics are injected into the caudal canal to control perineal pain following operations on the rectum, prostate, penis, bladder, vagina and cervix as well as for labour and delivery. The risk of hypotension is low. The caudal canal is located between the sacral cornua at the lower end of the spine. Caudal blocks are easy to insert and effective. Use strict asepsis, and carefully prepare the skin for this block because the area is intrinsically dirty. Do not use indwelling catheters because of the danger of infection. Position the patient on his side with his legs tucked up as far as possible, or prone with a pillow under his hips and legs slightly apart. The drugs used are the same as for epidural block and their duration is similar. In adults the typical volume to use is 10 to 20 ml.

In children a volume of $\dfrac{(\text{age in years} + 2)}{10}$ is needed to block one segment. As the sacral canal is highly vascular, significant amounts of the local anaesthetic solution may be absorbed so watch for signs of toxicity.

Intercostal blocks

Intercostal blocks provide pain relief after thoracotomy and upper abdominal operations such as cholecystectomy. The patient lies with the side to be blocked uppermost and 2–3 ml of local anaesthetic with adrenaline are infiltrated behind each rib into the neurovascular groove. Local anaesthetic freshly mixed with adrenaline will prolong the block to give pain relief for 8 or more hours. To every 20 ml ampoule of bupivacaine add 0.1 ml of 1 in 1000 adrenaline. This makes up a solution of 1 in 200 000 adrenaline. The two main dangers are accidental puncture of the pleura causing a pneumothorax, and intravascular injection of local anaesthetic causing toxicity.

Thoracic paravertebral blocks

Thoracic paravertebral blocks are useful to relieve the pain of thoracotomy. A catheter is placed in the paravertebral space and may be left in for up to five days. The risk of infection is less than in the epidural space.

Brachial plexus blocks

Brachial plexus blocks provide analgesia for upper limb surgery. There are two approaches, the axillary and the supraclavicular. Both are effective, but the supraclavicular approach carries a high risk of a pneumothorax and nerve damage. With a fully successful block the patient loses all muscle power in his arm. Since biceps flexion is sometimes spared, warn the patient not to bend his arm or try to look at his hand because it might fly out of control and hit him in the face. Bupivacaine should only be used for long periods of analgesia, because it causes the block to last for 24 hours, or more. Warn the patient not to worry about this, and protect his arm with a sling.

Intrapleural blocks[31]

20 ml of 0.5 % bupivacaine with adrenaline injected into the pleural space give good pain control for fractured ribs; and moderate pain control for thoracotomy, cholecystectomy, renal surgery, and following breast surgery. This technique is insufficient alone, but useful in combination (multimodal anaesthesia) with other forms of pain relief such as opioids. Contraindications include adhesions, pleural injury, emphysema and bleeding diathesis. Do not use higher doses of bupivacaine because it is taken up rapidly from this space, and there is a risk of convulsions Pneumothorax occurs in about 2 per cent of patients. Insert a thoracic drain if the patient becomes distressed or breathless (see page 31).

Ilio-inguinal blocks

For ilio-inguinal nerve blocks inject 20 ml of 0.25 per cent bupivacaine with 1 in 200 000 adrenaline just beneath the external oblique aponeurosis (that is the first fascial layer) a finger breadth medial to, and a finger's breadth below the anterior superior iliac spine. A subcutaneous vein runs close to the injection site, so be careful not to inject local anaesthetic intravenously. Problems are few, but inadvertent block of the lateral cutaneous nerve of the thigh may occur. Keep well away from the testicular artery, which is an end artery.

Intra-articular local anaesthetics

Arthroscopies can be painful and intra-articular bupivacaine is useful for analgesia. Sometimes morphine 1–5 mg is instilled with or without the local anaesthetic. Patients should not be discharged until one hour after intra-articular injection of bupivacaine, because peak plasma levels are delayed by slow absorption from the joint[32], and any side effects may take this long to become apparent.

Regional and local blocks in children

All the adult regional techniques can be scaled down and used for children. Penile blocks and caudal analgesia are particularly useful for small boys having circumcisions. Don't be too surprised if a boy, whom you are sure has an adequate block, begins to scream. If he peeps into his pants and glimpses the povidone (Betadine®) prep he will assume he has been mutilated. A small dose of morphine will allay his anxiety.

Penile blocks

Penile blocks are used for circumcision, but a caudal block is more effective. Many surgeons are using topical lignocaine gel around the wound with good effect.

Precautions when using local anaesthetic blocks

- Keep all drugs and equipment for resuscitation immediately available.
- Always secure intravenous access before commencing the block.
- Be sure of the maximum recommended dose of the local anaesthetic you are using.
- Never use adrenaline-containing solutions near end arteries, or on the nose, ears, fingers, toes or penis.
- Patients with cardiac, hepatic or renal disease will clear drugs more slowly, so reduce doses and use longer dose intervals.
- Inject the drugs slowly, and aspirate often to make sure the local anaesthetic is not entering a blood vessel.
- Use the lowest effective concentration, and dose needed for the purpose. With repeated injections the drug may accumulate to cause toxicity. Reduce the drug dose by at least a third in the elderly, acutely ill or very young patients. Give it slowly.
- Decrease the maximum dose by one third in smaller patients.

- Do not use increased maximum doses in larger patients, especially if they are obese.
- Do not use regional blockade if there is sepsis in the area.
- Be wary of using epidural, or regional nerve blockade if the patient is septic, and do not leave a catheter in place because it will become a focus for infection.
- Consider options other than regional blockade if the patient is suffering from a coincidental neurological condition.
- Epidural and spinal anaesthesia commonly cause hypotension, so be prepared to treat it. Always have a good intravenous infusion running.
- Avoid regional anaesthesia in patients with a genetic predisposition to malignant hyperthermia.
- Do not stick needles into anticoagulated patients.

WARNING

Peripheral vasodilation caused by sympathetic blockade after spinal or epidural anaesthesia can cause severe hypotension in patients who are unable to increase their cardiac output. Do not vasodilate patients with aortic or mitral stenosis, hypertrophic obstructive cardiomyopathies, cardiac tamponade, or restrictive pericarditis. Consider alternative management in patients with severe bradycardias, cardiomyopathies, cardiac conduction disturbances, and digitalis intoxication.

Local anaesthetics used for regional anaesthesia
Hints:
- Local anaesthetic solutions seem to work faster, and last longer if they are warmed to body temperature before they are used[33]. Carry the solution around in your pocket for a few minutes to warm it up.
- When testing the efficacy of the local block do not prick the skin with a needle, because it is not reliably painful and damages the skin. Instead use a piece of ice to test the analgesia. The sensation for cold is carried in the same nerves as the sensation for pain, (the A delta and C fibres). If the sensation of pain has gone, so will have the sensation to cold.

Do not exceed maximum dose of:

Lignocaine	3 mg/kg	plain
Lignocaine	7 mg/kg	with adrenaline
Procaine	5 mg/kg	plain
Prilocaine	5 mg/kg	plain
Prilocaine	8 mg/kg	with adrenaline

Bupivacaine   2 mg/kg   plain or with adrenaline
Ropivicaine   4 mg/kg   plain or with adrenaline

Table 12.4

PROPERTIES OF LOCAL ANAESTHETIC AGENTS				
Drug	% needed	Onset (min)	Duration (min)	Toxicity*
Lignocaine	I	10–15	60–180	I
Prilocaine	I	10–20	60–180	0.5
Procaine	I	15–30	60–180	I
Bupivacaine	0.5	20–30	220–300	4
Ropivicaine	0.5	20–30	220–300	2

Compares to lignocaine, e.g. bupivacaine is 4 times as toxic as lignocaine.

Toxic Reactions and Treatment

Warning signs of an accidental intravascular injection of local anaesthetic are ringing in the ears, and numbness around the face and mouth. Vision may dim and the patient feels light headed. Sometimes the patient speaks in a confused babble. If the dose is large the patient may lose consciousness, convulse and stop breathing. An initial tachycardia is followed by bradycardia and hypotension. Treat the convulsions with either thiopentone or diazepam. Safeguard the airway by intubating, and ventilating the patient with 100 per cent oxygen. Treat ventricular irritability with bretylium. Cardiac arrest, if it occurs is difficult to treat. Persist with external cardiac massage for as long as possible to allow the local anaesthetic drug to detach from the receptor sites on the myocardial cell membrane.

Table 12.5

TOXICITY OF LOCAL ANAESTHETICS		
Stage	Signs	Treatment
I.	Numbness of face, visual disturbances, confusion.	• Give oxygen by mask; • encourage deep breathing; • diazapam 2–5 mg IV.
2.	Coma	• summon help; • turn into coma position; • clear airway, assist breathing; • attach pulse oximeter and ECG; • check pulse and blood pressure.
3.	Convulsions	• diazepam 5–10 mg IV
4.	Hypotension	• give IV fluids, ionotropes

Prilocaine, when used in excess of 10 mg/kg will cause methaemoglobin (see page 151).

Epidural Anaesthesia

Abdominal and thoracic operations can be very painful. To control postoperative pain the anaesthetist may insert a fine catheter into the epidural space to give, either local anaesthetic drugs, or opioids, or sometimes both. The drugs can be given at intervals or continuously infused. Local anaesthetic agents such as bupivacaine anaesthetize the somatic nerves as they leave the spinal cord, while the opioids interrupt the transmission of pain impulses in the spinal cord itself. This provides analgesia for the incision, the nearby skin, and muscle, and will almost completely relieve postoperative pain. Ill-defined deep visceral pain from the underlying organs may persist, because these impulses are transmitted through the vagus nerve, and do not travel in the spinal cord. If deep visceral pain becomes distressing, a small dose of opioid will relieve it. Do not use opioids systemically if they are being given into the epidural space because of the risk of severe, unpredictable respiratory depression.

Thoracic epidurals are used to provide postoperative analgesia for upper abdominal operations. Lumbar epidurals are used for lower abdominal, vascular and gynaecological surgery. Sometimes lumbar epidurals are used for lower limb surgery, and are continued into the postoperative period to provide analgesia. Epidurals reduce postoperative myocardial ischaemia by reducing cardiac preload and afterload, and reducing adrenergic effects[34]. Whether it is safe to use epidurals in patients who are taking aspirin is controversial[35].

Advantages of epidural analgesia include:

- At the most the patient should have only minor discomfort, with little need for opioids.
- Postoperative drug induced nausea and vomiting is minimal.
- Epidural blockade minimizes the bad effects of postoperative stress syndrome helping wounds to heal faster, reducing wound infection and lowering the metabolic insults caused by surgery.
- It reduces the incidence of deep vein thromboses and pulmonary emboli because blood flow through the lower body and legs is increased, preventing formation of clots.

Disadvantages of epidural analgesia

- An intravenous infusion is essential to treat hypotension which can occur after top-ups.
- Regional blockade in a patient who has received substantial doses of

opioids may cause respiratory depression, because these side effect of the opioids will no longer be antagonized by the pain.
• Sometimes, for reasons that are not clear, epidural analgesia skips segments so that an area may be not be anaesthetised yet everything around it will be pain free. Skipped areas are more common in patients who have previously had an epidural anaesthetic, probably due to scarring in the epidural space preventing the anaesthetic from spreading around.

Risks in epidural anaesthesia
The main risks arising during the insertion of epidural injections are
1. Toxicity;
2. Accidental dural puncture;
3. Hypotension.
4. Respiratory depression with opioids (see page 189).

1. Toxicity
Before injecting any local anaesthetic into the epidural space it is essential to ensure that the injection is not intravascular, and is not sub-arachnoid. Give a small test dose of lignocaine 30–50 mg with 1:200 000 adrenaline and wait for 2 minutes. If the epidural is inside the sub-arachnoid space the patient will report the onset of block; and if it has found its way into an epidural vein then the pulse rate will rise by 30–40 beats per minute. (For a description of toxicity see page 211.)

2. Accidental dural puncture (dural tap).
If the epidural needle is advanced too far it will puncture the dural membrane and allow cerebrospinal fluid to escape into the epidural space. This results in severe headache, the so called post-spinal headache. If the headache does not resolve with simple measures such as hydration and analgesia[36], then stop the leak with a blood patch.

If the dural tap is not recognized, and a large volume of local anaesthetic is accidentally injected into the cerebrospinal fluid it causes total spinal anaesthesia. The patient collapses, loses consciousness and becomes hypotensive. He will need intubation, ventilation and ionotropic support with dopamine to maintain his blood pressure. Uneventful recovery can be anticipated, but it may take up to 24 hours.

*The recovery room must be equipped
to handle complications of regional anaesthesia.*

> ## BLOOD PATCH FOR CONTROL OF HEADACHES[37]
>
> Although dural puncture during epidural anaesthesia is rare in experienced hands, there is an overall incidence of 1–4 per cent. When it occurs cerebrospinal fluid leaks into the epidural space causing a severe headache. This sometimes develops in the recovery room. The anaesthetist may decide to place a blood patch over the hole in the dura. Ten to twenty millilitres of blood is taken from the patient's arm and injected into the epidural space at the level of the hole. Lie the patient flat for 2 hours. Ideally the blood will clot over the hole to block the leak. In most cases the headache eases almost immediately.
>
> Two operators are needed to carry out the procedure, one takes blood from the patient's arm, while the other locates the epidural space. It is essential that the procedure is carried out with strict sterile precautions. If the clot becomes infected in the epidural space, an abscess will develop and irreversible paraplegia may follow.

3. Hypotension

Sympathetic blockade with hypotension and bradycardia if the block extends to T_4 or above. Vasodilation in the lower body causing hypotension will respond to a colloid load, or more likely to a small dose of ephedrine. Lie the patient flat, give oxygen and infuse 250–500 ml of colloid such as polygeline. If the blood pressure does not rise give ephedrine. Dilute ephedrine 30 mg in 10 ml of sterile saline and give 3 mg (1 ml) increments every 2 minutes until the blood pressure returns to a safe level. Monitor the blood pressure frequently to ensure the hypotension does not recur. An automated non-invasive blood pressure machine is a useful monitor in these patients.

Care of Epidural Lines

Insertion of the epidural catheter

This is a sterile procedure requiring, gloves, gown, drapes and a mask. Position the patient comfortably on his side with his legs tucked up. Do not use epidural, or caudal analgesia if the patient has a bleeding tendency or is anticoagulated. It is acceptable to establish the epidural before anticoagulants have been given, but not after.

Precautions with epidural lines

Once established, epidural catheters rarely cause any problems. The worst, but fortunately rare complication, is infection in the epidural space. To help avoid this small bacterial filters are fitted to the end of the catheters, and these should not be disconnected for any reason. Protect the catheter and filter as a neat package in a sterile plastic bag, wrapped in a sterile drape. Do not leave catheters in place for more than 36 hours, because of the risk of infection.

Top-ups

Intermittent administration of drugs through the epidural catheter are called top-ups. Only specifically instructed staff should top-up the epidural catheter with local anaesthetic. It is a sterile procedure, and needs proper skin preparation, drapes, gloves and mask. Hypotension is common after top-ups. It occurs within 10–15 minutes and may require treatment.

Local anaesthesia wears of abruptly,
be ready to top it up.

Continuous infusion

To avoid the inconvenience of continually having to top up the epidural use a volumetric pump to infuse epidural opioids when the patient returns to the ward. This can be set up in recovery room.

Removal of the catheters

Ease the catheters out gently. If you meet resistance, then call for skilled assistance. Rarely, these fine catheters break off in the epidural space while being removed. For this reason carefully inspect them after removal to make sure the catheter is intact, and the record this fact in the patients' notes. Usually the piece left behind causes no problems, but the patient must be warned in writing of the danger of it becoming a focus for infection.

AGENTS USED IN EPIDURAL ANAESTHESIA

Bupivacaine and epidural opioids are the agents most frequently used for epidural analgesia. Lignocaine is sometimes used, but it is too short acting for postoperative analgesia.

Bupivacaine

Epidural bupivacaine (Marcain®) is the most commonly used drug.
Useful facts about bupivacaine.
* Bupivacaine takes 10–20 minutes to work and its effect lasts 3–6 hours.
* Some anaesthetists speed the onset and prolong the duration of bupivacaine by alkaliinizing the solution. Use 0.05 ml of 8.4% sodium bicarbonate for every 10 ml of bupivacaine.

Table 12.6

EFFECTS OF EPIDURAL BUPIVACAINE		
	Motor effects	Analgesia
Bupivacaine 0.5%	blocks all movement	deep analgesia
Bupivacaine 0.375%	weak motor function	good analgesia
Bupivacaine 0.25%	moderate motor function	good analgesia
Bupivacaine < 0.2%	moving, no weight bearing	moderate analgesia

• Weaker concentrations are more suitable in elderly patients, where it is important to keep the total dose low.
• Bupivacaine, with commercially added adrenaline, does not have a significantly longer duration of action than the plain solution, but it does reduce the incidence of toxic symptoms by retarding absorption, and it does warn of accidental intravascular injection. If you add fresh adrenaline (see page 208) to the solution it will greatly increase not only the duration and intensity of the block, but also its spread.
• 20 ml of 0.5 per cent bupivacaine contains 100 mg of bupivacaine. The toxic dose of bupivacaine is about 2 mg/kg of lean body mass. Do not exceed this dose in any given top-up period as it may produce convulsions, ventricular arrhythmias and cardiac failure.
• Age is one of the most important factors influencing the spread of the block. Minimal spread occurs in 20-year-olds, and only half the volume is needed for 70–80-year-olds. From 20–40 years about 1 ml of local anaesthetic is needed to block each dermatome. Taller patients need about 10 per cent more solution.
• The dose of bupivacaine required for effective analgesia depends on the level of the tip of the epidural catheter, normally between 8–12 ml for a catheter inserted in the lumbar region and between 3–8 ml for a catheter inserted in the thoracic region. A rapid injection will extend the spread of the block, but this is difficult to achieve through a fine catheter and bacterial microporous filter. Always use the same technique and you will soon discover the optimal dose and spread of the drugs. If you continually change your catheter size, needles' gauge and solutions strength, you will become confused.
• A common problem with epidural anaesthesia is an inadvertent block of the sympathetic supply to the heart (T_1-T_4) reducing the cardiac output and cause the blood pressure to fall.

Ropivicaine is similar to bupivacaine but more potent. It causes less cardiotoxicity, and a less reliable motor block. It is also slightly shorter acting[38].

Epidural Opioids

Epidural opioids do not interfere with motor function or cause as much hypotension as local anaesthetics agents. However opioids do cause:
• respiratory depression;
• itching;
• urinary retention.

Fentanyl

Fentanyl works quickly and lasts 2–4 hours. Draw up 100 micrograms of fentanyl in a 10 ml syringe and make up to 10 ml with saline. Use a volume of 0.1 ml/kg of estimated lean body mass.

Fentanyl provides good analgesia by blocking pain pathways in the spinal cord without affecting the sensations of touch or pressure. Motor pathways are left intact, in contrast to the local anaesthetics, this allows the patient to move about. Fentanyl will not cause sympathetic blockade, or peripheral vasodilation, and so the blood pressure should remain unaffected.

If the blood pressure falls after epidural fentanyl
—the patient may be hypovolaemic.

Pethidine

Pethidine works quickly and lasts for 3–4 hours. Draw up 100 mg of pethidine in a 10 ml syringe and make up to 10 ml with saline. Use a volume of 0.1 ml/kg of estimated lean body mass.

Morphine

Draw up 10 mg of morphine in a 10 ml syringe and make up to 10 ml with saline. Use a volume of 0.1 ml/kg of estimated lean body mass. Morphine takes about 15 minutes work and is effective for 4–8 hours or even longer. An unsettling and irritating itch can be a problem. Try promethazine 0.125 mg/kg If this doesn't work, naloxone will but it will also reverse the analgesia.

Mixtures of opioids and local anaesthetics agents

Mixtures of opioids and local anaesthetics agents are clearly superior to either agent used alone. The advantages are a low incidence of motor blockade, shivering, and urinary retention[39]. Some infusion packs containing fentanyl and bupivacaine are available commercially. They contain 0.1 per cent bupivacaine and fentanyl 100 micrograms in 100 ml of saline with a usual rate of infusion of 10–20 ml per hour. For larger volumes take a bag of 500 ml of saline, and withdraw 120 ml of the saline. Then add 100 ml of 0.5 per cent bupivacaine and 200 microgram of fentanyl. For a thoracic epidural start with 4–6 ml per hour, and a lumbar epidural 8–16 ml per hour. Titrate an initial loading dose until the pain is relieved. Morphine and bupivacaine are sometimes used, The dose of bupivacaine is 0.1 per cent at 3–4 ml/hour with morphine 0.3–0.4 mg/hour. Pethidine and bupivacaine are also effective, and have the advantage of not causing an itch, but the incidence of vomiting and urinary retention is higher.

Patient Controlled Epidural Analgesia (PCEA)

PCEA is gaining popularity in some centres in the United Kingdom and Scandinavia. The principle is similar to the patient controlled analgesia used for intravenous opioid infusions.

Precautions with Epidural and Intrathecal Opioids

Respiratory depression

There have been a number of reports of profound respiratory depression, occurring up to 2 hours after a single of epidural fentanyl[41]. Patients should be kept under close observation for at least 3 hours after epidural fentanyl.

Respiratory depression can occur from any time from 30 minutes to 18 hours after commencing an epidural opioid infusion[42]. The onset of respiratory depression is not sudden. Typically the respiratory rate falls slowly to 6–8 breaths a minute (or even less) over an hour or more. The patient becomes drowsy, sweaty, and even cyanosed. Severe respiratory depression occurs if any additional systemic opioids are given (either intramuscularly, subcutaneously, or intravenously) in conjunction with the epidural opioids. Respiratory depression typically outlasts the analgesia. Put a warning sign DO NOT GIVE OPIOIDS on the patient's drug sheet, and bed head.

Epidural opioids exclude the use of systemic opioids.

The respiratory depression can be reversed with small doses of naloxone 0.1 mg intravenously at intervals of one minute up to a total dose of 0.8 mg. If respiratory depression is not relieved by this dose, then it is unlikely to be due to the opioids, so consider other causes. For established opioid induced respiratory depression use a naloxone infusion, it will require about 10 micrograms/kg/hour intravenously. This dose reverses the analgesic effects of morphine, but not necessarily the analgesia of epidural fentanyl[43]. A stat order for naloxone must always be written in the drug sheet in case it is needed for emergency use.

Give naloxone intravenously
if the respiratory rate is less than 8 breaths per minute,
OR
the patient is sweaty and drowsy in the absence of pain.

Before returning to the ward record the following in the patient's notes:
• the site of the infusion;
• the total volume of the infusion;
• the concentration of the drug;
• time of commencement;
• the rate of infusion in millilitres an hour;
• instructions about what to do if set limits of respiratory rate and blood pressure changes are exceeded;
• orders for an antidote and the doses needed;
• name and signature of the doctor supervising the infusion;
• where and how the doctor can be contacted.

Epidural opioids require a stat order for naloxone
and provision for an infusion.

Epidural clonidine
Epidural clonidine is being used in clinical trials and shows promise as an agent to augment the action of opioids and local anaesthetic agents.

Intrathecal opioids
Small doses of a variety of drugs have been introduced into the cerebrospinal fluid in conjunction with spinal anaesthesia. The major risk with opioids used in this way is respiratory depression, which has been reported to occur from 30–45 minutes after injection, to peak at 3–6 hours,

but may be delayed as late as 18 hours. This event can be catastrophic if not noticed in the ward. If the patient has received an intrathecal opioid, warn the ward nurses about this. Continuous infusion of intraspinal drugs is not advised, because of the risk of nerve damage.

1. Harmer M. (1991). *Anaesthesia,* 46: 167–8
2. Donovan M., Dillon P., *et al.* (1987). *Pain,* 30: 69–78
3. Weis O. F., Sriwatanakul K., *et al.* (1983). *Anesthesia and Analgesia,* 62: 70–4
4. Merskey H., Albe-Fessard D. G., *et al.* (1979). *Pain,* 6: 249–52
5. Editorial Lancet (1985) (1). 1018–9
6. Kehlet H. (1989). *British Journal of Anaesthesia,* 63: 189–95
7. Hughes S. C. (1989). *Current Opinion in Anesthesiology,* 2: 295–302
8. Aun C., Houghton T., *et al.* (1988). *Anaesthesia and Intensive Care,* 16: 396–404
9. Weis O. F., Sriwatanakul K., *et al.* (1983). *Anesthesia and Analgesia,* 62: 70–4
10. Anesthesiology Clinics of North America (1991). Vol. 9, No. 4
11. Anand K. J., Hickey P. R. (1987). *New England Journal of Medicine,* 317: 1321–9
12. Williams N., Kapila L. (1993). *British Journal of Surgery,* 80: 1231–6
13. Wall P. D. (1988). *Pain,* 33: 289–90
14. Katz J., Kavanagh B. (1992). *Anesthesiology,* 77: 439–46
15. Plezia P. M., Lindford J., *et al.* (1988). *Anesthesiology,* 69: A364
16. Koetntop D., Redman J., *et al.* (1986). *Anesthesia and Analgesia,* 65: 227–32
17. Wride S. R., Smith R. E. (1989). *Anaesthesia and Intensive Care,* 17: 374–7
18. Mather L. E., Owen H. (1986) *Anaesthesia and Intensive Care,* 16: 427–47
19. Gaukroger P. B., Tompkins D. P., *et al.* (1991). *Anaesthesia and Intensive Care,* 19: 134
20. Gaukroger P. (1992). *Australian Anaesthesia,* (ed D. Kerr, J. Thirlwell) pp. 11–14
21. Parker R. K., Holtman B., *et al.* (1992). *Anesthesiology,* 76: 362–7
22. Tyler D. C., Woodham M. *et al.* (1995). *Anaesthesia and Analgesia,* 80: 14–19
23. Dahl J. B., Kehlet H. (1991). *British Journal of Anaesthesia,* 66: 703–12
24. Tonkin A. L., Wing L. M. H. (1988). *Clinics of Rheumatology,* 2: 455–83
25. Sommer P., Kromann-Andersen B., *et al.* (1989). *British Journal of Urology,* 63: 4–6
26. McGlew I. C., Angliss D. B., *et al.* (1991). *Anaesthesia and Intensive Care,* 19: 40–5
27. Murray M. D., Brater D. C. (1990). *Annals of Internal Medicine,* 112: 559–60
28. Maze M., Tranquilli W. (1991). *Anesthesiology,* 74: 581–605
29. De Cock M., Lavandhomme P. (1994). *Anaesthesia and Intensive Care,* 22: 15–21
30. Bennet F., Boico O., *et al.* (1990). *Anesthesiology,* 72: 423–7
31. Murphy D. F. (1993). *British Journal of Anaesthesia,* 71: 426–34
32. Katz J. A., Kaeding C. S., *et al.* (1988). *Anesthesia and Analgesia,* 67: 872–5
33. Heath P. J., Brownlie G. S., *et al.* (1990). *Anaesthesia,* 45: 297–30
34. Breslow M. J., Jordan D. A. (1989). *Journal of the American Medical Association,* 261: 77–81
35. Paull J. (1994). *International Journal of Obsetric Anaesthesia,* 3: 1–2
36. Stride P. C., Cooper G. M. (1993). *Anaesthesia,* 48: 247–55
37. Carrie L. E. S. (1993). *British Journal of Anaesthesia,* 71: 177–81
38. Katz J. A., *et al.* (1990). *Anaesthesia and Analgesia,* 70: 16–21
39. Westmore M. D. (1990). *Anaesthesia and Intensive Care,* 18: 292–300
40. Periss B. W., Latham B. V. (1990). *British Journal of Anaesthesia,* 64: 355–7
41. Brockway M. S., Noble D. W., *et al.* (1990). *British Journal of Anaesthesia,* 64: 243–5
42. Knill R., Clement J., *et al.* (1981). *Canadian Anaesthetic Society Journal,* 28: 537–41
43. Gueneron J. P., Ecoffey C. (1988). *Anesthesia and Analgesia,* 67: 35–41

13. POSTOPERATIVE NAUSEA AND VOMITING

For the patient, postoperative nausea and vomiting (especially after day surgery) can turn an otherwise successful operation into a disaster. In many cases surgical patients fear postoperative nausea and vomiting (PONV) more than pain. The severity ranges from mild queasiness through to a distressing, prolonged, life-threatening illness needing resuscitation with intravenous fluids. The incidence ranges roughly from 10–45 per cent (or even more) of patients having a general anaesthetic. It is probable that patients are willing to accept drowsiness, increased pain, increased cost, and even dysphoria, to avoid postoperative nausea and vomiting[1].

Postoperative nausea and vomiting delays the patient's discharge from the recovery room, and increases the nurses' work load. Just under one per cent of patients have to stay in hospital overnight because of uncontrollable nausea and vomiting. Hospital admission after day case surgery is an expensive complication.

Vomiting

Vomiting (*emesis*) is a protective reflex for removing ingested toxins from the body. It is an active process producing either solid or liquid matter. The patient usually realizes that they are about to vomit, and it then begins with a deep inspiration. The glottis closes, the diaphragm and abdominal muscles contract violently, and these involuntary movements eject the stomach contents.

Nausea

Nausea is an unpleasant feeling of the need to vomit. It is accompanied by sweating, pallor, bradycardia, and salivation. If a patient is nauseated, it means that he feels as though he wants to vomit. On the other hand if a patient is nauseous, it means the patient is so vile and repulsive that he makes you feel sick. On the whole, patients are nauseated, and rarely nauseous. It is easy to remember! Consider the statement 'people are poisoned, and rarely poisonous'.

Vomiting is hazardous because it can cause:
- aspiration into the lungs with fulminating chemical pneumonitis;
- damage to the cornea if it gets into the eyes,
- damage to facial skin flaps;

- raised intraocular pressure;
- physical exertion that may tear suture lines;
- bradycardia in patients with ischaemic heart disease;
- hypotension in patients with peripheral vascular disease;
- if prolonged, it leads to hypokalaemia and saline depletion;
- tearing and rupture of the oesophagus in a few susceptible individuals.

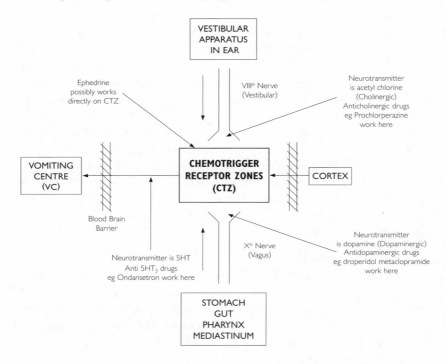

Fig 13.1 Simplified diagram illlustrating inputs that cause nausea and vomiting

Mendelson's syndrome

Mendelson's syndrome is a peculiarly vicious, and sometimes fatal, aspiration pneumonitis of pregnancy. The term is occasionally used (incorrectly) for all aspiration pneumonitis.

Regurgitation is a passive process where fluid matter refluxes up the oesophagus from the stomach. It occurs without warning, and can cause aspiration pneumonitis in a comatose or obtunded patient. Regurgitation is likely to occur in a patient with:

- hiatus hernia;

- distended abdomen;
- intestinal obstruction;
- ascites;
- pregnancy.

PHYSIOLOGY OF VOMITING

Nausea and vomiting is an adaptive reflex to protect against ingested toxins. There are three components to the vomiting reflex: emetic detectors, co-ordinating centres, and motor outputs.

Emetic detectors are stretch receptors in the gut wall that respond to distension; and polymodal chemoreceptors in the mucosa of the stomach and duodenum that monitor the intraluminal environment. The stimulus is carried by the afferent fibres of the vagus nerve to the brain stem.

Co-ordinating centres. The centres co-ordinating vomiting in the brainstem have neural inputs from the stomach, the vestibular apparatus in the ear, emotional centres, in the cortex and from direct stimuli by toxins carried in the blood.

The *vomiting centre* lies inside the blood brain barrier in the lateral reticular formation of the medulla. It co-ordinates the control of the complex vomiting reflex. Rich in cholinergic receptors, it receives incoming signals from the pharynx, gastrointestinal tract and mediastinum via the vagus nerve; and from the vestibular portion of the eighth cranial nerve and the chemotrigger receptor zone. It is interconnected with other centres that control various aspects of the autonomic nervous system, such as salivation, sweating, bradycardia and blood pressure control.

The *chemotrigger receptor zone* (CTZ), on the other hand lies outside the blood brain barrier in the medulla, where it is exposed to circulating toxins. It is rich in dopaminergic, opioid and 5-HT_3 receptors. Stimulation of the chemotrigger receptor zone triggers the vomiting centre to co-ordinate vomiting.

Motor output. Sweating, skin vasoconstriction, pupillary dilation, and tachycardia are mediated by sympathetic nerves; while salivation is mediated by parasympathetic nerves. The ejection phase consisting of retching and vomiting, involves vilent contractions of the abdominal wall and diaphram. The effort may be strong enough to fracture ribs in the elderly.

CAUSES OF NAUSEA AND VOMITING

Postoperative nausea and vomiting occurs in all types of patients, and with all types of operations and anaesthetics[2]. There are, however, certain groups of people, and certain types of procedures where vomiting is more likely[3].

Surgical Factors

- intra-abdominal operations where the peritoneum is stretched;
- biliary surgery;
- thyroid surgery;
- gynaecological surgery;
- ophthalmic operations, especially squint surgery;
- ENT surgery, especially tonsillectomy, adenoidectomy, and middle ear surgery;
- urological surgery, especially if the spermatic cord is involved;
- emergency surgery, especially for fractures;
- laparoscopy.

Patient Factors

Children are more likely to vomit than adults. The incidence is low in infants (about 5 per cent) and increases through childhood reaching a peak of 30–50 per cent in the 6–16-year age group[4]. Women (especially during the last half of their menstrual cycle[5]) are two to four times more likely to vomit than men[6]. Elderly patients (over 70 years) do not often vomit. Obese patients are often thought to be more likely to vomit than thin patients, but the evidence is slim. Obese patients have a high risk of regurgitation, because they often have hiatus hernias. Patients who get motion sickness are at high risk. There is also a strong psychological factor; those patients who think that they are likely to vomit, or who have a history of doing so, are three times more likely to vomit after subsequent operations.

Drugs as a Cause of Vomiting

Opioid drugs are a potent cause of nausea and vomiting. They directly act on the brainstem centres; and are more likely to cause vomiting if the patient is ambulant. They sensitize the vomiting centres to input from the vestibular apparatus; in effect opioids make you sea-sick. Opioids given as premedication, and during operations more than double the incidence of vomiting. All opioids are approximately equivalent in this respect.

All the inhalational anaesthetic agents; and many induction agents, such as thiopentone, methohexitone, ketamine, and particularly etomidate, cause nausea and vomiting. Propofol is the least likely of the induction agents to cause nausea and vomiting. Benzodiazepines, and muscle relaxants have no effect on the incidence of nausea and vomiting[7].

Anaesthetic Technique

Patients who breath spontaneously during the operation are less at risk, than those who are ventilated, but this could be related to the increased use of opioids in the ventilated group. The way in which patients are ventilated before intubation also plays a part. An experienced anaesthetist is unlikely to put air into the stomach, and therefore causes less vomiting. Neostigmine, given at the end of surgery, contracts the stomach and may cause vomiting on waking. Patients who have been hypotensive during their anaesthetic are also susceptible, but the reason for this is unknown.

Spinal and epidural anaesthesia cause less vomiting than general anaesthesia, providing the block does not cause hypotension.

Factors in the Recovery Room

In the recovery room nausea and vomiting may be induced by:
• pain which tends to produce nausea rather than vomiting;
• hypotension;
• hypoxia;
• hypovolaemia;
• anxiety;
• early mobilization;
• swallowed blood;
• acute water intoxication.

Nausea or vomiting after epidural, or spinal anaesthesia may be a sign of hypotension that needs immediate treatment.

MANAGEMENT OF NAUSEA AND VOMITING

Conscious patients will often dry retch before vomiting. They become pale and sweaty with a weak pulse, and their blood pressure falls. They find it easier to vomit while sitting up.

*If the patient is fully conscious
and about to vomit—help him sit up.*

Immediate Management

1. In a semiconscious patient; roll him onto his side, take his pillow away, and suck out his mouth and pharynx with a wide bore sucker. Be gentle, or you will stimulate further vomiting.

2. Patients who are expected to be susceptible to either regurgitation, or vomiting usually leave the theatre with a nasogastric tube draining freely. Be aware that a nasogastric tube will not prevent regurgitation, nor reduce the risk of aspiration pneumonia.
3. Most children only vomit once or twice following anaesthetics, and recover quickly. Side effects from the anti-emetic drugs are severe in children, and it is better to withold drug therapy and wait.
4. Moving patients around after giving an opioid is a potent cause of nausea and vomiting postoperatively[8]. Sit your patients up, and face them forward when transporting them on their trolleys. Turn the trolley from the foot end, so as not to swing the head in a wide arc when turning corners. We have found these simple measures reduce vomiting in the first hour after returning to the ward by about half[10].
5. Try to work out the cause of the vomiting and select the appropriate antiemetic drug.

Table 13.1

GROUPING OF ANTI-EMETICS			
GROUP	DRUG	DOSE	MAIN SITE OF ACTION
Antihistamines	Cyclizine	0.75–1 mg/kg	vestibular input + central action
	Promethazine	0.2–0.4 mg/kg	central action
Phenothiazines	Prochlorperazine	0.1–0.2 mg/kg	vestibular input
	Trifluperazine	0.05–0.1 mg/kg	vestibular input + central action
	Perphenazine	0.1 mg/kg	vestibular input + central action
Benzamides	Metoclopramide	0.15 mg/kg	vagal input + gut receptors
Butyrephenones	Droperidol	10–20 µg/kg	vagal input + central action
5-HT antagonists	Ondansetron	60 µg/kg	central action + gut receptors
Catecholamine	Ephedrine	0.5 mg/kg I/M	? central action ? antihypertensive

ANTI-EMETIC DRUGS[10]

There are many controlled studies of the efficacy of antiemetic drugs, but they often contradict each other. It is difficult to compare these studies to arrive at valid conclusions.

The following facts emerge:
- Antidopaminergic anti-emetics seem to work best against inputs from the vagus nerve.
- Anticholinergic drugs appear to work best against cholinergic input from the labyrinth (vestibular apparatus) in the ear.
- Antiseritonin (5-HT$_3$) antagonists work well against both.

If the drug you have given is not effective,
try one from another group.

Anti-cholinergic Drugs

Anti-cholinergic drugs block the cholinergic muscarinic receptors in the brain, and in the periphery. Centrally acting anticholinergic drugs block input from the vestibular apparatus in the ear to the chemotrigger receptor zone; so they are effective against motion sickness.

Scopolamine

Scopolamine is an anticholinergic drug, used in premedication of children and young adults. Its anti-emetic effects last about an hour, which is not long enough to cover the postoperative period. It gives patients a dry mouth and prevents them sweating; this is not a good thing in a hot climate. Other side effects include drowsiness, blurred vision, and urinary retention. Scopolamine causes disorientation, and confusion in the elderly. Treat this with physotigmine.

Antihistamines

Antihistamines block H$_1$ receptors, in the brain and periphery. Their antiemetic effect is probably due to their anticholinergic muscarinic blocking activity. Although they are less effective than scopolamine in alleviating motion sickness, they are also less sedating. The cyclizine and promethazine are two phenothiazines without significant antidopaminergic activity.

Cyclizine

Cyclizine (Valoid®, Marezine®), a piperazine phenothiazine, is an effective anti-emetic against opioid induced vomiting. It is less sedating than other phenothiazines, and deserves to be more popular. The adult dose is 50 mg intramuscularly, and it works for about 4 hours.

Promethazine

Promethazine (Phenergan®), an aliphatic phenothiazine, is sometimes used, but makes patients drowsy, delays emergence, and can drop their blood pressure by causing peripheral vasodilation. It works mainly through its antimuscarinic action on the chemotrigger receptor zone. The adult dose is 12.5–25 mg intramuscularly, 4–6 hourly.

Phenothiazines

Phenothiazines work primarily because they are dopaminergic D_2 antagonists acting on the chemotrigger receptor zone. Because of their slow total body clearance, they are all long acting with a half life of more than 30 hours. In elderly or debilitated patients they are prone to cause hypotension, agitation, apprehension, and sleep disturbance.

EXTRAPYRAMIDAL SYNDROME

Children, young adults, and debilitated elderly patients are susceptible to extrapyramidal syndrome (dystonia and nystagmus). This is frightening for the patient, who develops muscle rigidity, and marked oscillations of the eyes, (nystagmus) known as an oculogyric crisis. With phenothiazines the incidence is about 0.3%, but a quarter of these reactions occur after a single parenteral dose. Treat this with benztropine (Cogentin®) 1 mg IV, and repeat in 10 minutes if necessary.

Prochlorperazine

Prochlorperazine (Stemetil®) is a widely prescribed for postoperative nausea and vomiting, and morphine induced symptoms, particularly if the input is coming from the vestibular apparatus in the ear. The dose is 0.1–0.2 mg/kg intramuscularly, because of its long action, do not repeat the dose in less than 6 hours. Thiethylperazine (Torecan®) , and perphenazine (Fentazin®) are similar, but even longer acting drugs. They both delay emergence from anaesthesia.

Benzamides

Metoclopramide and dromperidone are dopamine D_2 antagonists that have a peripheral action on the gut, as well as a central action similar to the phenothiazines. They are superior to the phenothiazines if the stimulus to vomit is coming from the gut. They are useless against motion sickness that is triggered by the vestibular apparatus in the ear, and are not as effective against opioid induced vomiting as the phenothiazines.

Metoclopramide

Metoclopramide (Maxolon®, Reglan®) seems useful for symptoms induced by handling of the bowel, or uterus and ovaries, or swallowed blood. It is an overused, and largely ineffective drug. Surprisingly 50 per cent of studies have found metoclopramide to be no more effective than placebo in the treatment of postoperative nausea and vomiting[11]. It is ineffective against opioid induced vomiting, and is useless against motion sickness. The dose is 0.15 mg/kg intramuscularly, 4–6 hourly as needed. Higher doses are more effective, but are more likely to cause side effects. Severe bradycardia can occur with intravenous metoclopramide, so give it slowly over one minute. Metoclopramide can cause an unpredictable *extrapyramidal syndrome*, particularly in children and young women. Keep the dose below 0.5 mg/kg/day.

Since it is a dopamine antagonist, do not give metoclopramide to a patient whose blood pressure is being supported by a dopamine infusion.

Dromperidone

Dromperidone (Motilium®) is similar to metoclopramide, but since it is not available for injection, it is not widely used for postoperative nausea and vomiting. It has the advantage, unlike metoclopramide, of not passing the blood–brain barrier, and therefore does not cause extrapyramidal symptoms. Large doses can cause cardiac arrhythmias. Suppositories are useful in children.

Butyrephenones

The butyrephenones have strong antidopaminergic activity, and work in a similar manner to the phenothiazines and benzamines on the chemoreceptor trigger zone. They are also alpha blockers, and in larger doses cause postural hypotension.

Droperidol

Droperidol (Droleptan®, Inapsine®), a potent neuroleptic agent, is certainly effective, but the side effects of agitation, anxiety, and sometimes severe dysphoria are unpleasant if higher doses are used. The patient outwardly appears calm and tranquil, and inwardly feels miserable, and fearful. It is not a drug to use in day case surgery[12]. It is more effective in smaller, rather than larger doses, with the most effective dose being about

10–20 microgram/kg[13]. Doses of up to 75–100 microgram/kg intravenously are sometimes given during the anaesthetic. In this dose range, it is a long acting drug, and may cause sedation or dysphoria for up to 6 hours, or more, postoperatively.

5-Hydroxytryptamine (Serotonin) Antagonist

Ondansetron

Ondansetron (Zantron®) is a specific antagonist of the 5-HT$_3$ receptor in the vomiting centre, and is effective in controlling nausea and vomiting. 5-HT$_3$ is a neurotransmitter involved in activating vagal afferent pathways. Give 4 mg intravenously over 90 seconds. Apart from an annoying headache, it has few side effects, and does not cause extrapyramidal syndrome. It is an expensive drug, and about twice as effective as metoclopramide for prophylaxis of postoperative nausea and vomiting in gynaecological surgery[14].

Catecholamine

Ephedrine

In day case surgery ephedrine 0.5 mg/kg intramuscularly, is thought to be as effective as droperidol, but without the side effects. It probably acts by preventing postural hypotension in ambulant patients, but there may be a central mechanism.

Acupressure and Acupuncture

Acupuncture and acupressure have been advocated for the control of postoperative vomiting[15]. It is sometimes effective, and worth trying. The pressure point (P6 or Neiguan point) is in the midline on the anterior aspect of the left forearm about a Chinese inch above the proximal skin crease of the wrist.

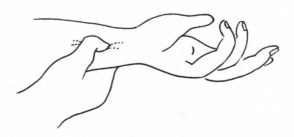

Fig 13.2 Acupressure at point P6

A Chinese inch is the length of the interphalangeal joint of the thumb. Probe about with your thumb until you find a point of deep ache. (It has to cause an ache to be effective.) Press firmly here and the nausea may abate, let go and it will return. Instruct the patient to find his own pressure point.

If acupressure is successful in relieving the nausea a more prolonged effect can be obtained by acupuncture. Insert a fine 26 G needle at the point directing it straight down at right angles to the skin to a depth of 1.5 cm. Twist the needle about its axis several times and then leave it for 5 minutes before withdrawing it. Stimulation of the of the P6 point by transcutaneous electrical stimulation does not work well[16].

CLINICAL IMPRESSIONS ABOUT VOMITING

- Some patients will be nauseated and vomit, and often there is not much you can do about it.
- Nausea after a spinal or epidural anaesthetic is a warning sign of worryingly low blood pressure. Use ephedrine or phenylepherine to restore the blood pressure.
- When the input for nausea or vomiting is coming from the abdomen, or mediastinum via the vagus nerve then try metoclopramide. Ondansetron is better, but expensive.
- When the input is coming from the vestibular apparatus, or is opioid induced, try prochlorperazine.
- Metoclopramide is ineffective against opioid induced vomiting.
- Patients do not like the butyrephenones, and find their side effects unpleasant.
- If one of a group of anti-emetic drugs does not work, try a drug from a different group.
- Acupressure is noninvasive, and many patients favour it. We have not found it useful once vomiting has started. Acupuncture is better, but transcutaneous electrical stimulation is ineffective.
- Transport your patients sitting up, and facing forward.
- Children are likely to get dystonic side effects from the anti-emetic drugs. As children usually only vomit once or twice, it is best to avoid these drugs. If it is necessary to use an antiemetic in children; try droperidol 20 μg/kg I/M, This often stops vomiting, and will not cause prolonged sedation.
- Lignocaine 2 mg/kg IV used in place of succinylcholine for intubation in children undergoing strabismus surgery, reduces postoperative vomiting[17].
- Hunger is a good sign of a functioning gut, but thirst is not. If a patient is hungry he will probably tolerate fluids and food without vomiting. Usually this occurs about an hour or so after day case surgery, and 4–6 hours after non-abdominal surgery. If it is safe, and the patient feels hungry, feed the patient a

small sandwich, and a glass of clear fluid. This often reduces nausea and vomiting.

- In hot weather, start intravenous fluids and keep the patient fasting until he feels up to tolerating 60 ml of cold clear fluid. Wait 15–30 minutes to see what happens, then gradually increase the oral fluids.
- Prolonged preoperative fasting aggravates postoperative vomiting.
- It is easier to prevent nausea and vomiting, than to treat it. Preoperatively, teach your patient about acupressure, give prophylactic anti emetics in the operating theatre, control his pain, do not move him roughly, and sit him up as soon as possible after he has regained consciousness.

1. Orkin F. K. (1992). *Anaesthesia and Analgesia,* (Suppl) 74: S225
2. Watcha M. F., White P. F. (1992). *Anesthesiology,* 77: 162–84
3. Rabey P. G., Smith G. (1992). *British Journal of Anaesthesia,* 69: (Suppl. 1) 40S–5
4. Cohen M. M., Cameron C. B., *et al.* (1990). *Anesthesia and Analgesia,* 70: 160–7
5. Kenny G. N. (1994). *Anaesthesia,* 49: (Suppl) 6–10
6. Lerman J. (1992). *British Journal of Anaesthesia,* 69: (Suppl. 1) 24S–32S
7. Forrest J. B., Beatties W. S., *et al.* (1990). *Canadian Journal of Anaesthetists,* 37 (Suppl.): S90
8. Muir J. J., Warner M. A., et al. (1987). *Anesthesiology,* 66: 513–8
9. Tronson M. *Unpublished data*
10. Rowbotham D. J. (1992). *British Journal of Anaesthesia,* 69: (Suppl. 1) 46S–59
11. Rowbotham D. J. (1992). *British Journal of Anaesthesia,* 69: (Suppl. 1) 46S–59
12. Melnick B., Sawer R., *et al.* (1989). *Anesthesia and Analgesia,* 69: 748–751
13. Pandit S., Kothary S. (1989). *Anesthesia and Analgesia,* 68: 798–802
14. Malins A. F., Field J. M., *et al.* (1994). *British Journal of Anaesthesia,* 72: 231–33
15. Dundee J. W., Young J., *et al.* (1990). *Lancet,* (i) 541
16. Ho R. T., Jarwan B., *et al.* (1989). *Anaesthesia,* 45: 327–9
17. Warner L. O., Rogers G. L., *et al.* (1988). *Anesthesiology,* 68: 618–21

14. THE CARDIOVASCULAR SYSTEM

PHYSIOLOGY

The Heart and the Circulation

Most anaesthetics depress the cardiovascular system, and these effects continue in the recovery room. General anaesthesia depresses myocardial function. Local or regional techniques cause peripheral vasodilation, so the heart needs to increase its output to maintain the blood pressure. In a poorly planned anaesthetic, the patient on waking may be abruptly assaulted with varying combinations of severe pain, hypoxia, fluid imbalance, muscle weakness, and increased oxygen demand from shivering. Under such an assault it is not surprising that his physiological alarm mechanisms go into overdrive. More than 80 per cent of patients over the age of 65 years have myocardial ischaemia, arrhythmias or degrees of heart failure in the first few hours after general anaesthesia[1]. These events warn of the possibility of postoperative heart failure, myocardial infarction or even death, in the first week after surgery.

THE RESPONSE TO STRESS

At rest the body is running at a *basal metabolic rate*, producing just enough energy to keep it going. *Stress* occurs as soon as the body takes part in an activity. The body's response, is usually proportional to the stress causing it, and brings into action two sets of coping mechanisms. The first is the autonomic nervous system (*or neural*) response, and the other is a hormonal (*or humoral*) response. The neural response, controlled by the hypothalamus, works instantly; but the various hormonal responses take time to achieve their effect. The autonomic nervous system has two components; a sympathetic (adrenergic) system, where the effector neurotransmitter is noradrenaline, and a parasympathetic (cholinergic) system where the neurotransmitter is acetyl choline. The endocrine response is principally mediated through adrenaline produced by the adrenal medulla, and cortisone produced by the adrenal cortex. In the USA, they call noradrenaline, *norepinephrine*; and adrenaline *epinephrine*. and cortisone is called *cortisol*. (Greek. Epi = centre, nephros = kidney)

Noradrenaline and adrenaline are members of a group of compounds called catecholamines. Other catecholamines used as drugs, mimic the effects of

---

noradrenaline or adrenaline; these include ephedrine, metariminol, phenylephrine, dopamine, and dobutamine.

The sympathetic nervous system (SNS) is part of the body's *fight and flight response*. Noradrenaline prepares the body for brief intense effort (to fight); and adrenaline dilates muscle vasculature, preparing the body for a sustained effort to run away (flight). In other words noradrenaline is the neurotransmitter for unavoidable life threatening situations: such as haemorrhage, heart failure, and the pain of surgery; while adrenaline is a hormone secreted predominantly for exercise and other metabolic activities. There is considerable overlap of these two catecholamines and their functions.

Those drugs that increase the heart rate, and its force of contraction, are known as beta (β) agonists. Those that cause peripheral vasoconstriction in skin, muscle, kidney and gut are called alpha (α) agonists. Most of the adrenergic drugs have varying degrees of both alpha and beta effects. Noradrenaline has predominantly alpha effects causing peripheral vasoconstriction raising the blood pressure. Adrenaline has mixed alpha and beta effects increasing the heart rate and its force of contraction; but also causing vasoconstriction in the kidney, skin and gut, and vasodilation in muscle.

The parasympathetic nervous system's action on the heart is to slow down the rate of discharge of the sinoatrial node, this in turn, slows the heart rate. Drugs that augment the action of acetylcholine cause a bradycardia; they include neostigmine, and physostigmine. Atropine blocks the effects of acetylcholine on the heart, causing a tachycardia.

Table 14.1

EFFECT OF STIMULATING ADRENERGIC RECEPTORS

Receptor	Heart	Arterioles	Lungs	Other
α1	-	constricts	-	reduces gut mobility
β1	increase rate increases strength	dilates coronary arteries	-	glycogenolysis
β2	increases rate increases strength	dilates most arteries	bronchodilation	tremor, tocolysis, hypokalaemia
β3	-	-	-	lipolysis

MONITORING THE HEART AND CIRCULATION

Importance of Blood Pressure

Blood pressure is the pressure generated by the heart as it pushes the blood around the body against the resistance of the arterioles. If these arterioles dilate the blood pressure falls. Because the arterial flow is *pulsatile* it is the overall average *(mean)* blood pressure, (not the systolic pressure), that determines tissue perfusion. The pressure in the veins, returning blood to the heart, is not pulsatile and is much lower than in the arteries.

Table 14.2

BLOOD PRESSURES		
	Systemic circulation	**Pulmonary circulation**
Systolic pressure	120 mmHg	22 mmHg
Mean blood pressure	93 mmHg	14 mmHg
Diastolic pressure	80 mmHg	8 mmHg
Pulse pressure	40 mmHg	8 mmHg
Venous pressure	3–7 mmHg	< 3 mmHg

Arterial Blood Pressure

Measure arterial pressure either, by using a sphygmomanometer, or an *intra-arterial catheter.* The mean arterial blood pressure (MAP) can be roughly calculated viz:

$$MAP = \text{diastolic blood pressure} + \frac{(\text{pulse pressure})}{3}$$

where the pulse pressure = (systolic pressure − diastolic pressure)

If you are using an intra-arterial cannula and a transducer, you can display the pulse form on a monitor screen. Two important wave forms are *pulsus alternans* and *pulsus paradoxus*. Pulsus alternans occurs where a bigger pulse wave alternates with a smaller pulse wave. It is a sign of a failing left ventricle. Pulsus paradoxus is a sign that the patient may be volume deplete. The height of the pulse wave rises on expiration. If the patient is on a ventilator, the reverse may occur, where the pulse wave rises on inspiration.

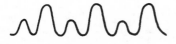

Pulsus Alternans

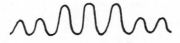

Pulsus Parodoxus

Fig 14.1 Pulse forms

Pulse Rate

Heart rate is partly controlled by sympathetic nerves, which speed it up; and the parasympathetic nerves, which slow it down. Adrenaline, a hormone, also increases the heart rate. This combined neural and hormonal response to stress is called a *neurohumoral response*.

Tachycardia (See page 251)

Bradycardia (See page 252)

Perfusion Status

It is important to assess the perfusion status, because this measures how effectively the heart is pumping blood through the tissues. It also gives some indication of the activity of the sympathetic nervous system.

Observe:

- conscious state;
- skin colour, temperature, and sweating;
- pulse rate;
- blood pressure.

Table 14.3

PERFUSION STATUS			
Observation	**Adequate**	**Poor**	**No perfusion**
Conscious state	Alert, oriented in time and place	Obtunded, confused, anxious or agitated	Unconscious
Skin	Warm, pink, dry	Cool, pale, clammy sweating	Cool/cold, pale +/- sweating
Pulse	60–100/min	Either < 60/min or > 100/min	Absent or feeble pulse
Blood pressure	> 100 mmHg	< 100 mmHg	Unrecordable

Other signs of poor perfusion are:

- dyspnoea;
- chest pain;
- poor capillary return in fingernail beds;
- peripheral or central cyanosis;
- acidosis;
- ECG signs of ischaemia, infarction or the onset of arrhythmias;
- abdominal pain.

Most pulse oximeters also measure skin perfusion by registering changes in capillary blood flow (plethysmography). The skin blood flow is exquisitely sensitive to the activity of the sympathetic nervous system. Cold hands, poor perfusion, or sweating, are excellent indicators that the body's alarm mechanisms are responding to a stress. Do not ignore these signs.

Cold hands are a warning sign
that something is wrong.

Electrocardiograph (ECG)

The ECG records the millivolt electrical activity of the heart, and displays it on a screen. It warns of cardiac ischaemia and disturbance of cardiac rhythm. Some monitors have arrhythmia detection and ST segment analysis built into them. These monitors are better at detecting abnormalities than trained staff who just glance at the monitor screens now and again. (See page 385 for hints on how to use your monitor.)

Central Venous Pressures (CVP)

The internal jugular veins act as a convenient manometer to measure the filling pressure of the right atrium. This information can guide fluid replacement or warn of right heart failure. The internal jugular veins are not always easy to see. To overcome this difficulty use a central venous catheter (see page 380). For reliable information about left heart function use a pulmonary flotation catheter. (see page 379).

HYPOTENSION

Hypotension in the recovery room is benign unless the fall is more than 20 per cent of the preoperative blood pressure. If hypotension becomes severe enough to jeopardise tissue oxygenation the patient is shocked. You need an accurate diagnosis of the cause of hypotension to treat it properly.

Causes of Hypotension

Heart rate problems
Too slow:
- sinus bradycardia (see page 252);
- heart blocks (see page 261);
- drugs, such as neostigmine and β-blockers (see page 247);

Too fast:
- sinus tachycardia (see page 251);
- atrial flutter or atrial fibrillation (AF) (see page 259);
- paroxysmal supraventricular tachycardias (PSVT) (see page 256);
- ventricular tachycardias (VT) (see page 268);
- drugs, such as adrenaline, and atropine.

Pump problems
- myocardial ischaemia or infarction (see page 276);
- heart failure (see page 281);
- valvular heart disease (see page 288);
- cardiac tamponade (see page 287);
- pulmonary, or air embolism (see page 140);
- drugs that depress cardiac contractility.

Blood volume problems
Absolute loss of blood volume:
- haemorrhage (see page 349);
- extracellular fluid loss, as seen in anaphylaxis and burns (see page 142);
- adrenal insufficiency (aldosterone).
Relative loss of blood volume:
- epidural or spinal anaesthesia (see page 214);
- tension pneumothorax (see page 339);
- sepsis (see page 177);
- adrenal insufficiency (cortisol) (see page 177);
- central nervous system damage;
- drugs that dilate peripheral vessels.

Table 14.4

INTERPRETATION OF CENTRAL VENOUS PRESSURE		
Central venous pressure*	Blood pressure	Causes
Low (hypovolaemia)	Low	hypovolaemia shock
High (normovolaemia)	Low	low cardiac output cardiac failure cardiac tamponade pulmonary embolism vasodilation
High	High	fluid overload

Pulmonary artery wedge pressures give an even better guide.

Use the central venous pressure, and blood pressure to help you determine whether there is an absolute or relative loss of blood volume.

Management of Hypotension

Relative loss of blood volume

Pain tends to keep the blood pressure up. The main causes of hypotension are the residual effects of general anaesthesia; or the vasodilation caused by spinal or epidural blocks. Most fit patients will tolerate a systolic blood pressure of 80–90 mmHg, unless they are elderly, or have myocardial or cerebrovascular disease. If the patient has warm hands, and a urine output greater than 60 ml per hour, a pulse rate with a regular rhythm between 50–100 beats per minute, a normal ECG and a normal pulse oximeter reading, there is no need to worry.

Severe hypotension is likely if the vasodilatory effects of spinal or epidural anaesthesia are combined with drugs that depress the heart. If a patient complains of nausea, feels dizzy, or shows signs of ST changes on his ECG monitor, then treat the hypotension. Raise the patient's legs on pillows, give oxygen by mask, and attach an ECG and pulse oximeter. Give 200–500 ml of polygeline (Haemaccel®) rapidly. At the same time give ephedrine in 5 mg increments intravenously over 30 seconds. Wait 2 minutes and repeat the dose of ephedrine until the blood pressure rises. Some patients respond more readily to ephedrine than others. The effect lasts 10–15 minutes, and may be repeated.

Exclude hypotension as a cause of nausea
in a patient with an epidural or spinal anaesthetic.

Absolute loss of blood volume

If hypovolaemia is the cause of the hypotension, the patient will be pale, with cold hands, a tachycardia, and a poor urine output. This patient clinically is now in shock. Check the perfusion status and record it in the patient's notes. (See page 347 for management.)

HYPERTENSION

Chronic hypertension

Chronic hypertension is endemic in the community. Do not suspend the patient's antihypertensive therapy preoperatively, they should take all their cardiac medication on the day of surgery. Acute β-blocker withdrawal causes an unopposed sympathetic response to swing into action, with the development of hypertension, tachycardia, sweating, ventricular arrhythmias, and possibly sudden death.

PHYSIOLOGY OF HYPERTENSION

Hypertension is due to, either an elevated cardiac output, or an increased peripheral resistance, or both. Most hypertension in the recovery room is caused by increased levels of circulating catecholamines, arising from activation of the sympathetic nervous system in response to an actual, or perceived stress. The elevated blood pressure increases cardiac work, which in turn, increases the heart's need for oxygen and nutriment. The heart is only perfused during diastole. Tachycardias shorten diastolic time, and reduce both coronary blood flow and cardiac oxygen supply. If a tachycardia (which reduces coronary perfusion) accompanies hypertension (which increases cardiac oxygen demand), the combination becomes a potent cause of cardiac ischaemia.

Acute hypertension

Acute hypertension is common in the recovery room. Hypertension can be defined as a systolic blood pressure greater than 160 mmHg, or a diastolic blood pressure greater than 95 mmHg; or a systolic blood pressure that is 20 per cent higher than the preoperative base-line blood pressure.

Causes of acute hypertension include:
- pain;
- hypoxia;
- CO_2 retention;
- full bladder;
- over transfusion;
- vasopressors;
- ketamine anaesthesia;
- obstructed airways;
- shivering;
- hypoglycaemia;
- phaeochromocytoma;
- tetanus, carcinoid.

Risks associated with hypertension in the recovery room include:
- myocardial ischaemia, myocardial infarction;
- cardiac failure;
- arrhythmias;
- strokes; subrachnoid, or cerebral haemorrhages;
- bleeding from the operative site.

The patient with a tachycardia and hypertension
is at risk from myocardial ischaemia.

Pain, or fluid overload, frequently causes normal healthy patients to be hypertensive while they are in the recovery room. Treat the hypertension if it is sustained (for more than 10 minutes) or associated with:
• a systolic pressure above 180 mmHg;
• a diastolic over 105 mmHg;
• ventricular premature beats;
• a deteriorating conscious state.

The elderly, or those with pre-existing heart disease, are at risk of cardiac ischaemia and arrhythmias, especially if they also develop a tachycardia. If you see ventricular premature beats (extrasystoles), suspect myocardial ischaemia. Controlling the hypertension usually resolves the extrasystoles.

Haemorrhage, or a rapid infusion of intravenous fluids can cause unexpectedly large swings in blood pressure in patients with chronic hypertension. Myocardial infarction and cerebrovascular bleeds, are a constant risk in these patients.

Fulminating (malignant) hypertension can occur if the blood pressure acutely rises beyond 220/120 mmHg. Control the blood pressure urgently if the patient shows signs of developing cerebral oedema, such as:
• headache;
• deterioration in mental state;
• an up-going plantar (Babinski) response;
• drowsiness;
• disorientation;
• nystagmus;
• muscle weakness.

Features of cardiac ischaemia, and failure, may accompany this hypertension with signs of a gallop rhythm, rales in the lung bases, and retrosternal chest pain. Unexpected fulminating hypertension can occur with undiagnosed phaeochromocytoma, tetanus, carcinoid syndrome, or spinal cord damage.

Principles of Management of Hypertension

Use one or more of the following groups of measures to reduce blood pressure:
• achieve peripheral vasodilation with glyceryl trinitrate, hydralazine, or nitroprusside;

- improve myocardial oxygen supply with oxygen and glyceryl trinitrate;
- reduce sympathetic nervous system drive with opioids, β-blockers, regional or local anaesthetic blockade; or
- reduce the power of heart contraction with β-blockers, or nifedipine.

ANTI-HYPERTENSIVE DRUGS

Nitroprusside (SNP) (Nipride®) is a potent ultra-short-acting vasodilating drug. It is the best drug for the control of fulminating hypertension. It causes a reflex tachycardia, and is a cerebrovascular dilator. Cyanide is released as SNP is metabolized, and it in turn is metabolized to thiocyanate. Thiocyanate toxicity causes hypoxia, disorientation, muscle spasms, and tinnitus. The toxic level of thiocyante in the blood is 1725 μmol/litre. Although cyanide toxicity is possible with prolonged administration, it is rare. It is unlikely to be a problem in the recovery room.

Nitroglycerine (GTN) is a short-acting drug that dilates vascular smooth muscle and improves myocardial oxygenation. It is a better drug than sodium nitroprusside for those with ischaemic heart disease, or where you wish to dilate the pulmonary vasculature. Tachyphlaxis will occur. To achieve pulmonary vasodilation GTN 5 μg/kg/min is equivalent to SNP 2 μg/kg/min. Its effect wears off in 5–8 minutes.

Nifedipine is a calcium channel blocker with a 2 minute onset if it is absorbed through mucosa; but it takes 15–20 minutes to act if given orally. Its main use is as a coronary and peripheral vasodilator. It rarely aggravates cardiac failure, because the reduction in peripheral resistance offsets the decrease in myocardial contractility.

Hydralazine is a direct acting peripheral arteriolar vasodilator. It causes a reflex tachycardia, with increased cardiac contractility, so it may cause cardiac ischaemia. The diastolic blood pressure responds to a greater extent than the systolic pressure.

β-blockers should not be used as first line therapy of hypertension in the recovery room. Both α and β receptor stimulation cause hypertension. Leaving α_1 stimulation unmodified to cause peripheral vasoconstriction, while reducing myocardial contractility with β-blockade aggravates tissue ischaemia, and cardiac failure.

Phentolamine is a short acting α_1 blocker that causes arteriolar vasodilation. The dose is 0.1 mg/kg IV stat. Its effects wear off after 6–10 minutes.

Labetalol is a combined selective α_1 blocker and a non-selective β-blocker. It has a greater β-effect than a effect so bradycardia may become a problem when larger doses are used. It reduces blood pressure by reducing cardiac output and heart rate, and decreasing the peripheral vascular resistance. The half life is between 3.5 and 6.5 hours. depending on the dose given. The adult dose is 50 mg given intravenously over at least one minute, repeat it 5 minutes later if necessary. We find it easier to control blood pressure, and pulse rate with nifedipine than labetalol.

> # WARNING
>
> Peripheral vasodilation to reduce blood pressure can cause severe hypotension in patients who are unable to increase their cardiac output.
>
> Do not vasodilate patients with
> * aortic or mitral stenosis;
> * hypertrophic obstructive cardiomyopathies;
> * cardiac tamponade;
> * restrictive pericarditis;.
> * head trauma;
> * hypovolaemia;
> * epidural or spinal anaesthesia;
> * closed angle glaucoma.

CLINICAL MANAGEMENT OF HYPERTENSION

1. Reassure the patient, give oxygen, attach an ECG, pulse oximeter and automated blood pressure monitor. It may help to sit him up.
2. Uncontrolled pain is the usual cause of acute hypertension. First eliminate hypoxia, hypercarbia and hypoglycaemia as a cause.
3. If the patient is showing signs of myocardial ischaemia, with either chest pain or ST changes on the ECG, use sublingual nifedipine. With a needle, prick the end of 10 mg capsule of nifedipine, and squeeze the contents into the patient's mouth. Give a small sip of water to aid its dispersal. Nifedipine acts within a couple of minutes, and the effects last for about an hour. If reflex tachycardia becomes a problem, consider controlling it with a β-blocker, such as metoprolol 5–20 mg intravenously slowly over two minutes.
4. If the patient is hypertensive without a tachycardia, try a sublingual (or an intranasal spray) of glyceryl trinitrate (Anginine®). This works for about 10 minutes, and will give you time to set up a glyceryl trinitrate (GTN) infusion to control the blood pressure. Start the GTN infusion with an initial drip rate of 10 micrograms/minute , but you may need to increase in steps of up to as much as 200 micrograms/minute. The hypotensive effects take 3–4 minutes to occur, and wears off in about 8–10 minutes. Headaches may be a problem with glyceryl trinitrate.
5. Hydralazine 5–20 mg slowly intravenously will reduce blood pressure, but it takes about 15–20 minutes to reach maximum effect, and works for about 3–4 hours. If necessary repeat the hydralazine within 4–5 hours, use about two thirds of the dose. As its effects are unpredictable, dilute it and give in 5 mg increments every 5 minutes. Consider

controlling any reflex tachycardia with a small dose of propanolol 0.01 mg/kg intravenously.

6. In severe or fulminating hypertension where the blood pressure is greater than 220/120 mmHg, sodium nitroprusside (SNP) is the drug of choice. As with all potent infusions use a separate intravenous line, so that it does not mix with anything else. Insert an arterial line for continuous blood pressure monitoring. Start the infusion of SNP at 0.5 microgram/kg per minute and increase the dose by 5 micrograms per minute every 3 minutes until the blood pressure falls. The dose range is 0.3–0.6 microgram/kg per minute. A response should be seen within 30 seconds. Aim for a diastolic pressure of 90–110 mmHg. The blood pressure will return within 2–4 minutes of turning off the SNP.

7. To prevent cyanide toxicity keep the infusion rate below 10 micrograms/kg per minute . The maximum total dose should not exceed 70 mg/kg in a patient with normal renal function. Cover the diluted SNP with light proof paper, because it deteriorates to release cyanide. If the solution turns a blue colour, it means it has broken down, and you should discard it.

CARDIAC ELECTROPHYSIOLOGY

See the end of this chapter for a summary of normal electrophysiology.

ABNORMAL CARDIAC ELECTROPHYSIOLOGY

There are two mechanisms that cause arrhythmias, *abnormal impulse generation*, and *abnormal impulse propagation*.

Abnormal impulse generation. Arrhythmias may arise at any point in the impulse's journey from the SA node to its final extinction in the ventricles. Ischaemic, irritated, or inflamed myocardial cells will discharge spontaneously. These stray, or *ectopic beats*, may arise anywhere in the heart to set off unco-ordinated, inefficient contraction. Examples of such abnormal heart rhythms are atrial fibrillation; and premature atrial, or ventricular contractions. Some drugs, such as digoxin, and quinidine make the heart irritable and cause arrhythmias. Other causes include hypoxia, and electrolyte disorders, especially hyperkalaemia, and hypomagnesaemia.

A tachycardia or a bradycardia can arise in the SA node. The SA node can be driven faster by sympathetic impulses, or slowed down by parasympathetic impulses. Hormones, such as thyroxine, and many drugs can also affect the heart rate.

Normally SA or AV node pacemaker activity is sufficiently rapid to trigger the myocardial cells before they have the chance to spontaneously fire themselves. However, if an impulse from a pacemaker does not arrive soon enough, a group of myocardial cells will, as if becoming impatient, spontaneously discharge to become an *ectopic pacemaker*. If the SA node stops firing, the AV node will become the heart's pacemaker having *escaped* the influence of the SA node. It sets a ventricular rate of about 35 per minute, a phenomenon called *AV nodal escape*.

If not stimulated by an impulse arriving from elsewhere, the ventricles will adopt their own rate of about 20–35 per minute. This is called the ventricles' *intrinsic rate*.

If ectopic beats arise from a single source (*unifocal ectopics*), the danger is not as great as it is when large parts of the heart are sick, and impulses are arising from all over the place (*multifocal ectopics*).

Abnormal impulse propagation occurs when the electrical impulse is blocked, or delayed, or goes the wrong way. If a group of myocardial cells becomes hypoxic, or part of the heart muscle dies, impulses are diverted from their usual path. This upsets the normal sequence of cardiac contraction. Impulses blocked from passing through the AV node cause heart blocks. If impulses are blocked in the major branches of the bundle of His, this causes right or left bundle branch blocks. Damage to the minor branches of the bundle of His causes right or left hemiblocks.

ARRHYTHMIAS

Arrhythmias are common and occur in up to 6 per cent of patients in the recovery room[2]. Most arrhythmias are simple tachycardias or bradycardias.

The patient may complain of one or more of:
- palpitations;
- chest pain;
- nausea;
- light headedness;
- shortness of breath.

You may notice:
- slow, fast, irregular, or even absent pulse;
- hypotension;
- changes in mental state;
- collapse;
- sweating.

Causes of arrhythmias in the recovery room include patient factors, surgical factors and anaesthetic factors.

1. Patient factors:
- pain;
- hypoxia;

- cardiac ischaemia;
- hypercarbia;
- hypertension or hypotension;
- electrolyte imbalance, especially of potassium and magnesium;
- drugs, such as tricyclic antidepressants, and digoxin.

Ischaemia and electrolyte imbalance
are the commonest causes of arrhythmias.

2. Surgical factors:
   - thoracic operations, especially if the pericardium has been damaged;
   - unrelieved pain, particularly from upper abdominal surgery;
   - operations on the eyes, ears, and upper jaw;
   - drugs, such as adrenaline, or cocaine, used to reduce bleeding;
   - developing shock.
3. Anaesthetic factors:
   - residual effects of drugs, such as fentanyl, or neostigmine causing bradycardias; or atropine causing tachycardias;
   - hypothermia.

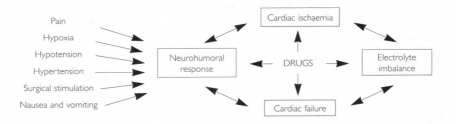

Fig 14.2 Priniciple causes of arrhythmias in the recovery room

Principles of Management of Arrhythmias

1. Check the pulse by feeling the carotid artery in the neck.
2. Take a 12-lead ECG and a long rhythm strip. Look at the rhythm. It will either be regular, or irregular. If you are unsure, mark the position of a series of three R wave peaks on the edge of a strip of paper, (or better still use geometery dividers). Slide the paper along to another series of three peaks. Do they match? If they do match the rhythm is regular.
3. Measure the width of the QRS complexes. Supraventricular tachycardias

are either wide complex or narrow complex tachycardias (see table 14.5 page 273).

4. Look for causes of the arrhythmia.
   • Treat hypoxia, hypercarbia, and hypotension.
   • Correct electrolyte imbalance, particularly potassium and magnesium.
   • Withdraw arrhythmogenic drugs, such as catecholamines and aminophylline.
5. Control rate and if possible revert to sinus rhythm with:
   • anti-arrhythmic drugs;
   • cardioversion;
   • overdrive pacing.
6. Follow-up persistent, or dangerous arrhythmias. They will need monitoring in a high dependency unit until they resolve. This may take three or four days.

Give patients with arrhythmias high flow oxygen.

ANTI-ARRHYTHMIC DRUGS

ATRIOVENTRICULAR CONDUCTION BLOCKERS

Adenosine[3] an endogenous purine nucleoside, is a potent atrioventricular blocking agent. This is the drug of choice for supraventricular tachycardias arising in the SA or AV node. It is not much use for atrial flutter. If available adenosine is the best treatment for both wide-complex regular tachycardias and narrow-complex supraventricular tachycardias. Its therapeutic effect persists for 20–30 seconds. Titrate the dose starting with 50 μg/kg IV, and then give incremental doses of 50 μg/kg IV every two minutes. The mean dose required to revert AV nodal re-entry arrhythmias ranges from 100–250 μg/kg. Side effects of dyspnoea, chest pain, hypotension, nausea and headache are very common, but they only last for about 30 seconds. Adenosine is antagonised by aminophylline, and markedly potentiated by dipyridamole. Adenosine is metabolized by erythrocytes and vascular endothelium.

BETA BLOCKING DRUGS[4] ('β-BLOCKERS'[6])

Beta blockers block the effects of catecholamines, such as, noradrenaline and adrenaline. By slowing the rate of the SA node and the AV node, they slow the heart rate. They make the heart contract less powerfully, which is useful in hypertension, and ischaemic heart disease. They are also useful to control supraventricular tachycardias. Many β-blockers are available, and all are approximately equally effective. The two most useful and widely available are propanolol, and metoprolol. If you understand the pharmacology of these two drugs, you will be able to cope with most circumstances.

All β-blockers:
- slow the heart, induce myocardial depression, and may precipitate heart failure;
- are effective antihypertensives. They reduce cardiac output, and alter baroreceptor sensitivity;
- can cause heart block;
- relieve the symptoms of angina by reducing cardiac work;
- often cause bronchoconstriction, and make asthma worse;
- mask the signs of hypoglycaemia, hypovolaemia, and hypercarbia;
- control the pulse rate in patients with phaeochromocytoma; however, you will also need an α blocker, such as phentolamine to control the rise in blood pressure.

Cardioselectivity refers to drugs that have fewer vascular, respiratory and metabolic effects, and yet still have a β-effect on the heart. Cardioselective β-blockers are less likely to cause bronchoconstriction.

Metoprolol is a cardioselective β-blocker, which is less likely to cause asthma, than propanolol. The dose is 0.1–0.15 mg/kg IV. Give it over 2 minutes. It has a half life of 3–4 hours, and is metabolized by the liver.

Esmolol is an expensive, short acting, cardioselective β-blocker that is especially useful to control rapid ventricular rates in patients with atrial fibrillation or flutter. It works in less than 5 minutes, and has an elimination half life of 9 minutes. Use a 10 mg/ml solution, and give a loading dose of 500 μg/kg over one minute. Follow this with a four minute maintenance infusion of 50 μg/kg/min. It may be necessary to modify the maintenance dose to get the effect you want. If this is effective continue the maintenance dose. If the ventricular rate does not fall and the blood pressure remains stable, then repeat the loading dose, and increase the maintenance dose in steps of 50 μg/kg/min to a maximum of 200 μg/kg/min. Once the heart rate is under control it can be maintained with another agent, such as digoxin.

Esmolol must not be used with verapamil as it may cause fatal bradycardias and asystole.

Sotalol is useful in treating atrial fibrillation and flutter, arrhythmias in Wolff–Parkinson–White syndrome, ventricular tachycardia, and ventricular premature beats. Unlike other β-blockers it only slightly depresses the heart's contractility, but may cause sinus bradycardia. The dose is 0.5–1.5 mg/kg IV over 10 minutes. It is excreted by the kidney and the effect lasts about 6 hours. Use atropine 0.6–2.4 mg IV if there is excessive bradycardia causing symptoms, such as hypotension, dyspnoea, or mental state changes. Bradycardia and heart block are more likely if the patient is hypokalaemic.

PROLONGATION OF REFRACTORY PHASE

Once a myocardial cell contracts, it takes a short time to recover before it can contract again. This is called the *refractory phase*. Amiodarone and sotalol are drugs that prolong the refractory phase, and are useful for suppressing abnormal depolarization in irritable myocardial cells.

Amiodarone is the most effective drug in the acute arrhythmias. However, it is often recommended (in theory) to reserve it as 'the drug of last resort' for patients with refractory ventricular arrhythmias and poor left ventricular function. If you have the facilities to supervise and monitor the patient for a few days postoperatively, then use amiodarone; if not then use the other antiarrhythmics first. It unlikely to cause a significant fall in cardiac output. Vasodilation, causing troublesome hypotension occurs if amiodarone is given too rapidly to patients in heart failure. It is only useful in the acute situation, because side effects preclude long term maintenance. Make up 300 mg in 50 ml of 5% dextrose. (It is not compatible with 0.9% saline). The oily vehicle causes thrombophlebitis, so infuse it into a central vein. The initial loading dose is 4–5 mg/kg (about 0.7–0.8 ml/kg) over 20 minutes. The maintenance dose is 0.3–0.4 mg/kg/hr for the next 24 hours. If the rate control remains poor give an extra 1 mg/kg over one hour, repeat if needed. As amiodarone is a non-competitive adrenoceptor antagonist, it will potentiate the effects of β-blockers or calcium channel blockers increasing the risk of hypotension and bradyarrhythmias.

CARDIAC GLYCOSIDES

Digoxin usually slows the ventricular rate in atrial fibrillation, however it does not revert the heart to sinus rhythm. Its beneficial effect in atrial fibrillation is to increase myocardial contraction, and slow the rate of impulse transmission through the AV node. The loading dose is up to 10–15 µg/kg IV, given over 20 minutes and a further 5 µg/kg after 6 hours. Use the lower range in the elderly. Never give digoxin I/M, because it causes massive muscle necrosis.

CALCIUM BLOCKERS

Verapamil's main action is to slow AV node conduction. It is useful to control atrial fibrillation and flutter, but vasodilation may cause the blood pressure to fall. It does not revert the heart to sinus rhythm. It is likely to cause severe bradycardia, heart block, or even asystole if used with β-blockers. Give 0.1–0.2 mg/kg IV over 10 minutes. If an infusion is needed then continue at 5 µg/kg/min (see page 462).

MEMBRANE STABILIZERS

Lignocaine is useful for management of ventricular ectopics, and to help stabilization of the myocardium in ventricular fibrillation. It may also decrease cardiac output and reduce blood pressure. Give a bolus dose of 1.0–1.5 mg/kg stat, followed by an infusion if needed. Infuse at 0.05 mg/kg/min for 1 hour, followed by 0.025 mg/kg/min for 2 hours and then 0.0125 mg/kg /min.

Other useful membrane stabilizers are procainamide and bretylium.

Diagnosis and Management of Arrhythmias

Medical and nursing staff who have direct responsibility for patient care in the recovery room should be able to recognize on the ECG trace, and treat the following arrhythmias.

1. Sinus tachycardia.
2. Sinus bradycardia.
3. Premature atrial contractions (PAC).
4. Paroxysmal supraventricular tachycardia (PSVT).
5. Atrial flutter.
6. Atrial fibrillation (AF).
7. Junctional rhythms.
8. Atrioventricular blocks of all degrees.
9. Premature ventricular contractions (PVC).
10. Ventricular tachycardias (VT) including Torsade de pointes.
11. Ventricular fibrillation (VF).
12. Asystole (cardiac standstill).

If arrhythmias occur they will cause the pulse to slow,
or speed up, or become irregular.

Normal Rhythms

Sinus arrhythmia

This is a normal variant in young people. The heart speeds up during inspiration and slows down during expiration.

RHYTHM	irregular, rate faster on inspiration, and slower on expiration
P WAVE	normal
P:QRS	1:1
P–R INTERVAL	0.12–0.2 sec
ATRIAL RATE	bradycardia or normal sinus rhythm
QRS SHAPE	normal
QRS WIDTH	less than 0.12 sec
VENTRICULAR RATE	bradycardia up to 100 per minute

Sinus bradycardia

Is normal in fit young athletes who may have pulse rates as low as 45 beats per minute.

ABNORMAL RHYTHMS

1. Sinus Tachycardia

A tachycardia is a pulse rate greater than 100 per minute. Never ignore tachycardia, it is warning sign that all may not be well. Try to find and treat the cause, do not just treat it symptomatically.

Children's heart rates vary with age. A tachycardia in children is a rate more than 20 per cent above the base-line. (see page 67)

Sinus tachycardia

RHYTHM	regular
P WAVE	normal position, but can be merged with previous T wave
P:QRS	1:1
P–R INTERVAL	0.12–0.2 sec
ATRIAL RATE	100–150/min
QRS	normal shape
QRS WIDTH	less than 0.12 sec
VENTRICULAR RATE	10–150/min

If you cannot see the P waves, and the rhythm is regular, then it is probably a paroxysmal supraventricular tachycardia.

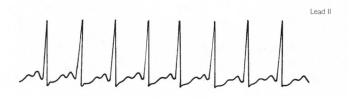

Lead II

Fig 14.2 Sinus tachycardia

Causes of tachycardia include:
- pain;
- hypoxia;
- hypercarbia,
- airway obstruction
- agitation, restlessness;
- shivering, shaking;
- hypovolaemia; bleeding
- drugs, such as atropine, adrenaline, pethidine, ephedrine, ketamine;

- heart failure;
- cardiac arrhythmias;
- hypoglycaemia;
- hyperthermia;
- pneumothorax;
- following thyroid surgery.

Tachycardias and bradycardias reduce cardiac output.

The heart is only perfused during diastole, and tachycardias shorten diastolic time. This means that tachycardias reduce coronary blood flow and may render the myocardium ischaemic. Consider treating a pulse rate above a value of [200 minus the patient's age in years]. For instance in a 60 year old this would be 140 beats per minute. Treat a tachycardia if the ECG shows signs of ischaemia, the patient's perfusion falls, or there are signs of cardiac failure, such as breathlessness.

2. Sinus Bradycardia

A bradycardia is a pulse rate of less than 60 per minute. It is a common arrhythmia. It may be normal in a fit young athletic person.

Bradycardia may be a sign of critically dangerous hypoxia.

Causes of bradycardia include:
- extreme fitness in young people;
- hypoxia, this is a grave sign;
- intraoperative fentanyl; especially if propofol has also been given;
- nausea;
- residual neostigmine;
- beta blockers, calcium channel blockade;
- painless urinary retention causing a distended bladder;
- hypothermia;
- reflex secondary to hypertension;
- myocardial ischaemia, and especially after antero-inferior infarction;
- raised intracranial pressure;
- spinal cord injury;
- airway suctioning;
- carotid artery surgery;
- myxoedema.

Lead II

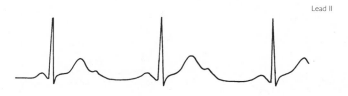

Fig 14.3 Sinus bradycardia

RHYTHM	regular, or slightly irregular
P WAVE	normal position and shape
P:QRS	1:1
P–R INTERVAL	0.12–20 sec
ATRIAL RATE	less than 60/min
QRS	normal shape
QRS WIDTH	less than 0.12 sec
VENTRICULAR RATE	less than 60/min

Do not treat a sinus bradycardia if the pulse rate is above 45 per minutes, and the patient has warm hands, a good urine output, and is comfortable. If the pulse rate is less than 60 per minute, monitor the patient with a pulse oximeter until you are sure the cardiovascular state is stable. If the pulse rate is below 45 per minute, attach a pulse oximeter, and an ECG and check the rhythm. Myocardial ischaemia, hypotension, an escape rhythm or poor perfusion requires treatment. A sinus bradycardia will respond to a small dose of atropine 0.01 mg/kg intravenously, and its effects last about 10 minutes. If it does not work immediately repeat it after 2 minutes. If the bradycardia persists, then consider the possibility of heart block. This may require an adrenaline infusion, at a rate of 1–10 micrograms per minute, or a pacemaker.

3. Premature Atrial Contractions (PAC)

Premature atrial contractions arise from an ectopic atrial focus, and consequently shows an abnormally shaped P wave. Sometimes they occur with right or left bundle branch blocks. Causes include sympathetic stimulation (pain, agitation, hypoxia), myocardial ischaemia and digoxin toxicity. Treat the cause and they usually resolve.

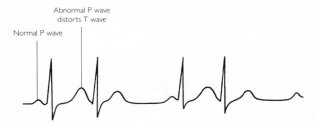

Fig 14.4 Premature atrial contractions

RHYTHM	irregular
P WAVE	P waves look different from normal sinus P wave
P:QRS	1:1
P–R INTERVAL	0.12–0.2 sec
ATRIAL RATE	varies depending on underlying rhythm
QRS	normal shape
QRS WIDTH	less than 0.12 sec
VENTRICULAR RATE	varies depending on underlying rhythm

Multifocal atrial tachycardia (MAT)

Multifocal atrial tachycardia is characterized by irregular and different forms of P waves (chaotic P waves) with a ventricular rate of greater than 100 beats per minute. It is a rhythm usually seen in elderly patients who have severe ischaemic heart disease.

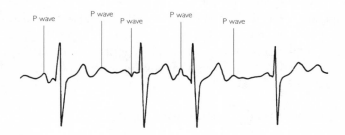

Fig 14.5 Multifocal atrial tachycardia

RHYTHM	irregular
P WAVE	forms differ with chaotic P waves that may be on top of T waves
P:QRS	P waves may arrive faster than QRS

P–R INTERVAL   variable
ATRIAL RATE   150–200/min
QRS   usually normal in shape unless altered by P wave
QRS WIDTH   usually less than 0.12 sec
VENTRICULAR RATE   depends on AV conduction

MAGNESIUM[5]

Magnesium is an essential co-factor for the production of ATP in biochemical reactions. It is a physiological calcium antagonist. Magnesium deficiency is associated with cardiac arrhythmias, cardiac failure and sudden cardiac death. It can precipitate refractory ventricular fibrillation. Magnesium supplementation may decrease the incidence of post-ischaemic arrhythmias. Suspect magnesium deficiency in patients who have been on diuretics, have had large intestinal fluid losses, or who are hypokalaemic. Because magnesium spreads evenly through out the extracellular fluid, it needs a large loading dose. Magnesium is rapidly excreted by the kidney, therefore to maintain blood levels, follow the loading dose with a constant intravenous infusion. It works mainly by presynaptic inhibition of neurotransmitter release in peripheral nerves, or by direct inhibition of cardiac muscle, or by vascular smooth muscle dilation. Magnesium also blocks the vagus nerve causing a tachycardia. Apart from its antiarrhythmic activity it is a bronchodilator, a tocolytic, and has renal vasodilatory activity. Calcium is an effective antagonist of magnesium's effects.

TREATMENT

Treat MAT with magnesium sulphate 10 mmol (5 ml of 49.3% solution) intravenously over 5 minutes. Repeat if necessary.

4. Supraventricular Tachycardias (SVT)

In a fit young person the maximum rate the ventricles can respond to the SA node is about 220–240 per minute. This ability decreases with age. As a rule of thumb, treat tachycardias when the perfusion status is inadequate, or the rate rises too high.

The maximum acceptable heart rate = (200 − patient's age)

Supraventricular tachycardias usually have a rate of 150–250 per minute. The QRS look normal, or may have a wide QRS complex. Any cardiac failure is aggravated by a decrease in coronary blood flow that occurs with tachycardias. More than half the patients will have hypotension, with associated oliguria and deteriorating oxygenation.

Supraventricular tachycardias are the most common arrhythmias causing cardiovascular instability in infancy and childhood. SVT may produce heart rates near 240 beats per minute, but it may be as high as 300 beats per minute. Any tachycardia with wide QRS complexes (greater than 120 milliseconds) should be assumed to be a ventricular arrhythmia.

Paroxysmal supraventricular tachycardia (PSVT)

Paroxysmal supraventricular tachycardia is the most common of the supraventricular tachycardias. It usually begins and ends abruptly. Patients often describe sensations of fluttering (palpitations) in the chest. If the paroxysm is prolonged cardiac perfusion becomes impaired resulting in ischaemia, angina, a fall in cardiac output, hypotension, poor peripheral perfusion and oliguria. Immediate cardioversion is seldom needed if the pulse rate is less than 150 beats per minute.

Causes include:
- usually occurs in otherwise fit young people;
- Wolff–Parkinson–White syndrome. (WPW);
- ischaemic heart disease;
- rheumatic heart disease.

RHYTHM	regular
P WAVE	within the QRS or on T wave
P:QRS	1:1
P–R INTERVAL	not visible
ATRIAL RATE	170–250/min
QRS	normal
QRS WIDTH	less than 0.12 sec
VENTRICULAR RATE	170–250/min

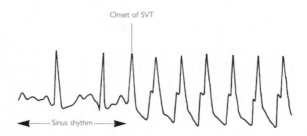

Fig 14.6 *Paroxysmal supraventricular tachycardia (PSVT)*

MANAGEMENT

Vagal manoeuvres. Paroxysmal supraventricular tachycardias can often be abruptly terminated with vagal stimulation. Attach an ECG, pulse oximeter and non-invasive blood pressure cuff. To start with, try putting an ice-cold sloppy wet towel on the patient's face. If this fails try gentle carotid sinus massage. The carotid sinus is close to the bifurcation of the common carotid artery, adjacent to the angle of the jaw. With the head turned to one side put your thumb over the point of maximum pulsation and firmly massage up and down along the length of the carotid artery by pressing it against the spine for no longer than 10 seconds. Try the right side first, and then the left side, but never both sides together. Keep your other hand on the radial pulse, and listen with a stethoscope over the apex of the heart. Carotid sinus massage may convert the rhythm to sinus rhythm, or slow the pulse rate down. If carotid sinus massage fails, treat the patient as a narrow complex tachycardia. It is unwise to do carotid sinus massage in patients with cerebrovascular or carotid artery disease.

If the vagal manoeuvres are unsuccessful, the patient's blood pressure is within normal limits, and he is not on β-blockers; then try verapamil 5 mg intravenously over 2 minutes. Wait 15 minutes and repeat verapamil 10 mg intravenously.

If the patient is unstable, or has a low blood pressure, use synchronized cardioversion 75–100 joules. Increase this to 200 joules and then 300 joules. If the rhythm fails to revert do not use further cardioversion; in this case a pacemaker may be needed. Meanwhile try amiodarone or digoxin.

WOLFF–PARKINSON–WHITE SYNDROME.

Wolff–Parkinson–White (WPW) syndrome is caused by an abnormal conduction pathway (called the bundle of Kent) between the atria and the ventricles, through which impulses take a shortcut to the ventricles, bypassing the AV node. The ECG shows a characteristically short PR interval that often fuses with the QRS complex. This is called a fusion beat Sometimes the impulse re-enters the atria through another pathway setting up a rapid feed back on itself stimulating a fast ventricular response. The pulse rate can rise to 200/min or more. Patients with Wolff–Parkinson–White syndrome sometimes spontaneously go into supraventricular tachycardia or atrial fibrillation.

Atrial fibrillation in these patients is life threatening because the rapid atrial rate is not delayed at the AV node, and it may stimulate the ventricles up to 400 times per minute. The QRS complexes are widened (>120 msec), and can trigger ventricular fibrillation. Do not use digoxin, verapamil, or adenosine. These drugs slow transmission through the AV node, so then more impulses will take the short cut, and paradoxically increase the ventricular rate. Procainamide will sometimes slow the conduction through the aberrant pathway.

Do not use digoxin, verapamil or adenosine in patients with WPW syndrome, treatment is defibrillation

Restrict the use of verapamil to patients with narrow complex PSVT who have normal blood pressures. Do not use verapamil in patients with wide QRS complexes, it may be lethal.

RHYTHM	regular
P WAVE	may merge with QRS
P: QRS	1:1
P–R INTERVAL	less than 0.12 sec
ATRIAL RATE	bradycardia or normal sinus rhythm
QRS SHAPE	normal
QRS WIDTH	less than 0.12 sec
VENTRICULAR RATE	60–100/min

P wave with short PR interval

Fig 14.7 Wolff–Parkinson–White (WPW) syndrome

5. Atrial Flutter

Atrial flutter is easily recognized because of the saw-toothed pattern of the P waves on the ECG. The causes are similar to atrial fibrillation.

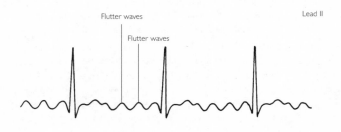

Flutter waves   Lead II

Flutter waves

Fig 14.8 Atrial flutter

RHYTHM	regular or irregular
P WAVE	saw-toothed pattern
P:QRS	more P waves than QRS complexes. The complexes may come in a fixed ratio in which case the ventricular rate will be regular.
P–R INTERVAL	difficult to measure
ATRIAL RATE	250–350/min
QRS	normal complex
QRS WIDTH	less than 0.12 sec
VENTRICULAR RATE	depends on AV conduction ratio.

TREATMENT

Treat it as a narrow complex irregular rhythm (see table 14.5).

6. Atrial Fibrillation (AF)

Atrial fibrillation is a common arrhythmia, and is usually a result of long standing ischaemic heart disease. It may arise in recovery room following:

• thoracotomy, especially if the pericardium has been damaged;
• oesophagectomy;
• following thyroid surgery;
• pulmonary embolism.

Since atrial contraction contributes up to 25 per cent of the cardiac output the onset of atrial fibrillation can cause the cardiac output to fall enough to precipitate heart failure in patients with poor cardiac reserves.

RHYTHM	irregular
P WAVE	no formed P waves, just chaotic fibrillation waves
P:QRS	more fibrillation waves than QRS complexes
P–R INTERVAL	none
ATRIAL RATE	greater than 350/min
QRS	normal
QRS WIDTH	less than 0.12 sec
VENTRICULAR RATE	varies, but in uncontrolled fibrillation is greater than 100/min

TREATMENT

Treat atrial fibrillation as a narrow complex irregular arrhythmia (see Table 14.5). Aim to, either revert the fibrillation to sinus rhythm, or failing that, to bring the ventricular rate to under 100 beats per minute. If the rhythm starts in recovery room, and the patient's perfusion is falling, then consider cardioversion. Start with 1.0 joule/kg. Only attempt

3 countershocks. If this fails to convert the heart to sinus rhythm, then control the ventricular rate with verapamil and digoxin.

Lead II

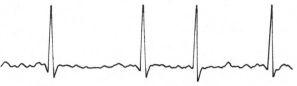

Fig 14.9 Atrial fibrillation

7. Junctional Rhythms

Junctional arrhythmias arise at, or near, the atrioventricular node.

Nodal or junctional escape rhythms

If the sinus node fails, the AV node usually takes over as the pacemaker for the heart. This takeover mechanism protects the patient from asystole.

Causes include:
- hypoxia;
- myocardial ischaemia;
- pain, especially visceral pain from the abdomen travelling via the vagus nerve;
- residual halothane.

RHYTHM	regular
P WAVE	before, during, or after the QRS complex, inverted
P:QRS	P waves less than, or equal to the number of QRS complexes
P–R INTERVAL	if present, less than 0.12 sec
ATRIAL RATE	cannot always see the P waves
QRS	normal
QRS WIDTH	less than 0.12 sec
VENTRICULAR RATE	40–60/min

TREATMENT

Eliminate hypoxia and myocardial ischaemia as a cause.

If the patient is not hypoxic, and has a good perfusion status, no treatment is necessary. If the patient has cold hands, is cyanosed, or has a blood pressure less than 80 mmHg, then treat it with atropine 0.01 mg/kg intravenously. Repeat the atropine at 2 minute intervals if needed.

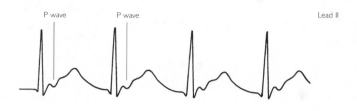

Fig 14.10 Nodal rhythm

8. Atrioventricular Blocks

Heart blocks occur when transmission of the cardiac impulse, is either blocked, or delayed on its normal journey through the heart. In recovery room always suspect myocardial ischaemia as the cause.

These include:
- right bundle branch block (RBBB);
- left bundle branch block (LBBB);
- first-degree heart block;
- second-degree heart block;
- complete heart block.

Exclude hypoxia or myocardial ischaemia if heart block occurs.

Causes include
- myocardial ischaemia and infarction;
- valvular disease;
- myocarditis;
- heart surgery;
- sometimes congenital.

MANAGEMENT

Aim to reduce cardiac work, and improve cardiac oxygenation. Give oxygen, control hypertension, and pain. If the cardiac output falls, causing hypotension, shortness of breath, or changes in mental state then treat the block. Drugs that temporarily increase cardiac output are atropine 0.6 mg intravenously, repeated as necessary; or if atropine fails then give an adrenaline infusion of 1–10 micrograms per minute. These measures will allow time for a pacemaker to be inserted.

Right bundle branch block (RBBB)

Right bundle branch block is not usually a serious concern. If it occurs acutely consider myocardial ischaemia, infarction or pulmonary embolism.

RHYTHM	Can occur with any rhythm
P WAVE	before QRS complex if the rhythm is sinus
P:QRS	1:1 if sinus rhythm, otherwise depends on underlying rhythm
P–R INTERVAL	depends on underlying rhythm
ATRIAL RATE	depends on underlying rhythm
QRS	often notched
QRS WIDTH	greater than 0.12 sec in right chest leads, and aVR and III
VENTRICULAR RATE	depends on underlying rhythm

Lead V₁

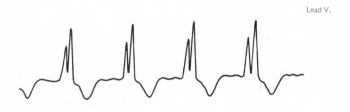

Fig 14.11 Right bundle branch block (RBBB)

Left bundle branch block (LBBB)

Left bundle branch block is usually a sign of severe heart disease. If it occurs acutely the patient has probably had a myocardial infarction.

RHYTHM	can occur with any rhythm
P WAVE	before QRS complex if the rhythm is sinus
P:QRS	1:1 if sinus rhythm, otherwise depends on underlying rhythm
P–R INTERVAL	depends on underlying rhythm
ATRIAL RATE	depends on underlying rhythm
QRS	may be notched
QRS WIDTH	greater than 0.12 sec in left chest leads, and I and II
VENTRICULAR RATE	depends on underlying rhythm

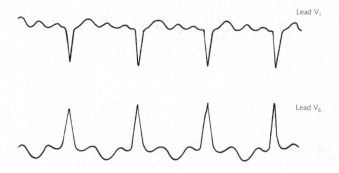

Lead V₁

Lead V₆

Fig 14.12 Left bundle branch block (LBBB)

First-degree AV block

First-degree AV block, occurs if the PR interval is longer than 0.2 seconds, which is one large box on normal ECG paper. It means the impulse is delayed, usually at the AV node, and is a sign of myocardial ischaemia. It may progress to second- or third-degree heart block.

RHYTHM	regular
P WAVE	uniform shape
P:QRS	1:1
P-R INTERVAL	prolonged more than 0.2 sec.
ATRIAL RATE	any sinus rate
QRS	normal complex
QRS WIDTH	less than 0.12 sec
VENTRICULAR RATE	any sinus rate

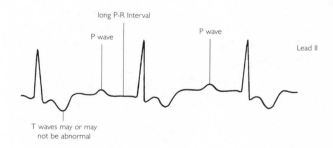

long P-R Interval

P wave

P wave

Lead II

T waves may or may
not be abnormal

Fig 14.13 First-degree block

Second-degree AV block – Möbitz Type I

Second-degree AV block, Wenckebach block (Möbitz Type I) occurs where the SA node fires at a regular rate, with a progressively longer PR interval until a ventricular beat is dropped. It is a sign of AV node ischaemia, and will respond to atropine. It is often transient, and may stop spontaneously.

RHYTHM	irregular
P WAVE	each QRS complex preceded by P wave, but some P waves do not trigger a QRS complex
P:QRS	more P waves than QRS complexes
P–R INTERVAL	prolonged more than 0.2 sec.
ATRIAL RATE	any sinus rate
QRS	normal complex
QRS WIDTH	less than 0.12
VENTRICULAR RATE	any sinus rate

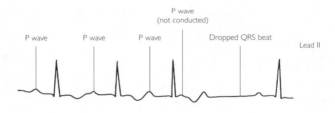

Fig 14.14 Second-degree AV block, Wenckebach block (Möbitz type I)

Second-degree AV block – Möbitz type II

Second-degree AV block, Möbitz type II block occurs when there are missed atrial beats. The P–R interval is normal, but the sick SA node is firing at irregular intervals. It may progress without warning to complete heart block. It is a sign of severe myocardial ischaemia, or anteroseptal myocardial infarction. Avoid atropine, because the SA node is already malfunctioning, and it may stop, making the block worse.

RHYTHM	irregular
P WAVE	each QRS complex preceded by P wave, but some P waves do not trigger a QRS complex
P:QRS	more P waves than QRS complexes
P–R INTERVAL	varies
ATRIAL RATE	greater than the ventricular rate

QRS	less than 0.12 sec
QRS WIDTH	normal
VENTRICULAR RATE	any sinus rate

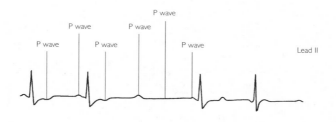

Fig 14.15 Second-degree AV block, Möbitz type II

Third-degree Heart Block

Complete heart block occurs where the ventricles are not triggered by the SA node, and the atria and ventricles are contracting independently of each other. This results in poor perfusion, and a fixed cardiac output and may cause the patient to feel dizzy or collapse. Often it is accompanied by transient junctional escape rhythms.

TREATMENT

If the complexes are wide, avoid atropine. If the complexes are narrow then, in order try:
• atropine 0.5–1 mg (repeat in 3–5 minutes to a total dose of 0.04 mg/kg.
• transcutaneous pacemaker (TCP) is a stop gap measure.
• dopamine infusion at a rate of 5–20 micrograms/kg per minute
• adrenaline infusion at a rate of 2–10 micrograms/kg per minute.
These measures will give you time to organize the insertion of a pacemaker.

RHYTHM	regular atrial and ventricular rhythm
P WAVE	uniform shape
P:QRS	more P waves than QRS complexes
P–R INTERVAL	varies
ATRIAL RATE	greater than ventricular rate
QRS	normal or widened
QRS WIDTH	less than 0.12 sec if pacemaker cell is in the A.V. junction greater than 0.12 sec if pacemaker cell is in the ventricles

VENTRICULAR RATE   40–60 per minute if escape pacemaker is in the AV junction. 20–40/min if the escape pacemaker is in the ventricles.

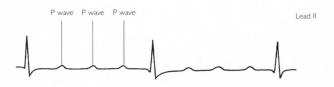

Fig 14.16 Third-degree AV block (complete heart block)

9. Premature Ventricular Contractions (PVCs)

Premature ventricular contractions are also called ventricular premature beats (PVB), ventricular ectopic beats (VPBs) or ventricular extrasystoles (VEs). They are premature contractions arising from some irritable, ectopic focus in the ventricles that come earlier than expected in the cardiac cycle.

Causes include:
• occur in 50 per cent of the healthy population and are aggravated by caffeine, alcohol, and tobacco consumption;
• hypertension;
• neurohumoral response to pain, anxiety or fear;
• drugs, such as digoxin, adrenoceptor agonists, tricyclic antidepressants and aminophylline;
• diuretics causing hypokalaemia, and hypomagnesaemia increase myocardial irritability;
• underlying cardiac disease, such as ischaemia, mitral valve prolapse, cardiomyopathy and aortic valve disease.

RHYTHM	regular, until interrupted by ectopic beat, and then followed by a compensatory pause
P WAVE	none with premature beat
P:QRS	less P waves than QRS complexes
P–R INTERVAL	none for premature beat
ATRIAL RATE	normal for sinus beats
QRS	abnormal complex is wide and frequently in opposite direction to ST segment and T wave.
QRS WIDTH	abnormal beat is wide, others less than 0.12 sec
VENTRICULAR RATE	depends on underlying rhythm.

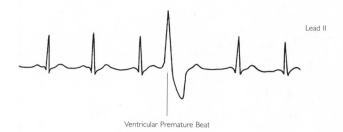

Lead II

Ventricular Premature Beat

Fig 14.17 Ventricular premature beats

TREATMENT

Eliminate hypoxia, or myocardial ischaemia as a cause. If the blood pressure, and pulse rate is within normal limits, the patient's perfusion is normal, and there are less than 5 ectopics per minute, no treatment is necessary. More than 5 abnormal beats per minute are a minor predictor of serious sequela, such as, postoperative myocardial infarction, pulmonary oedema or ventricular tachycardia[6]. Treat as for bigeminy (see below).

Bigeminy

Bigeminy occurs when a normal beat is followed by a ventricular ectopic beat, to be followed by a compensatory pause before the next cycle is started. Bigeminy signals more severe damage than the occasional ectopic beat. It is a sign of irritable myocardial muscle, due to one or more of: myocardial hypoxia, hypertension, digoxin toxicity, high catecholamine levels, hypokalaemia or hypomagnesaemia. Bigeminy usually either resolves spontaneously, or progresses to a ventricular tachycardia.

RHYTHM	irregularly regular, two beats close together followed by a compensatory pause and then two beats close together. Sometimes called coupling.
P WAVE	none with premature beat
P:QRS	half the number of P waves as QRS complexes
P–R INTERVAL	normal for normal beats, absent for premature beats
ATRIAL RATE	60–100/min
QRS	normal beat followed by premature ventricular beat which is opposite in direction to ST segment and T wave
QRS WIDTH	normal for normal beat, greater than 0.12 for premature contraction
VENTRICULAR RATE	60–100/min

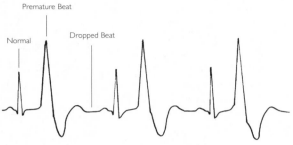

Fig 14.18 Bigeminy

TREATMENT

The arrhythmia may resolve with treatment of any hypoxia, or hypertension. Otherwise try lignocaine 1.5 mg/kg intravenously, or if the patient has a tachycardia use a β-blocker, such as propanolol or metoprolol. Treating the arrhythmia does not prevent it from progressing to a ventricular tachycardia. Using lignocaine is like covering a wound with a bandage, it only hides the underlying problem.

Cardiac Failure and VPBs

A patient with ventricular ectopic activity in the presence of myocardial ischaemia, and poor left ventricular function, is at high risk of sudden death. Following myocardial infarction, a β-blocker reduces ectopic activity, and may improve prognosis. Hypertension causes myocardial ischaemia, and you may see ventricular ectopic beats. If you suspect myocardial ischaemia, then aim to improve myocardial oxygen supply, and to decrease myocardial work. Give oxygen, treat pain, reduce blood pressure if it is elevated, improve cardiac perfusion with nitroglycerine, or calcium channel blockers, and consider cautiously slowing the heart rate with a β-blocker.

10. Ventricular Tachycardia (VT)

Ventricular tachycardia is a life threatening arrhythmia, generally occurring in patients with poor left ventricular function. If it is sustained the patient rapidly becomes hypotensive, with poor peripheral perfusion. Ventricular tachycardia is defined as three, or more ventricular premature beats in succession.

Causes include:
• myocardial ischaemia and infarction;
• hypotension;
• inflammation;
• drug toxicity.

RHYTHM	regular
P WAVE	absent
P:QRS	absent
P–R INTERVAL	none
ATRIAL RATE	cannot be determined
QRS	often notched or bizarre, and opposite in direction to ST segment and T wave
QRS WIDTH	greater than 0.12 sec
VENTRICULAR RATE	100–250+/min

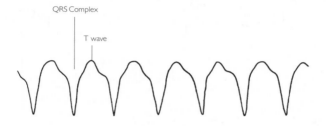

Fig 14.19 Picture of ventricular tachycardia

TREATMENT

A precordial thump may convert ventricular tachycardia to sinus rhythm. If the patient has a poor or absent perfusion status, do not delay, immediately use DC synchronized cardioversion. Pulseless VT should be treated as ventricular fibrillation. The patient who is alert with a good perfusion status, may revert with lignocaine 0.75–1.5 mg/kg intravenously given as a bolus. Because of the sluggish circulation allow up to 3 minutes for the drug to reach the heart. If you have given the drug into an arm vein, then elevate the arm to hasten venous return. This dose may be repeated at 5–10 minute intervals to a total of lignocaine 3 mg/kg. Follow this with a lignocaine infusion if needed (see page 461). If this fails try procainamide 20–30 mg per minute.

Patients with severe left ventricular dysfunction sometimes get a paradoxical response to antiarrhythmics, and the drug makes the rhythm, or its rate, worse. If this happens stop the antiarrhythmic drugs, and use cardioversion.

Do not give verapamil to a patient with a
wide complex tachycardia—it can be lethal.

Torsade de pointes (polymorphic VT)

Torsade de pointes means *twisting about a point*. This is a type of rapid ventricular tachycardia with rapidly changing QRS morphology. It looks as though the QRS complexes are revolving, as a spiral, around a baseline axis. It may occur in patients on quinidine, and is often fatal.

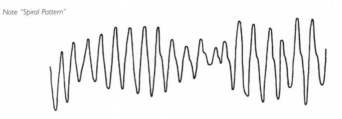

Note "Spiral Pattern"

Fig 14.20 Torsade de pointes

RHYTHM	regular or irregular
P WAVE	none
P:QRS	absent
P–R INTERVAL	absent
ATRIAL RATE	cannot be determined
QRS	alternating positive and negative deflection
QRS WIDTH	greater than 0.12 per sec
VENTRICULAR RATE	cannot be determined

MANAGEMENT

First use DC countershock, and then give magnesium sulphate 2 gm intravenously over 2 minutes. Other antiarrhythmics are ineffective, and if the patient is hypotensive he usually will not survive long. Isoprenaline may be useful.

11. Ventricular Fibrillation (VF)

Ventricular fibrillation is chaotic quivering of the ventricles. There is no cardiac output, and it is lethal.

RHYTHM	none
P WAVE	none
P:QRS	absent
P–R INTERVAL	none
ATRIAL RATE	cannot be determined

QRS	irregular chaotic electrical activity with bizarre shapes
QRS WIDTH	coarse or fine waves
VENTRICULAR RATE	cannot be determined

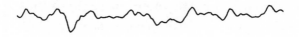

Fig 14.21 Ventricular fibrillation

TREATMENT

Immediately defibrillate and manage as for a cardiac arrest according to your protocol.

12. Asystole (Cardiac Standstill)

This is usually fatal, and responds poorly to resuscitation efforts. The ECG shows a flat line with no carotid pulse detectable.

Line may wave slightly

Fig 14.22 Asystole

RATE	none
RHYTHM	none
P WAVE	none
P:QRS	none
P–R INTERVAL	none
ATRIAL RATE	none
QRS	slowly fluctuating base-line
QRS WIDTH	none
VENTRICULAR RATE	none

TREATMENT

Immediately commence CPR, and ensure adequate oxygenation, and ventilation. Try to find out the reason. Exclude hypoxia, hypovolaemia, tension pneumothorax, and cardiac tamponade. Give 1 mg (1 ml of 1:1000) adrenaline intravenously. Follow the adrenaline with 20 ml of saline and lift the arm to hasten the drug to the central circulation. If there is no response within 3–5 minutes then double the dose of adrenaline. If there is still no response consider a small dose of sodium bicarbonate 0.25 mmol/kg given over 2 minutes. This is a lethal arrhythmia, with a poor prognosis.

Practical Points in the Treatment of Arrhythmias

It is often difficult to distinguish between sinus tachycardia, ventricular tachycardia, supraventricular tachycardia and a paroxysmal supraventricular tachycardia even with the help of a 12-lead ECG trace. It is almost impossible to separate these arrhythmias on a recovery room monitor screen.

The following points are critically important.
• Treat the patient, not the monitor.
• If the patient is hypotensive, or has poor peripheral perfusion, prepare for immediate cardioversion.
• If the tachycardia complex appears wide (>120 milliseconds) and you are unsure of its nature, then treat the rhythm like a ventricular tachycardia.
• Never give verapamil to a patient with a wide complex tachycardia. It can be lethal.
• If you cannot provide oxygen to the heart you are unlikely to succeed in treating the arrhythmia.
• Just because the ECG shows electrical activity, this does not mean the heart is contracting. Pulseless electrical activity (PEA) is also called electromechanical dissociation (EMD).

Cardioversion

With acute onset of an SVT causing life threatening hypotension, consider immediate cardioversion. Pre-treatment with a β-blocker increases the chance of success. The patient will require a small dose of induction agent and airway support during this procedure.

Defibrillation does not jump start the heart. It produces momentary asystole, and by depolarizing all the myocardium provides an opportunity for the natural pacemakers to resume normal activity.

Try the following settings to start with:

Any patient on digoxin	0.1 joule/kg
Atrial flutter	0.1 joule/kg
Ventricular tachycardias	0.5 joule/kg
Atrial fibrillation	1.0 joule/kg

Table 14.5

SUMMARY OF THE TREATMENT OF TACHYCARDIAS		
ECG rhythm	**Broad complex** **QRS > 120 msec**	**Narrow complex** **QRS < 120 msec**
Irregular ECG rhythm	Usually a ventricular tachycardia with fusion beats.	Usually: • Atrial fibrillation • Atrial flutter
Management	If the blood pressure and perfusion is good then try one of: • esmolol • sotalol, • propanolol, • metoprolol. and then • amiodarone. If the blood pressure is low, then use cardioversion. Avoid adenosine Avoid verapamil Avoid digoxin.	Try, in order: • adenosine, • verapamil • digoxin. Treat new onset arrhythmias associated with poor peripheral perfusion with cardioversion.
Regular ECG rhythm	Usually a ventricular tachycardia	Usually a supraventricular tachycardia.
Management	Try lignocaine 1.5 mg/kg IV push. Wait 5–10 minutes before repeating. Then use adenosine 6 mg stat IV over 1–3 seconds. Wait 1–2 minutes Then try procainamide IV 20–30 mg/minute. If that fails use synchronized cardioversion. Avoid verapamil.	If on a β-blocker, or has a poor cardiac output, then use cardioversion. If the patient's perfusion and blood pressure is good, and he is not on β-blockers, try adenosine, and if that fails then verapamil. May need to stabilize later on digoxin, with or without a β-blocker

Place the paddles to maximize the current flow through the myocardium. Place one paddle just to the right of the sternum under the clavicle, and the other to the left of the nipple with the centre of the paddle in the mid clavicular line. Take care the gel or electrode paste is not smeared between the paddles on the chest, otherwise the current will just flow along the chest wall and bypass the heart. Do not use a non-conductive jelly (such as KY Jelly®) or water because the current will cause deep burns.

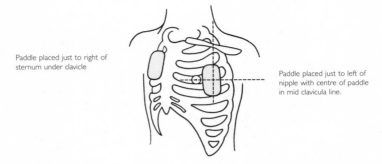

Paddle placed just to right of sternum under clavicle

Paddle placed just to left of nipple with centre of paddle in mid clavicula line.

Fig 14.22 Diagram of where to place the paddles for cardioversion

MYOCARDIAL ISCHAEMIA AND INFARCTION

In developed countries about 12–20 per cent of patients have preoperative evidence of ischaemic heart disease. Perioperative myocardial infarction is the most common cause of death in non-cardiac surgical patients. Be alert for the possibility of myocardial ischaemia or infarction in a patient known to have coronary artery disease. Myocardial ischaemia during the operation, or in the first few hours after operation put the patient at risk of arrhythmias, ischaemic episodes, or cardiac failure in the first postoperative week.[7] Most postoperative infarcts occur on the second or third postoperative day[8].

Risk factors are:

- coronary artery disease;
- congestive cardiac failure;
- emergency surgery;
- current, or ex-smoker;
- vascular disease;
- hypertension;
- diabetes;

- painful surgery over age 45 years;
- prolonged surgery of more than 3 hours;
- vascular surgery;
- BP unstable during anaesthetic;
- lung disease;
- polycythaemia;
- hyperlipidaemia.

Attempts to quantify risk factors have been made. The widely quoted is the Goldman Risk Index[9] does not specifically assess risks or complications that occur in the recovery room.

The surgical patients who are likely to infarct postoperatively are:

- those who have had a myocardial infarct in the past six months, and especially in the past 3 months;
- those with unstable preoperative angina, congestive cardiac failure at the time of surgery[10].
- prolonged, or emergency surgery in a patient with other risk factors;
- intraoperative tachycardia, hypotension or hypertension in patients with other risk factors.

DEMAND AND SUPPLY INDUCED ISCHAEMIA[11]

Heart muscle can become hypoxic in two main ways. Firstly, not enough oxygen reaches the heart, because the patient is hypoxic, anaemic, hypotensive, or the coronary arteries are blocked This is sometimes called *demand induced ischaemia*. Secondly the heart may be working so hard that its oxygen demands outstrip its oxygen supply. This is called *supply induced ischaemia*.

If the heart muscle does not receive enough oxygen, it may:
* fail to contract hard enough to maintain an adequate cardiac output;
* become irritable and contract prematurely causing ectopic beats;
* give rise to ischaemic pain;
* infarct and die.

Variables affecting myocardial blood and oxygen supply include:
1. Heart rate
2. Preload
3. Afterload
4. Heart size.

1. Heart rate is important, because the heart muscle is only perfused when it is not contracting; that is, during diastole. During systole blood flow to the myocardium almost ceases. As the heart rate increases during a tachycardia, diastole gets shorter, leaving less time for perfusion of the heart muscle. Bradycardia too, can be dangerous, particularly in the elderly. It is common following an anaesthetic where propofol and fentanyl have been used.

2. Pre-load is the pressure filling the ventricle. It is measured by the pulmonary artery wedge pressure. A high pre-load may be associated with pulmonary oedema; and may be a sign of *diastolic dysfunction*. (See page 284.)

3. High afterload causes ischaemia by making the heart work harder to eject blood through a tight valve, or against a high systemic blood pressure. An enlarged ventricle, caused by hypertension or previous myocardial infarction causes *systolic dysfunction*. (See page 281.) Hypertensive patients are at high risk from cardiac ischaemia, particularly if they develop a tachycardia or arrhythmia. A high afterload causes endocardial ischaemia by partially squashing the blood vessels supplying oxygen to the myocardial tissues lining the ventricles. This can be detected by T-wave inversion on the anterior leads of the ECG.

4. Heart size is a factor, because the harder the heart works, the more oxygen it consumes. Big hearts need more oxygen than little hearts, because the myocardium has to contract more strongly to achieve the same pressure within the ventricle. Hearts can enlarge because the myocardium is damaged by infarction and the ventricular walls become thin, dilated and floppy; or the myocardium can hypertrophy because of the extra effort needed to pump blood through a tight valve, or to maintain hypertension.

Emergence from anaesthesia is characterized by physiological turmoil. The resultant adrenergic stress contributes to ischaemia by:

* changing calibre of myocardial vessels, so-called spasm;
* changing blood viscosity;
* increased blood coagulability.

DIAGNOSIS OF ISCHAEMIA AND INFARCTION

Patients are sometimes maximally stressed as they emerge from anaesthesia, and so it is not unusual for ischaemia to occur for the first time in the recovery room. If it remains unrecognized by the staff, the patient will return to the ward at risk of suffering a myocardial infarct. About half postoperative myocardial infarcts are clinically silent and deaths are frequent. Excellent pain relief reduces the risk.

The diagnosis of ischaemia and infarction depends on two features:
1. Chest pain.
2. ECG changes.

It is almost impossible clinically to distinguish between myocardial ischaemia and myocardial infarction in the recovery room. Myocardial ischaemia may, or may not, proceed to infarction.

1. Chest Pain

Angina

Ischaemic chest pain is called *angina*. It feels like a crushing pain behind the sternum, usually described by the patient 'as though someone is sitting on my chest', or 'a tight band around my chest'. It may be accompanied by a pain down the arm or in the jaw. Angina is a late sign of ischaemia, and indicates that one or more of the major coronary arteries are obstructed. In the recovery room it is a grave warning sign of impending acute myocardial infarction. In the immediate postoperative phase it is often symptomless[12]; this is so-called *silent angina*. The patient does not complain of pain, but looks and feels unwell. The patient may present with one or more of a combination of baffling signs. The patient may: sweat, appear grey, have a poor perfusion status, feel nauseated, become hypotensive, feel anxious, shake, become short of breath, complain of dizziness, or have an arrhythmia.

Angina in the recovery room may be precipitated by:

Demand induced ischaemia
• pain,
• hypertension,
• emotional stress.

Supply induced ischaemia
• hypotension,
• tachycardia,
• bradycardia,
• hypoxia, anaemia.

Tachycardia increases the risk of cardiac ischaemia.

Myocardial infarction

If the ischaemia is not relieved the patient will progress to myocardial infarction with the death of heart muscle. There is clear evidence that repeated episodes of ischaemia cause myocardial infarction[13]. The crushing central chest pain may radiate to the neck, jaw or arms. It is often accompanied by sweating, breathlessness, hypotension, hypertension, nausea or arrhythmias. If the patient is able to speak he may report that he feels 'alarmed' or 'terrible', and the pain is the worst he has ever experienced. The pain is diagnostically not relieved by glyceryl trinitrate. Insidiously these signs may be absent in the immediate postoperative period, and the infarct may be clinically silent with no pain, but just ECG signs of ST elevation or depression. Suspect silent infarction if a patient becomes hypotensive, has an irregular pulse, starts to sweat or develops pulmonary oedema with wheezing, and basal crepitations in the lung.

2. ECG changes

Monitoring may reveal arrhythmias and ST and T wave changes[14].

- Left axis deviation, (indicating a left anterior hemiblock) in an otherwise healthy patient, suggests ischaemia;
- With ischaemia the ST segments first become prolonged (greater than 0.12 seconds), and then depressed. J point depression with up-sloping ST segment may be the earliest sign of ischaemia. Later, the ST segment may also be depressed below the isoelectric line, but remain horizontal;
- Down sloping ST depression represents profound myocardial ischaemia, and may be associated with T wave inversion. ST segment elevation occurs with severe transmural ischaemia, but also with hyperkalaemia.
- T wave changes alone occur in up to 20 per cent of patients in their first hour in the recovery room, but these are not always a sign of ischaemia[15].
- Epicardial ischaemia is just one of the causes of inverted T waves. Although often missed, U wave inversion is a sign of myocardial ischaemia.
- Patients presenting for vascular surgery have a high incidence of coronary artery disease.
- Postoperative myocardial infarction is usually preceded by prolonged periods of ST depression[16].

Differential diagnosis of ST segment depression includes:

- ischaemia;
- bundle branch blocks;

- ventricular hypertrophy with strain;
- digoxin, and catecholamines;
- pericardial damage during surgery;
- hypokalaemia;
- hypomagnesaemia;
- alkalosis;
- changes in posture.

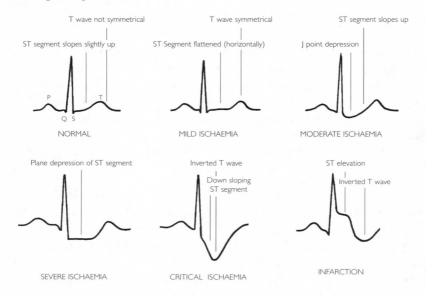

Fig 14.23 Progress of ST segment and T wave in ischaemia

Management of Ischaemia and Myocardial Infarction

In the early stages it is impossible to distinguish between reversible ischaemia, and irreversible myocardial infarction, because ST segment depression occurs in both. Myocardial ischaemia with acute ST elevation is potentially reversible, but if it is greater than 2 mm and does not resolve within 5–10 minutes then an infarct has probably occurred.

Principles of Therapy

With the hope of limiting the extent of the ischaemia, or infarct, the aims of treatment in the recovery room are:

Correct demand induced ischaemia:
- control the pain;
- treat hypertension;

- and reduce myocardial oxygen consumption.

    Correct supply induced ischaemia
- prevent hypoxia;
- correct hypotension;
- correct arrhythmias.

    Maintain adequate tissue perfusion, to prevent cardiac failure and tissue hypoxia.

Management of the Acute Ischaemic Episode

1. Reassure the patient. Sit him up. Give high flow oxygen by mask. Attach pulse oximeter, and ensure the oxygen saturation is greater than 95 per cent.

DRUGS USED IN TREATMENT OF ISCHAEMIA

Drug therapy is aimed at improving the supply of oxygen to the heart by causing coronary arteriolar vasodilation, and reducing the myocardial oxygen demands.

Nitroglycerine can be used topically, sublingually, or intravenously. It relaxes vascular smooth muscle. The notion that nitroglycerine is predominantly a venodilator is false. There is ample evidence that it is a vasodilator throughout the circulation, but predominantly for the coronary and pulmonary arteriolar vasculature[17]. If the patient is hypovolaemic nitroglycerine will cause profound hypotension. As it abolishes the hypoxic pulmonary vasoconstrictor response, it can open up vascular shunts in the lung causing hypoxia. It works for about 20 30 minutes when given sublingually, and for about 6–8 minutes intravenously. Side effects include headaches, flushing, dizziness, and postural hypotension. Vasodilation will cause severe hypotension in aortic stenosis, obstructive cardiomyopathies, mitral stenosis. Use glass or polyethylene containers as it loses potency if it comes in contact with polyvinyl chloride (PVC). Large dose of nitroglycerine will cause methaemoglobinaemia. Treat this with intravenous methylene blue 1 mg/kg.

Beta blockers reduces myocardial work, and limits myocardial infarction size[18]. (see page 247)

---

2. Attach ECG, and non-invasive blood pressure monitors. Computerized ST segment monitoring is good for detecting myocardial ischaemia. If you do not have this option available, use the modified CM_5 lead for detecting ST and T wave segment changes. Place the left arm electrode over the fifth left intercostal space in the mid-axillary line, and turn the *lead select* switch to Lead I. As soon as practicable, do a full 12-lead ECG.

3. Give the patient a glyceryl trinitrate tablet 600 micrograms under his tongue. Repeat this every 5 minutes to a maximum of three tablets, or the onset of side effects, such as hypotension or intolerable headache. Consider a nitroglycerine infusion if the pain remains uncontrolled. Start with a low dose of 0.5–1.5 microgram/kg per minute, and increase the dose by 1 microgram/kg per minute until the mean blood pressure is 95–100 mmHg.

4. Do not use prophylactic lignocaine in patients with ischaemia or infarction unless there are multiple ventricular premature contractions (see page 266). Even then it is probably better to use a β-blocker instead of lignocaine.

5. Give morphine 0.1 mg/kg intravenously slowly to relieve pain. Repeat in 5 minutes if necessary.

6. Control pain, hypoxia, hypertension, hypotension, tachycardia, bradycardia, anaemia, and emotional stress. These insults increase cardiac work, or decrease cardiac oxygen supply.

7. If the pulse rate is greater than 60 per minute consider cautiously giving a β-blocker, such as metoprolol 5–10 mg intravenously. Intravenous β-blockers decrease mortality by about 15 per cent;

8. If the blood pressure greater than 180/100 mgHg consider using nifedipine 5–10 mg orally, or alternatively, use an infusion of glyceryl trinitrate; start at 5 micrograms/kg per minute.

PULMONARY OEDEMA

Pulmonary oedema is a feature of low output left ventricular failure and occurs when fluid enters lung tissue. The pulmonary artery wedge pressure (PAWP) measures the blood pressure in the pulmonary capillaries. If this pressure rises beyond the colloid osmotic pressure of plasma (about 25–30 cm H_2O), fluid seeps from the circulation into the lung tissue (interstitial pulmonary oedema), and then into the alveoli (alveolar oedema). Interstitial pulmonary oedema makes the patient wheeze, cough and breathless, while alveolar oedema will cause frothy pink sputum. For the oedema to resolve the pressure in the pulmonary capillaries must fall below the colloid osmotic pressure of the blood.

Low pressure pulmonary oedema can occur where the lung tissue is damaged, such as in septicaemia, pneumonia, or adult respiratory distress syndrome.

Fluid in the interstitium of the lung, or in the alveolae quickly impedes the uptake of less soluble oxygen, but only in the late stages interferes with the transfer of carbon dioxide. Arterial oxygen pressures fall swiftly, but carbon dioxide does not accumulate until the patient is moribund.

CARDIAC FAILURE

Cardiac failure can be functionally classified into two groups, systolic dysfunction and diastolic dysfunction[19].

Systolic dysfunction is characterised by poor left ventricular contractility, with a left ventricular ejection fraction of less than 40%, and a dilated large heart displacing the apex beat. The ventricular dysfunction is usually due a previous myocardial infarction, and associated coronary artery disease; but it also may be due to alcoholic cardiomyopathy or hypertension. Recovery room management includes ionotropes, diuretics and vasodilators.

Diastolic dysfunction is characterized by normal left ventricular contractility, with a left ventricular ejection fraction greater than 40% and a normal sized heart. The ventricular dysfunction can be due to intermittent ischaemia; a hypertensive, or hypertrophic cardiomyopathy. Other causes include thyrotoxicosis, myxoedema and Paget's disease. Since the myocardium is contracting adequately, ionotropes are of no use. Control the cause, reduce the blood pressure if necessary, control the cardiac rate, and treat arrhythmias.

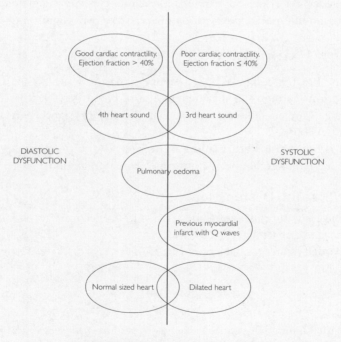

Fig 14.24 Relationship Between Signs of Heart Failure

There is some overlap between the two. A history of myocardial infarction, Q waves on the ECG and a third heart sound (S3 gallop) favour systolic dysfunction. Hypertension, a fourth heart sound (S4 gallop) and normal cardiac size favour diastolic dysfunction.

Pulmonary oedema can occur in either group.

9. If pain remains uncontrolled, or the patient has arrhythmias or hypotension, then consider the diagnosis of myocardial infarction. Treat pain with morphine to a maximum of 20 mg intravenously. Monitor the patient with a pulse oximeter to ensure oxygen saturation does not fall unnoticed. Take blood for baseline creatinine phosphokinase (CK-MB) isoenzyme. Use dobutamine for blood pressure support (see page 286). Transfer patient to the intensive care unit for further monitoring.

10. If pain resolves, and there are no arrhythmias, the blood pressure remains stable, and the ECG signs of ischaemia resolve; the patient may return to the ward after being pain free for one hour. Ideally monitor them for three to four days in an intensive care unit where arrhythmias, ischaemia, and cardiac failure can be detected early.

11. Aspirin will reduce myocardial mortality by up to 40 per cent, but the surgeon will need to consider the risk of postoperative haemorrhage.

12. Consider referring the patient for acute coronary angiography in preparation for angioplasty or coronary artery bypass grafting.

HEART FAILURE

The heart is composed of two pumps that feed each other. Usually they work in harmony so that the amount of blood they eject is virtually the same. Cardiac failure occurs when the left or right heart fails to maintain its output.

It is unusual for heart failure to occur as a result of coronary artery disease, unless there has been a prior myocardial infarction.

Acute Systolic Dysfunction

The common causes of acute systolic in the recovery room include:
• myocardial ischaemia;
• myocardial infarction, which may be painless;
• arrhythmias;
• drugs.

Diagnosis

With a failing left ventricle, the features of breathlessness and wheeze become dramatically worse if the patient lies flat. The patient will be restless, agitated, pale, cyanosed and sweaty. He will be wheezy and have moist sounds in his lungs (pulmonary oedema). His blood pressure may fall, and there may be a tachycardia. Urine output will be low and his perfusion status poor. If the failure is unrelieved he will go on to become

HEART SOUNDS IN CARDIAC FAILURE.

Listen to the chest over the apex beat, you may hear a *triple rhythm* (sometimes called a *gallop rhythm*). A triple rhythm is caused by an added heart sound. An extra sound in diastole may be *physiological* in pregnancy, or in children and young people. In older people it is usually *pathological*, and a useful sign of heart failure. Beware of drawing conclusions from an isolated sign. Look for further evidence, such as hypertension, fluid overload, dyspnoea, and so on.

Normally you will hear two heart sounds, the first heart and second heart sounds. Together they sound like 'LUB DUB'. It helps to say it while you listen, 'LUB DUB'. If a gallop rhythm starts it will probably be either a *third*, or a *fourth heart sound*. A third heart sound occurs with a floppy, dilated ventricle, and sounds like 'LUB DUBBA'. A fourth heart sound occurs when the atria are contracting forcefully, and sounds like 'daLUB DUB'. Occasionally you may even hear both. If you are having difficulty telling if the extra sound comes before, or after, the first and second heart sound, time the rhythm by feeling the carotid pulse. If there is a tachycardia it is difficult, or impossible to time the sounds; this is called a summation gallop. Practise actually singing aloud the gallops to yourself until they are familiar.

severely agitated and distressed, coughing up frothy pink sputum. Blood gases reveal a metabolic acidosis, with a low $PaCO_2$ and hypoxia. A chest X-ray will show pulmonary oedema, pulmonary vascular congestion and possibly cardiac enlargement.

*Painless myocardial infarction may
present with pulmonary oedema.*

Pulmonary Oedema

Acute left ventricular failure is often confused with an acute asthmatic attack. It is extremely unlikely, that an elderly patient will have her first acute asthma attack in recovery room. To help with the diagnosis, eliminate the possibility of fluid overload; or the possibility of an acute allergic reaction to a drug, blood or plasma expander.

All wheezes are not asthma.

MANAGEMENT OF PULMONARY OEDEMA
1. Reassure the patient. Sit him up as much as possible. Give high flow oxygen by mask. Attach ECG monitor, pulse oximeter and non-invasive blood pressure.
2. Give morphine 0.1 mg/kg intravenously slowly to relieve distress and slow breathing. Repeat in 5 minutes if necessary.
3. Investigations include chest X-ray, blood gases, and the cardiac enzymes CK-MB and LDH
4. Administer frusemide 0.5 mg/kg, and repeat it in 20 minutes if the urine output is less than 100 ml/hour.
5. Control arrhythmias if they are present.
6. Consider cardiac support with ionotropes, such as dopamine or dobutamine (see page 286). A direct arterial line for measuring blood pressure is needed is you are going to use ionotropes.
7. A GTN infusion (see page 460) will help reduce pulmonary vascular pressures.
8. Insert a urinary catheter to monitor the urine output, and prevent retention.
9. Arrange for eventual transfer to intensive care unit.

Low Output Cardiac Failure

Systolic failure may occur without pulmonary oedema initially. It may present with hypotension, shock, and signs of tissue hypoxia, such as, a metabolic acidosis. If these signs persist the patient is said to be in cardiogenic shock.

MANAGEMENT
1. Give high flow 100% oxygen. Attach ECG, blood pressure monitor and oximeter.
2. Adjust the patient's posture to make sure he is comfortable.
3. Start a dopamine or dobutamine infusion. If this fails consider adding an adrenaline infusion.
4. Consider moving the patient to an intensive care unit.

Acute Diastolic Dysfunction

Causes of acute diastolic dysfunction in the recovery room are:
• fluid overload;
• myocardial ischaemia;
• gas embolism;
• pulmonary embolism;
• arrhythmias.

Features of acute diastolic dysfunction are low blood pressure, nausea, vomiting, and dizziness. The jugular veins are distended and there is a progressive rise in central venous pressure. Peripheral perfusion is impaired, and the urine output low.

Acute pulmonary embolism, and gas embolism occur abruptly, causing great distress, hypoxia and collapse.

MANAGEMENT OF ACUTE DIASTOLIC DYSFUNCTION
1. Reassure the patient.
2. Sit him up.
3. Give high flow oxygen by mask.
4. Attach ECG monitor, and non-invasive blood pressure.
5. Exclude or treat pneumothorax (see page 339), air emboli (see page 140), or pulmonary emboli (see page 339).
6. If necessary, then treat pulmonary oedema. (See page 283).
7. Control arrhythmias if present.
8. Further investigations include chest X-ray, and blood gases.

CATECHOLAMINES USED IN SHOCK

Under conditions of physical or emotional stress, the alarm mechanisms in the body bring into action two catecholamines. These are adrenaline and noradrenaline.

Adrenaline (epinephrine) is a hormone of exercise. It is a most useful drug in the treatment of systolic dysfunction. Adrenaline is both an alpha and beta stimulator. Its many effects depend on the dose given. At low doses the effects are predominately beta but as the dose increases the alpha effects take over. In small doses of 0.1 microgram/kg $beta_1$, and particularly $beta_2$ effects prevail. The result is an increases in cardiac rate and force of contraction (β_1 effect) which raises the cardiac output, and vasodilation in skeletal muscle beds. As a result the systolic blood pressure rises, and as muscle blood flow increases, the diastolic blood pressure falls. The overall effect is an increase in pulse pressure. If the dose of adrenaline is increased, then alpha effects preominate with vasoconstriction, particularly in skin, gut, and kidney.

It is best to use a syringe pump. Dilute 3 mg of adrenaline in 5% dextrose and make it up to 50 ml (1 ml/hour = 1 microgram/minute). Infuse it into a central vein through its own dedicated line, because in this concentrated form it will necrose peripheral veins. In adults start with a dose of 1 microgram/minute and increase the dose by 0.5 microgram (0.5 ml/hour) every 3–5 minutes until the desired effect is achieved. The effective dose range is 1–20 micrograms/minute. On stopping the infusion the effects wear off in 6–8 minutes.

Nordarenaline (norepinephrine) is a neurotransmitter for the immediate response to threatening situations. It is useful for the treatment of conditions where peripheral resistance failure causes a falling blood pressure. It is predominately an alpha stimulator. It causes generalized vasoconstriction in most vascular beds and greatly increases peripheral vascular resistance so both the systolic and diastolic blood pressure rises. It increases blood pressure more than cardiac output.

Use a syringe pump. Dilute 3 mg of noradrenaline in 5% dextrose and make it up to 50 ml (1 ml/hour = 1 microgram/minute). Infuse it into a central vein through its own dedicated line, because in this concentrated form it will necrose peripheral veins. In adults start with a dose of 1 microgram/minute and increase the dose by 0.5 microgram (0.5 ml/hour) every 3–5 minutes until the desired effect is achieved. The effective dose range is 1–30 micrograms/minute. On stopping the infusion the effects wear off in 2–4 minutes.

Dopamine[20] is a biochemical precursor of noradrenaline synthesized in adrenergic nerve endings and the adrenal medulla. Dopamine stimulates two types of dopamine receptors (DA_1 and DA_2) as well as α_1 and α_2 and β_1 adrenergic receptors. DA_1 receptors are found in great number in mesenteric and renal vascular beds. Their stimulation causes smooth muscle relaxation and vasodilation. Dopamine is widely used for the treatment of acute cardiac failure and normovolaemic shock.

Dopamine has different effects depending on the dose given. At doses of 3 microgram/kg/minute its effects are mainly *dopaminergic*, improving cardiac output and renal blood flow, but with little effect on blood pressure or pulse rate. This dose is called *renal dose dopamine*. At doses of 5–15 micrograms/kg/minute it increases the rate and force of cardiac contraction to improve cardiac output. This is the *beta range* of dopamine. At doses greater than 15–20 micrograms/kg/minute dopamine cause vasoconstriction and increases cardiac work disproportionately. This is called the *alpha range* of dopamine.

Use a syringe pump. Dilute 300 mg of dopamine in 5% dextrose and make it up to 50 ml (1 ml/hour = 100 micrograms/minute). Infuse it into a central vein through its own dedicated line., because in this concentrated form it will necrose peripheral veins. In adults start with a dose of 2 micrograms/kg/minute and increase the dose by 1 microgram/kg/minute (1 ml/hour) every 3–5 minutes until the desired effect is achieved. The effective dose range is 200–1500 micrograms/minute. There is little to be gained by pushing the dose into the α range, instead combine it with adrenaline or even noradrenaline. On stopping the infusion the effects wear off in 2–4 minutes.

Dobutamine. The chemical structure of dobutamine resembles dopamine. Dobutamine is a good stimulator of cardiac contractility. In low doses dobutamine increases cardiac output, and decreases systemic and pulmonary vascular resistance. It does not maintain the blood pressure as effectively as dopamine, but has the advantage of increasing cardiac output without a parallel increase in heart rate. Since the heart rate is slower, and the blood pressure is slightly higher, then myocardial perfusion is better maintained than with drugs that increase the heart rate. This is a valuable asset for the ischaemic, failing heart. Dobutamine does not dilate the renal vasculature. At doses greater than 10 microgram/kg/minute the pulse rate starts to rise.

Use a syringe pump. Dilute 250 mg of dopamine in 5% dextrose and make it up to 41.5 ml (1 ml/hour = 100 micrograms/minute). In this concentrated form it will necrose peripheral veins, so infuse it into a central vein through its own dedicated line. In adults start with a dose of 2 micrograms/kg/minute and increase the dose by 1 microgram/kg/minute (1 ml/hour) every 3–5 minutes until the desired effect is achieved. The effective dose range is 2.5–15 micrograms/kg/minute. There is little to be gained by pushing the dose into the α range, instead combine it with adrenaline or even noradrenaline. On stopping the infusion the effects wear off in 4–6 minutes.

Dopexamine is a synthetic catecholamine dilating blood vessels in muscle and sphlanchnic beds by stimulating stimulating β_2 receptors. It causes renal vasodilation and improves renal blood flow by stimulating dopaminergic DA_1 receptors. It inhibits the neural reuptake of catecholamines and so increases the effects of endogenous adrenaline and noradrenaline. It increases the force of cardiac contraction and decreases peripheral resistance, this improves tissue blood flow.

Use a syringe pump. Dilute 50 mg of dopexamine in 5% dextrose and make it up to 41.5 ml (1 ml/hour = 20 micrograms/minute). In this concentrated form it will necrose peripheral veins, so infuse it into a central vein through its own dedicated line. In adults start with a dose of 20 micrograms/minute and increase the dose by 10–20 micrograms/minute (1 ml/hour) every 3–5 minutes until the desired effect is achieved.

The effective dose range is 0.5–60 microgram/kg/minute. On stopping the infusion the effects wear off in 20–30 minutes.

CARDIAC TAMPONADE

Cardiac tamponade occurs when blood, or fluid collects in the pericardial sac compressing the heart. The partly squashed heart cannot produce an adequate cardiac output. This is a complication of thoracic surgery, or following traumatic chest injury. A sudden bleed of 150–250 ml into the pericardial sac causes a major fall in blood pressure. Tamponade may accumulate more slowly, such as in renal failure, or with various infections, in which case the pericardial sac can distend to hold more than 1000 ml of fluid, before symptoms become severe. Clinically hypotension, tachycardia, dyspnoea, and distended neck veins give a clue. When the patient breathes in, the peripheral pulses may fall by more than 10 mmHg (pulsus paradoxus), and may even disappear altogether. Pulsus paradoxus is an important confirmatory sign. The ECG may show *electrical alternans* with alternating large and smaller QRS complexes. An increased cardiac shadow on chest x-ray, or decreased heart sounds are not reliable signs, because they are often absent. If in doubt, then confirm the diagnosis with an echocardiogram. If the effusion is causing symptoms it will need to be surgically drained, preferably as a formal procedure in the operating theatre.

VALVULAR HEART DISEASE

Patients with valvular heart disease, such as aortic and mitral stenosis or incompetence often have fixed cardiac outputs. The blood pressure falls precipitously, if either the cardiac output drops, or the patient vasodilates. Tachycardias are particularly hazardous, because there is not enough time for the ventricular contraction to eject the blood through a narrowed or incompetent valve. Sometimes valvular defects are associated with septal defects allowing blood to shunt between the left and right side of the heart. If the systemic vascular resistance rises, for instance, because of the sympathetic nervous response to uncontrolled pain, oxygenated blood may cross back into the pulmonary circulation. You need excellent pain control to help prevent this disaster.

Monitor these patients with an ECG, non-invasive blood pressure monitor, and a pulse oximeter. Probably the patient will have an arterial line, so you can see the pulse wave form. The anaesthetist should leave detailed and reasoned limits for acceptable heart rate, blood pressure, and oxygen saturation. Any breathlessness, anxiety, or deterioration in conscious state is a sign that the circulation may be decompensating. Keep the patient out of pain, because any autonomic stress will cause a tachycardia, or increase cardiac work and destabilize the circulation. Do not discharge the patient to the ward until he has a stable circulation, no pain, a good urine output and warm dry hands (that is, a good perfusion status).

CARDIOGENIC SHOCK

With cardiogenic shock the basic problem is that the myocardial damage is severe enough to overwhelm the neural, hormonal and vasoactive mechanisms that would normally maintain cardiac output and tissue perfusion pressure of the heart, kidney, gut, liver and pancreas. Skin and muscle circulation may almost cease. If a patient in cardiac failure has cold hands and feet, blood gases will show an acidosis, and this confirms the diagnosis of cardiogenic shock. Once the left ventricular function falls by about 30–40 per cent the physiological compensatory mechanisms become so intense that they aggravate the cardiac dysfunction leading to progressive tissue hypoperfusion. As the shock becomes worse, the pump failure becomes worse, and the patient's tissue perfusion further declines. This downward spiral inevitably results in death, unless there is therapeutic intervention (see page 290).

Low output cardiac failure

Systolic failure may occur without pulmonary oedema initally. It may present with hypotension, shock and signs of tissue hypoxia, such as metabolic acidosis. If these signs persist the patient is said to be in *cardiogenic shock*.

MANAGEMENT
1. Give high flow 100% oxygen.
2. Attach ECG monitor, pulse oximeter and non-invasive blood pressure.
3. Adujust the patient's posture so he is comfortable.
4. Insert an arterial line for direct measurement of blood pressure. Consider inserting a pulmonary artery flotation (Swan Ganz®) catheter.
5. Start a dopamine or dobutamine infusion. If the patient has ischaemic heart disease start with dobutamine. Adrenaline, or even noradrenaline, can be added as desperate measure if the blood pressure remains too low.
6. This condition is best managed in an intensive care unit.

CARDIAC ARREST

Conduct practice drills for cardiopulmonary resuscitation (CPR) at regular intervals. All staff need to be proficient at the management of cardiac arrest. Continual education and practice; and not the variations in different regimes, are the secret of successful resuscitation. There is no excuse for a disorganized or frenetic resuscitation. Have your trolleys and equipment prepared, and check them every day. Put your CPR flow chart on the wall where everyone can see it. Maintaining a clear airway, ensuring adequate ventilation and oxygenation, and giving immediate defibrillation are more important than administering drugs, or inserting intravenous lines.

A heart without oxygen,
will not respond to any form of therapy.

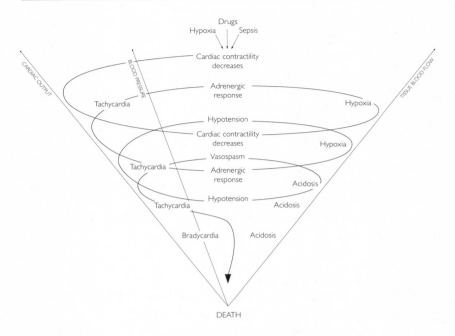

Fig 14.25 Cardiogenic spiral

SOURCES OF CARDIAC ARREST PROTOCOLS

There have been a number of changes to the *algorithms* (flow charts) for the management of cardiac arrest over the past few years. In the USA, the American Heart Association[21] has issued clear and comprehensive recommendations. These are the definitive word on cardiac arrest, but their length makes them difficult consult if you are in a hurry. In the UK and Europe, the European Resuscitation Council[22] has issued clear, brief and effective guidelines; these are highly recommended. You may be able to get a copy of their wall chart from Laerdal Medical Ltd. In Australia, the Australian Resuscitation Council[23] have published independent and slightly different guidelines. Obtain a copy of the guidelines applicable to your area.

Some Additional Points

A = AIRWAY
• Endotracheal intubation is the best way of maintaining the airway.
• Obturator airways are no longer recommended.
• It requires considerable skill, and constant practice to use a

self-inflating bag and mask confidently. Many staff are unable to use these devices effectively to deliver the necessary tidal volumes of 15 ml/kg per minute.

- Exclude cardiac tamponade, air embolism, and tension pneumothorax.

B = BREATHING

- Mouth-to-mouth ventilation in a non-intubated patient is easily taught and remembered, but understandably many staff are reluctant to use this. It achieves an inspired oxygen concentration of 16 per cent.
- Using a bag and mask to support a patient's breathing takes practice.
- If you are alone start the cycle of 2 breaths with mouth-to-mouth breathing followed by 15 sternal compressions.
- Once the patient is intubated give 5 sternal compressions for every breath.
- Give 5 initial breaths, preferably of 100 per cent oxygen, before starting cardiac massage to ensure good oxygenation.
- Try to achieve tidal volumes of at least 15 ml/kg, or as big breaths as you can achieve with the 1600 ml self-inflating bag.

C = CIRCULATION

- If you have no access to an ECG, remember that 90 per cent of cardiac arrest in adults is VF or VT; and early defibrillation is the key to survival. Use 200 joules, then 200 joules, and from then on 360 joules. Do not perform chest compressions while you recharge the defibrillator, reassessing the ECG trace, and feeling the carotid artery for a pulse, but do keep oxygenating the patient.
- Adrenaline 1 mg (1 ml of 1:1000 solution) is the first agent to use in cardiac arrest. Give subsequent doses at 3–5 minute intervals. Only use adrenaline after establishing oxygenation, commencing cardiac compression, and defibrillating the patient.
- To stabilize VT, or VF after defibrillation and adrenaline, try lignocaine 1.5 mg/kg intravenously and a further 1 mg/kg over the next half an hour. If lignocaine does not work, try bretylium 5 mg/kg intravenously.
- With asystole, if after 3 doses of adrenaline there is no electrical activity, try a supramaximal dose of adrenaline 5 mg intravenously.

D = DRUGS

- After giving any drug into a peripheral vein, raise the extremity and follow it with a 20 ml push of normal saline.
- 10% Calcium chloride, 5–10 ml intravenously, is only useful in hypocalcaemia, hyperkalaemia, or overdose of calcium channel blockers; otherwise do not use it.

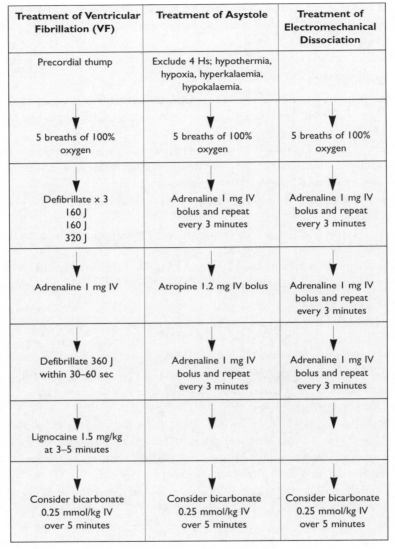

Treatment of Ventricular Fibrillation (VF)	Treatment of Asystole	Treatment of Electromechanical Dissociation
Precordial thump	Exclude 4 Hs; hypothermia, hypoxia, hyperkalaemia, hypokalaemia.	
5 breaths of 100% oxygen	5 breaths of 100% oxygen	5 breaths of 100% oxygen
Defibrillate x 3 160 J 160 J 320 J	Adrenaline 1 mg IV bolus and repeat every 3 minutes	Adrenaline 1 mg IV bolus and repeat every 3 minutes
Adrenaline 1 mg IV	Atropine 1.2 mg IV bolus	Adrenaline 1 mg IV bolus and repeat every 3 minutes
Defibrillate 360 J within 30–60 sec	Adrenaline 1 mg IV bolus and repeat every 3 minutes	Adrenaline 1 mg IV bolus and repeat every 3 minutes
Lignocaine 1.5 mg/kg at 3–5 minutes		
Consider bicarbonate 0.25 mmol/kg IV over 5 minutes	Consider bicarbonate 0.25 mmol/kg IV over 5 minutes	Consider bicarbonate 0.25 mmol/kg IV over 5 minutes

An example of a protocol for an adult cardiac arrest.

- Sodium bicarbonate is only indicated for hyperkalaemia, or acidosis after prolonged (10 minutes) arrest. It is a drug to use cautiously. Start with 0.1 mmol/kg intravenously, repeat at 2 minute intervals to a maximum of 0.5 mmol/kg.
- Adrenaline, lignocaine and atropine can be given down an endotracheal tube. Absorption is unreliable and about 2–3 times the intravenously dose is needed. Dilute the drug in 10 ml of normal saline.

- For intravenous access always try to use veins above the waistline. Follow peripheral drugs with a flush of 30 ml of fluid.
- Many other antiarrhythmics (such as magnesium, amiodarone, and sotalol) have been proposed for use in refractory VF; to date, there have been no trials to prove their usefulness.

When to stop?

In adults, survival is unlikely if the patient has failed to demonstrate a return to spontaneous circulation within 20 minutes, and is over the age of 45 years, and there is no evidence of drowning, drug overdose, local anaesthetic cardiotoxicity, or hypothermia.

Paediatric Cardiac Arrest

In children the following points may help[24]

Hypoxia and hypovolaemia are the commonest cause of cardiac arrest in the recovery room, and the prognosis is not good.

Cardiac arrest is usually preceded by:

- respiratory distress with tachypnoea, cyanosis, distress, and decreased breath sounds;
- poor perfusion with tachycardia, poor capillary return, cool or mottled peripheries;
- deterioration in conscious state, flaccidity.

Monitor all children with a pulse oximeter
while they in the recovery room.

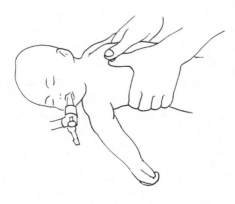

Fig 14.26 Position of thumbs on baby's chest for cardiac massage

Children under the age of 1 year of age are most at risk. There is less time to respond to apnoea in children, because they become hypoxic fast. Children nearly always (95 per cent) have asystole or bradycardia as the initial rhythm. When performing cardiac massage remember the heart is positioned under the lower third of the sternum in all children[25]. Compress the heart with either two thumbs or the heal of your hand, depending on the size of the child. Use about 80 compressions per minute.

Venous access is difficult in chubby infants. Try the external jugular or cubital veins. If this fails the intraosseous route is a valuable access for drugs and fluid. Use a short thick needle and screw it through the anteromedial surface of the proximal tibia, just below the level of the tibial tuberosity[26]. The brachial pulse is easier to feel in chubby children than the carotid. Neonates, infants and small children have short necks. Do not hyper-extend them, just lift the head forward a little (in a sniffing the morning air position). Insert a Guedal airway, use an appropriate mask, and ventilate at a rate of 40–60 per minute with puffs of 100 per cent oxygen.

Hypovolaemia

Hypotension is a late sign of hypovolaemia in neonates and infants. It usually does not occur unless the blood loss is more than 30 ml/kg. Initially restore blood volume with normal saline or Hartmann's solution. Give 20 ml/kg immediately and then reassess the situation. You can use a more appropriate fluid later, but the first priority is to expand the plasma volume.

Cardioversion

Cardioversion is in the sequence 2, 4, and 4 joule/kg. Over use of energy will damage the myocardium. Use paediatric paddles. Most modern defibrillators have a preset maximum dose of 100 joule when the paediatric paddles are connected.

To be successful it is far more important to restore vascular volume, maintain a clear airway, give adequate ventilation and oxygenation and use early cardioversion, than it is to use drugs.

Remember that small babies who have been stressed, or starved are at risk from hypoglycaemia, so check their blood sugar.

Drug treatment of cardiac arrest

- SVT rarely causes problems in children, but if it does use adenosine.
- Adrenaline is the best drug for treatment of asystole, electromechanical dissociation and bradycardia. The dose is at least 0.1–0.2 mg/kg.

- Adrenaline is the drug of first choice in cases of bradycardia. If this fails use atropine in doses of at least 20 micrograms/kg to avoid paradoxical bradycardia. Do not use isoprenaline.
- Bicarbonate is only indicated if there is hyperkalaemia. If you suspect acidosis, ventilate the baby rapidly with bag and mask.

When to stop?

The outcome of paediatric cardiac arrest is poor. Failure to achieve a return to spontaneous respiration after 15 minutes has a dismal outcome. The exceptions for this are arrests associated with hypothermia, hyperkalaemia, and bupivacaine toxicity. If in doubt phone a paediatrician for advice.

TERMINOLOGY

Asystole means the heart has stopped (cardiac arrest). The ECG shows a straight or gently undulating line with no electrical activity.

Atrial Ectopics occur when the impulse arises in odd places within the atria and not in the SA node.

Atrial Fibrillation (AF) occurs where the atrial excitation wave is unco-ordinated and atria ceases to contract. No P waves can be seen on the ECG and the ventricles contract irregularly. If the chest is opened the atria look as though they are shivering.

Atrial Flutter occurs where the atria are contracting ineffectively fast. It is seen as a saw-toothed picture between the QRS complexes.

Bradycardia is a heart rate less than 50 beats per minute.

Complete Heart Block is where no P waves can be seen and the ventricles beat at their intrinsic rate of about 25–35 per minute.

Ectopic Beats arise where they should not. They are 'out-of-place' beats.

Electromechanical Dissociation (EMD) occurs where a formed wave can be seen on the ECG, but there is no detectable peripheral pulse. This is usually fatal. Now called pulseless electrical activity (PEA).

Heart Block is where the P waves are further away from the QRS complex than normal. They might be a constant distance from the QRS complex (serious) or they may vary (dangerous).

Idioventricular Rhythm occurs when all the higher pacemakers are suppressed, and the ventricle contracts at its intrinsic rate of 25–35 per minute.

Multifocal Premature Beats (MPBS) are signs of a very irritable myocardium. Premature excitations are ectopic beats arising from many different sites in the ventricles. It needs urgent treatment.

Nodal Rhythms occur where the AV node triggers the beat instead of the SA node. The P waves are either absent (hidden in the QRS) or upside down.

Premature Atrial Contraction occurs when the atrial beat does not arise in the SA node, but somewhere else in the atria. Sometimes it is the result of an impulse in the AV node taking a U-turn.

Pro-arrhythmias are drug induced arrhythmias. They occur in about 10% of patients on antiarrhythmic agents.

R-on-T Phenomenon with the R wave snuggles right up next to, or even inside the T wave. This is a dangerous sign as the patient may flip into ventricular fibrillation, or a ventricular tachycardia. Treat this urgently.

Sick Sinus Syndrome is a condition of sinus bradycardia or even sinus arrest, following a supraventricular tachycardia. Sometimes this is known as the *tachycardia–bradycardia syndrome*.

Sinus Rhythm occurs when the sinoatrial node dictates the heart rate at a regular rhythm between 50–100 per minute.

Sinus Bradycardia is a bradycardia where the P waves are a normal distance from the QRS complex.

Sinus Tachycardia is where the heart rate is greater than 100 minute. The P waves and QRS waves are normal.

Supraventricular Arrhythmias arise in the atria.

Supraventricular Tachycardia (SVT) is a heart rate of 150–250 per minute. The P waves are usually, but not always, still visible. There are a number of causes.

Tachycardia is a heart rate greater than 100 per minute.

Tachycardia Bradycardia Syndrome—see Sick Sinus Syndrome

Torsades de Pointes (twisting of the points) is a very fine ventricular tachycardia with rapidly changing QRS shapes. It looks as though they are rotating about a baseline.

Ventricular Fibrillation (VF). If the chest is open the heart muscle is seen to be writhing like a bag full of earthworms, and there is no cardiac output.

Ventricular Premature Beats (VPBs) are wide, bizarre QRS complexes with a down sloping ST segment, and not preceded by a P wave. They indicate an irritable myocardium, where the ventricle has contracted without a normal triggering sequence. Sometimes these are known as ventricular ectopics, or ventricular extrasystoles (VEs), or even premature ventricular contractions (PVCs). Suspect myocardial ischaemia.

Ventricular Tachycardia (VT) occurs when there are runs of more than three VPBs together.

Wolff–Parkinson–White (WPW) Syndrome is one of the pre-excitation syndromes heart, where the ventricle is prematurely activated because the impulse has taken a shortcut through an accessory pathway. Usually the PR interval is short (0.1–0.2 second), and there is a wider QRS complex.

NORMAL CARDIAC ELECTROPHYSIOLOGY

When a myocardial cell contracts, sodium and calcium ions enter the cell and potassium leaves it. This ion flux is called *depolarization*. When the cell relaxes the ion flux is reversed, this is called *repolarization*. These ion exchanges generate a small wave of electrical current (called an *action potential*) that spreads from cell to cell, stimulating each cell to contract. All myocardial cells can spontaneously generate their own action potential, but normally do not do so. This is because their intrinsic rate is so slow that, before the cells get a chance to depolarize, they are triggered by an impulse arriving from elsewhere. The intrinsic rate of the ventricles is about 30 per minute.

There are two normal *pacemakers* in the heart, the *SA node*, high in the right atrium, near the entrance to the vena cava, is the dominant pacemaker setting the heart rate. If it fails the *atrioventricular (AV) node* will take over. The resting intrinsic rate of the myocardial cells in the SA node is about 70 per minute, and the AV node's intrinsic rate is about 40 per minute.

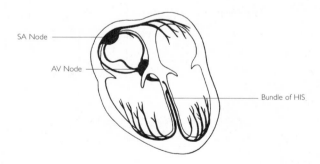

SA Node

AV Node

Bundle of HIS

Fig 14.28 Conduction system of the heart

Sympathetic (adrenergic) nerves stimulate the SA node pacemaker to fire faster, and parasympathetic vagal (cholinergic) nerves slow down the pacemaker.

When the SA node fires to generate its action potential the impulse spreads from cell to cell across the atrial muscle stimulating it to contract. This atrial contraction pushes blood through the atrioventricular valves into the ventricles. On reaching the *atrioventricular (AV) node*, the impulse is delayed slightly before fizzing, like a fast burning fuse, through the specialized conducting fibres of the bundle of His, down to the apex of the heart. Here the bundle of His divides into two main branches, going to the right and left ventricles respectively. Once in ventricles the impulse ignites a wave of contraction (*systole*) in the cardiac muscle that starts at the apex and spreads towards the base of the heart, squeezing the blood up through the valves into the arteries. For about 200 milliseconds after a myocardial cell has contracted, it cannot be stimulated to contract again. This period when the myocardial cell is recovering, is called the absolute refractory period. The ventricles then relax (*diastole*). The aortic and pulmonary valves close as blood starts to reflux back into the heart from the arteries, and then SA node fires to initiate atrial contraction again.

PR interval   0.12–0.20s

QRS complex   0.08–0.12s

QT interval   0.35–0.45s

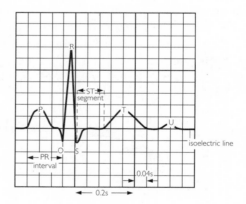

Fig 14.29 Normal ECG complex

How to interpret an ECG

Start by answering the following six questions:
1. What is the heart rate? 2. Is the rhythm regular? 3. Is there a P wave?
4. Is the QRS complex normal in both form and duration?
5. Is the rhythm dangerous? 6. Does the rhythm need treatment?

The heart rate can be calculated by counting the number of large

Table 14a.1

COMPONENTS OF AN ECG TRACE

Feature	Coincides with	Duration	Remarks
P wave	Atrial contraction	0.06–0.10 sec	Disappears in atrial fibrillation.
			Saw tooth pattern in atrial flutter.
			Typically upside down in nodal rhythms.
PR interval	Atrial relaxation	0.12–0.20 sec	Prolonged in heart block.
			Shortened in WPW syndrome.
QRS complex	Shows direction of impulse travel down bundle of his	0.08–0.12 sec	Abnormal patterns or broadened complexes suggest conduction abnormalities such as the various types of heart block.
ST segment	Continuous contraction of ventricular muscle	0.08–0.12 sec	If it is raised, depressed, or sloping, it indicates serious problems in the ventricular muscle such as ischaemia.
QT interval	Contraction and relaxation of ventricular muscle	0.35–0.45 sec	Prolonged in hypocalcaemia and patients at risk of developing Torsades de pointes.
			Shortened in hyperkalaemia.
T wave	Cardiac muscle recovery phase following contraction.		Narrow peaked T waves suggest hyperkalaemia.
			Flattened T waves may be hypokalaemia, but also may be non-specific.
			Inverted T waves may indicate endocardial irritation such as ischaemia or inflammation.
U wave	Small, but often absent		Prominent U waves occur in hypocalcaemia.

squares on the ECG paper that come between consecutive R waves, and dividing this into 300.

$$\text{Heart rate} = \frac{300}{\text{number of large squares in ECG paper}}$$

1. Breslow M. J., Jordan D. A., et al. (1989). Journal of the American Medical Association, 261: 3577–81.
2. Van Der Walt J. H., Webb R. K., et al. (1993). Anaesthesia and Intensive Care, 21: 650–2.
3. Aggarwal A., Waltier D. C. (1994). Current Opinion in Anesthesiology, 7: 109–22.
4. Louis W. J., Louis S., et al. (1994). Medical Journal of Australia, 161: 555–7.
5. James M. F. (1992). Anesthesia and Analgesia, 74: 129–36.
6. Goldman L., Caldera, D. L., et al. (1978). Medicine, 57: 357–61.
7. Roy W. L., Edelist G. (1979). Anesthesiology, 51: 393–7.
8. Ashton C. M., Petersen N. J., et al. (1993). Annals of Internal Medicine, 118: 504–10.
9. Goldman L., Caldera, D. L., et al. (1977). New England Journal of Medicine, 297: 845–50.
10. Mangano D. T., Browner W. S., et al. (1990). New England Journal of Medicine, 118: 504–10.
11. Cutfield G. (1992). Australian Anaesthesia 1992, pp 216–22, published by the Australian and New Zealand College of Anaesthetists, Melbourne, Australia.
12. Ashton C. M., Petersen N. J. et al. (1993). Annals of Internal Medicine, 118: 504–10.
13. Braunwauld E., Kloner R. A. (1982). Circulation, 66: 1146–9.
14. Hales P. (1992). Australian Anaesthesia 1992, pp 210–15, published by the Australian and New Zealand College of Anaesthetists, Melbourne, Australia.
15. Breslow M. J., Miller C. F., et al. (1996). Anesthesiology, 64: 398–402.
16. Landsberg G., Luria M. H., et al. (1993). Lancet, 20: 715–9.
17. Pearl R. G., Rosenthal M. (1982). Annals of Internal Medicine, 99: 9–13.
18. Frishman W. H., (1988). Medical Clinics of North America, 72: 37–75.
19. Goldsmith S. R., Candace D. (1993). American Journal of Medicine, 95: 645–55.
20. Murphy M. B., Elliot W. J., (1990). Critical Care Medicine, 8(1): S14–8.
21. Guidelines of Cardiopulmonary Resuscitation. (1992). Journal of the American Medical Association, 268: 2171–298.
22. Guidelines for Basic and Advance Life Support. European Resuscitation Council. (1992). Resuscitation, 24: 103–22.
23. The Australian Resuscitation Council Guidelines. (1993). Medical Journal of Australia, 159: 616–21.
24. American Heart Association. (1992). Journal of American Medical Association, 268: 2171–295.
25. Orlowski J. P. (1980). Pediatric Clinics of North America, 27: 495–512.
26. Spivey W. H. (1987). Lancet, 2: 1235–6

15. HYPOXIA AND RESPIRATORY PHYSIOLOGY

General anaesthesia causes respiratory depression, drying of secretions, and bronchial cilial dysfunction. The alveolar cells stop secreting a slippery detergent called *surfactant*, the epithelium sticks together and the alveoli collapse. The severity of lung dysfunction depends on the duration of anaesthesia, the preoperative state of the patient's lungs, and the site of the surgical incision. Respiratory depression, micro-alveolar collapse, and sputum retention can lead to pneumonia and respiratory failure. Good recovery room care lessens this risk.

The terms hypoxia and hypoxaemia do not mean the same thing.

Hypoxia

Hypoxia occurs when tissues do not receive enough oxygen to meet their metabolic needs. Tissues, such as brain, kidney and heart with a high metabolic rate are easily damaged by hypoxia; while others, such as skin, muscle and fat are more tolerant. Hypoxia quickly maims or kills; it is subtle, and often unpredictable[1]. It hides with many disguises, and is easy to overlook unless you understand how it occurs.

Hypoxaemia

Hypoxaemia, on the other hand, is something we measure. It occurs when the partial pressure in the arterial blood (PaO_2) falls below 60 mmHg (7.89 kPa), which is approximately an oxygen saturation of 90%. Hypoxaemia does not necessarily mean the tissues are hypoxic. And tissues can be hypoxic without hypoxaemia, for instance, if the patient is anaemic the PaO_2 and oxygen saturation can be normal, but because the blood is carrying little oxygen, the tissues become hypoxic.

PHYSIOLOGY OF HYPOXIA

A full list of terms, symbols and normal values are at the end of this section.

Each minute a resting adult uses about 250 ml of oxygen and produces about 200 ml of carbon dioxide. Every 100 ml of blood carries about 20 ml of oxygen bound loosely to haemoglobin inside the red cell. Without haemoglobin the same 100 ml of blood could only carry 0.3 ml of oxygen dissolved in the plasma.

From a physiological point of view, the most important task of the recovery room staff is to ensure that enough oxygen reaches the mitochondria in the cells. There are four components to this task:
1. Breathing. (Pumping oxygen into, and carbon dioxide out of, the lungs.)
2. Gas transfer between lungs and blood.
3. Oxygen supply to the tissues.
4. Mitochondrial oxygen supply. (How the cell obtains and uses oxygen.)

1. Breathing

Gas exchange in fish is easily achieved, water only has to flow past their gills. Land animals must actively use muscles to *breathe* exchange. The respiratory muscles are the diaphragm and the intercostal muscles. As these muscles contract, the intrathoracic volume increases, and air is sucked into the upper airways where it is humidified. The air passes on through the larynx to the lower airways, and into the alveoli where gas exchange occurs. If the patient has difficulty breathing, extra muscles are recruited to help move the air. These *accessory muscles of respiration* are the strap muscles in the neck and the abdominal muscles. If you see these muscles contract, it means that the patient is in severe respiratory difficulty.

The respiratory rate is normally about 12–15 breaths per minute. Each breath contains about 400 ml of air (called the *tidal volume*), and about half of this reaches the alveoli to give up part of its oxygen to the blood. At the same time, carbon dioxide leaves the blood, and is excreted in the expired air. The air remaining in the airways is called *dead space air.* Obviously if the tidal volume is less than the dead space, no fresh air will reach the alveoli, and no waste carbon dioxide can escape. As the tidal volume falls, the arterial level of carbon dioxide rises, and the patient is said to be *hypoventilating.*

At the end of a quiet expiration, about 3 litres of air remain in the lungs. This is called the *functional residual capacity* (FRC). This residual air continues to take part in the gas exchange. It acts as a small oxygen store when we breathe out. If it were not for the FRC acting as a residual store of oxygen, we would turn blue every time we breathed out, and pink when we breathed in again. As we age and our lungs lose their elasticity more gas remains in the lungs and the FRC gets bigger. Infants have proportionally the same FRC as an adult, but their oxygen consumption is twice an adult's rate, so hypoxia develops much faster in infants, and neonates than in adults. Many factors combine to lower FRC during and directly after anaesthesia. The patient is lying down, with his abdominal contents pushing the diaphragm up and reducing the functional (or useable) volume of the lungs. This is a major problem in the obese. Many alveoli close after abdominal and thoracic surgery, reducing the amount of useable lung.

A patient with a small FRC, does not tolerate a slow respiratory rate well.

Control of breathing

In effect you as a person with your emotions, reason, and free live in your cerebral cortex. Your brainstem on the other hand runs the second-to-second activities of your body, of which breathing is one aspect. Breathing is controlled by *respiratory centres* in the brain stem. Think of these centres as a biological computer that receives messages (input) from the periphery. It sorts them, then allots priorities (controller), and finally activates the nerves (output) that instruct muscles to contract. It controls the diameter of your airways, and makes you cough when you need to. This computer lets the cortex know what is going on if necessary. Your cortex too, can interrogate or instruct your brainstem, for instance, you can voluntarily take a deep breath, and hold it.

Input comes from sensors, these are:

- Chemoreceptors in the carotid sinus telling the respiratory centres about the levels of PaO2 in arterial blood. As the PaO_2 falls they progressively send stronger signals to the respiratory centres. Once the PaO_2 falls below about 55 mmHg (7.24 kPa) they become the main drive to respiration.
- Chemoreceptors in the brainstem are more sensitive to rises or falls in $PaCO_2$. The controller takes a lot of notice of these sensors, and small changes in $PaCO_2$ will cause a brisk response. These brainstem sensors are the ones that normally drive respiration to keep the level of carbon dioxide in the tissues at a constant level. Opioid drugs depress these receptors and therefore the response.
- Stretch receptors exist in the chest wall (muscle spindles) and in the lung tissue (J receptors). If you need to bring your intercostal muscles into action to help you breathe, the muscle spindles send a message to the respiratory centres which respond by telling you to feel short of breath (*dyspnoea*). Small amounts of fluid in the lung interstitium stretch the tissues, and this is registered by J receptors which lie near the alveola sacs and cause a similar response. Dyspnoea is an important warning sign that the work of breathing is increased.
- Epithelial receptors guard your airways, and signal the brainstem to cause sneezing, laryngospasm, and coughing.

Output drives the various muscles. Normally breathing is done by contraction of the diaphragm, but in times of respiratory difficulty the controller in the brainstem can recruit extra help from the *accessory respiratory muscles*. These are the intercostal muscles, and the strap muscles in the neck. Diseases, such as motor neurone disease and multiple sclerosis, will weaken the respiratory effort. Postoperatively the main cause of weakness is the residual effect of the muscle relaxants.

When you have a respiratory diagnostic problem, work through this scheme of input causes, processor causes, and output causes; as well as the problems involving the lungs themselves.

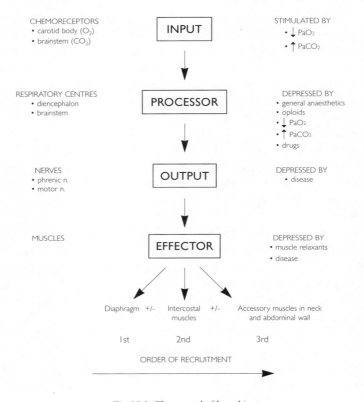

Fig 15.1 *The control of breathing*

2. Gas Transfer between the Lung and the Blood

For a healthy person breathing air (21 per cent oxygen), the normal arterial partial pressure of oxygen (PaO_2) is about 100 mmHg (13.3 kPa). This declines with age, and at 80 years will be about 80 mmHg (10.5 kPa).

Giving patients extra oxygen raises their inspired oxygen concentration. In a normal person if the inspired oxygen concentration increases, the partial pressure of oxygen in the arterial blood rises proportionally. This is not so in a patient with sick lungs. The reason for this is a process called *shunting*.

Shunting

In a patient with pulmonary disease, blood may miss out being oxygenated as it passes through diseased areas of the lungs. This occurs because the blood is shunted through capillaries serving un-aerated alveoli. In effect blood enters the pulmonary capillaries blue, and emerges blue at the other end to mix with red oxygenated blood from properly aerated alveoli. This *venous admixture* causes the arterial PaO_2 to fall. Unfortunately the more severe the lung disease, or cardiac failure, the greater is the effect of shunting, and the less effective is supplemental oxygen.

Give supplemental oxygen
to patients with lung disease.

CAUSES OF FAILURE TO OXYGENATE BLOOD

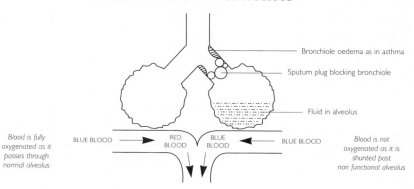

Fig 15.2 Shunting

There are many reasons for blood passing through un-aerated regions of the lungs. *Micro-atelectasis* is the random collapse of tiny segments of lung. It is thought that a reduction in the lungs' surfactant secretion during anaesthesia contributes to microatelectasis.

After abdominal and thoracic operations the diaphragm does not work properly. Encourage deep breathing and coughing to temporarily improve oxygen saturation by blasting open collapsed airways and alveoli.

Encourage deep breathing and coughing.
Ask the patient to take a deep breath and hold it for 3 seconds.

Hypoventilation as a cause of hypoxia

It is important to understand that patients receiving supplemental oxygen can hypoventilate without becoming hypoxic. By definition, the patient is said to be hypoventilating if the arterial $PaCO_2$ is raised. Although best considered as separate entities, hypoventilation and hypoxia are interrelated. As the alveolar PCO_2 rises, so the alveolar PO_2 falls. This conforms exactly to Dalton's Law of Partial Pressures, which states: the total pressure of a mixture of gases is the sum of the individual partial pressures.

How can we work out if the hypoxia is due to hypoventilation alone, or whether the lungs are damaged and unable to properly transfer oxygen to the haemoglobin in the red cells?

One way to calculate the *alveolar–arterial oxygen gradient* (ΔA-a). First measure the arterial blood gases to determine the PaO_2 and the $PaCO_2$. Now, using Table 15.1 below to find the partial pressure of inspired oxygen (PIO_2), calculate the alveolar partial pressure of oxygen (PaO_2).

Use the *alveolar air equation*

$$PAO_2 \quad = \quad PIO_2 - \frac{(PaCO_2)}{0.8}$$

Work out the A-a gradient

$$(\Delta\text{A-a}) \quad = \quad PAO_2 - PaO_2$$

If the A-a gradient is more than 10 per cent of the alveolar PAO_2 the lungs are not normal. Clinically it does not present a problem until there is at least a 20 per cent gradient.

Another much less accurate, but easier way of solving the problem is to simply add the arterial PO_2 and the arterial PCO_2 together. If their sum does not come within about 10–15 per cent of the inspired PO_2, then there are pathological changes in the lung.

Table 15.1

COMMON VALUES FOR THE ALVEOLAR AIR EQUATION				
Inspired oxygen concentration	PI O_2 mmHg (inspired PO_2)	$PaCO_2$ mmHg (arterial PCO_2)	PAO_2 mmHg (alveolar PO_2)	Abnormal gradient mmHg (ΔA-a)*
21%	150	40	100	> 10
28%	200	40	150	> 15
35%	250	40	200	> 20
60%	430	40	390	> 39
100%	713	40	663	> 66

*(Δ is the Greek letter delta, this symbol is used to indicate a gradient or difference.)

Diffusion hypoxia

Diffusion hypoxia is a particular hazard in the very young and the very old. For about 5–10 minutes after the end of a general anaesthetic, nitrous oxide diffuses back from the circulation into the lungs, diluting the inspired air and reducing the oxygen tension in the lung. This is one good reason to give high concentrations of oxygen for the first 10 minutes after discontinuing an anaesthetic.

3. Oxygen Supply to the Tissues

Oxygen diffuses across the epithelial lining cells of the lung, then into the red cell where, loosely bound to haemoglobin, the blood flow carries it to the tissues.

There are four factors involved in the supply of adequate oxygen to the tissues: healthy lungs, good cardiac function to pump the blood to the tissues, enough haemoglobin to carry the oxygen; and a variety of metabolic factors.

Lung function

Good lung function allows the haemoglobin to be fully saturated with oxygen. The haemoglobin oxygen saturation can be measured with a pulse oximeter. Respiratory failure or low inspired oxygen tensions causes *hypoxic hypoxia*.

Cardiac function

Cardiac output determines the speed at which the oxygen carrying haemoglobin reaches the tissues. In cardiac failure, blood is pumped more slowly through the tissues, and the oxygen supply falls. This type of hypoxia is called *stagnant hypoxia.*

Haemoglobin

Normally there is about 12–15 grams of haemoglobin in 100 ml of blood. Lack of haemoglobin causes *anaemic hypoxia.*

Metabolic factors

Each gram of haemoglobin carries about 1.34 ml of oxygen. Some metabolic disturbances, such as alkalaemia, and hypothermia, decrease the amount of oxygen carried by haemoglobin. These disturbances cause *metabolic hypoxia.*

Mathematically these four factors can be expressed as the *oxygen flux equation.* The equation is invaluable in helping to work out why patients suddenly deteriorate in the recovery room.

Oxygen supply to tissues	=	Cardiac output	×	Haemoglobin concentration	×	Haemoglobin saturation %	×	Oxygen carrying capacity of haemoglobin
1000 ml/min	=	5000 ml/min	×	14.5 g/100 ml	×	98.5/100	×	1.34 ml/g

Of the 1000 ml of oxygen normally carried to the tissues each minute only about 250 ml is used. Haemoglobin enters the tissues almost 100 per cent saturated and leaves about 75 per cent saturated, that is about three-quarters full.

Notice the multiplication signs. These show how the four components multiply together to cause tissue hypoxia. A failure of more than one component makes the oxygen supply many times worse. If the oxygen supply falls below about 400 ml per minute, the patient will probably die. This corresponds to an arterial PaO_2 of 25 mmHg (3.29 kPa) which is too low for survival. Such a low PaO_2 can occur insidiously in a sick patient. For example, a patient with a cardiac output of 4000 ml per minute, a haemoglobin of 8.5 g %, an arterial blood gas saturation of 90 per cent will have a tissue oxygen supply of 410 ml per minute and will be near death.

Oxygen supply to tissues	=	Cardiac output	×	Haemoglobin concentration	×	Haemoglobin saturation %	×	Oxygen carrying capacity of haemoglobin
410 ml/min	=	4000 ml/min	×	8.8 g/100 ml	×	90/100	×	1.34 ml/g

Yet any one of those factors on their own would not be an overwhelming threat to life.

Table 15.2

TISSUE OXYGEN SUPPLY AND PO₂ OF BLOOD ENTERING CAPILLARY BEDS		
Tissue oxygen supply	Haemoglobin saturation	PO₂ of blood entering capillary beds
1000 ml/min	100%	100 mmHg (13.3 kPa)
750 ml/min	75%	40 mmHg (5.3 kPa)
400 ml/min	40%	about 25 mmHg (3.3 kPa)*

* Acidosis allows haemoglobin to give up its oxygen more easily to hypoxic tissue (the Bohr effect). The Bohr effect occurs because the globule shape of the haemoglobin molecule is distorted by acidosis or alkalosis and this alters the way in which haemoglobin picks up, holds on to, and releases oxygen.

The haemoglobin oxygen dissociation curve

The curve's shape varies with the pH of the blood, and the temperature of the patient. To get oxygen into the tissues it has to be delivered both, in sufficient quantity, and with enough pressure. The haemoglobin saturation tells us about the quantity, and the PaO_2 about the pressure. The haemoglobin saturation just tells us how full of oxygen the haemoglobin molecule is. A saturation of 95 per cent means that the haemoglobin is 95 per cent full.

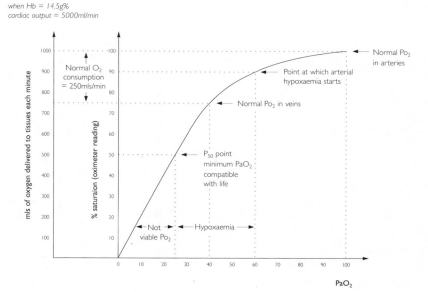

Fig 15.3 Haemoglobin oxygen dissociation curve

It is the partial pressure of oxygen (the PaO₂) in the capillary that provides the force to drive oxygen from the red cell into the tissues. If the PaO₂ falls below 60 mmHg tissue, the patient will probably develop a lactic acidosis. Patients in recovery room are often moderately acidotic and hypothermic. Acidosis causes the arterial PaO₂ to be higher than normal at a given saturation. This is a good thing, since the extra pressure increases tissue oxygenation. On the other hand hypothermia decreases tissue oxygenation, but also reduces the tissue's oxygen consumption.

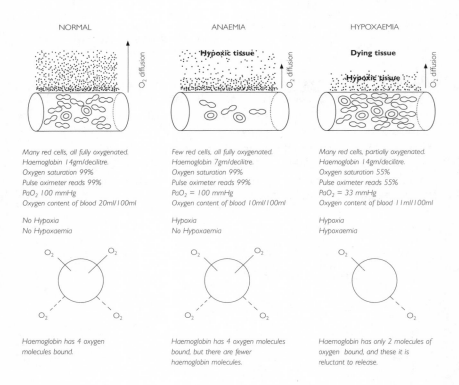

Fig 15.4 Tissue oxygen supply to normal, anaemic and hypoxic tissue

In summary the combination of two or more of the following may be lethal.
• anaemia;
• heart failure;
• poor lung function;
• hypothermia, alkalosis.

Extraction failure

Massive blood transfusion can lead to hypoxia. The freshly transfused red cells will pick up oxygen, but only release it reluctantly in the tissues. In patients dying from septicaemia, or severe shock, the cells are so sick that they cannot use oxygen even if it is delivered to them. The cells cannot extract oxygen from the haemoglobin. Comparing the oxygen content of arterial blood and mixed venous blood is the *extraction fraction* (Tx) gives an indication how much oxygen is being used by the tissues.

4. How the Cell Obtains and Uses Oxygen

Once in the tissues oxygen diffuses into the cell's mitochondria, where it is used for biochemical reactions involving *oxidative cellular metabolism*. In effect 80 per cent of the oxygen 'burns' with carbon (but in carefully graded steps so that not too much heat is released at once) to form carbon dioxide. The remaining 20 per cent of oxygen mops up hydrogen ions, and is converted into water. These processes release a lot of energy, most of which is stored in high energy phosphate compounds. These act like re-chargeable batteries, and are used all through the cell for fuelling chemical reactions.

At the arterial end of a capillary the PaO_2 is about 100 mmHg. As the red cell moves through the capillary it unloads oxygen, and picks up carbon dioxide. The PO_2 progressively falls so that by the time it has reached the venous end of the capillary the PO_2 is only about 40 mmHg. In technical terms the partial pressure of oxygen establishes a concentration gradient down which oxygen diffuses to reach the mitochondria inside the cells.

Put more simply, the partial pressure pushes oxygen from the haemoglobin on its microscopically long journey through membranes, and across fluid spaces to reach the mitochondria. The higher the pressure, the bigger the push, and the further the oxygen will diffuse. Cells close to the capillary receive a good oxygen supply, and those further away receive less.

The diagram below demonstrates this point. Around the capillary it is possible to describe a cylinder, known as a *Krogh cylinder*. Inside the cylinder cells are well oxygenated; but at the periphery of the cylinder the oxygen tension falls, and the cell's oxygen supply becomes more tenuous. To compensate for this the cylinders overlap one another so that the more peripheral cells get their oxygen supply from a number of adjacent cylinders.

Two things can jeopardize the oxygen supply. Firstly, the cylinders may be pushed apart by oedema fluid, as happens in cerebral oedema. The cells become hypoxic, and are unable to maintain their function. Secondly as the patient becomes hypoxic, the PaO_2 falls, then as the diameter of the Krogh cylinders contracts, the cells become hypoxic.

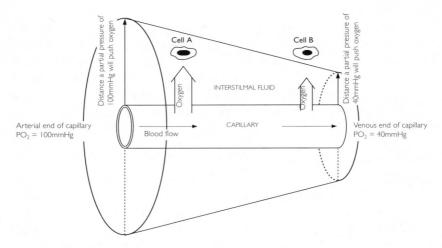

Cell A and Cell B are both the same distance from the capillary but the oxygenation of Cell A is much better than Cell B.

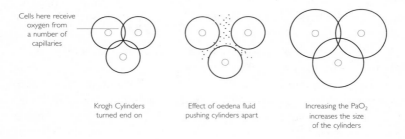

Fig 15.5 Krogh cylinder

By administering a higher concentration of inspired oxygen, we can increase the size of the Krogh cylinders, and improve tissue oxygenation. This is important after surgery where tissue trauma causes oedema. It is of crucial importance after head injury, where cerebral oedema jeopardises cells on the margins of the Krogh cylinders.

Once the oxygen supply falls the hypoxic cells, will for a short time, shift to anaerobic metabolism to provide the power to run their processes. However, if there is no oxygen to mop up the hydrogen ion produced by the cells, the hydrogen ion overflows into the tissue fluids and eventually causes acidaemia. As the hydrogen ion accumulates in the tissues its strong positive charge starts to bend proteins out of shape. Enzymes no longer function properly and this further upsets cellular function.

PROBLEMS WITH OXYGEN

Flammable material will burn briskly in oxygen, but oxygen itself will not burn. Keep naked flames and sources of electrical sparks at least 2 metres away from a source of oxygen.

Oxygen Sensitivity and Toxicity

Oxygen toxicity of the newborn

If exposed to high oxygen concentrations, premature babies and neonates (less than 1500 grams) are at particular risk from retrolental fibroplasia (also called retinopathy of prematurity or ROP), and will go permanently blind .

Table 15.3

OPTIMAL PAO$_2$ FOR THE NEWBORN			
Babies age	**PaO$_2$(mmHg)**	**PaO$_2$ (kPa)**	**Hb saturation %**
Pre term	40-60	5.3-8.0	70-90
Full term	50-70	6.6-9.2	84-92

Adult oxygen toxicity[3]

Older patients receiving 100% oxygen for longer than 4–6 hours run the risk of progressive lung damage. Many drugs including bleomycin, steroids and nitrofurantoin make the injury worse. With the chemotherapeutic drug bleomycin more than 28% inspired oxygen quickly causes inflamation, and later may progress to pulmonary fibrosis.

Carbon-dioxide resistant patients

In a normal person, a small rise in PaCO$_2$ will stimulate the respiratory centres to increase the rate and depth of breathing. Patients with chronic obstructive airway disease, and a chronically raised PaCO$_2$, (blue-bloaters), may stop breathing if given more than 28% inspired oxygen These patients have adapted to a high PaCO$_2$, and will no longer increase their respiratory effort if it rises. Instead, they depend on a low PaO$_2$ for their respiratory drive. Blue bloaters are easily recognized, because they almost invariably have pulmonary hypertension, with right heart failure (so called *cor pulmonale*). They are cyanosed, plethoric, can only say a few words between gasps, and frequently have swollen ankles. It is a common error to deprive them of supplemental oxygen, 'just in case they stop breathing'. To deprive them of oxygen will cause tissue damage. Watch them closely, and if their respiratory effort starts to fail, their oximeter reading falls, or they become drowsy (a sign of rising $PaCO_2$); then assist their breathing with a bag. This is a difficult problem, because once intubated and stabilized on a ventilator, these patients can be almost impossible to wean. Many physicians try to get by with other measures, for example an intravenous respiratory stimulant, such as doxepram.

Table 15.4

RESPIRATORY SYMBOLS AND DEFINITIONS

SYMBOLS

O_2	=	oxygen
CO_2	=	carbon dioxide
H_2O	=	water

Upper-case letters are used to describe substances in the gaseous phase.

P	=	partial pressure (tension) of a gas
A	=	alveolar
I	=	inspired gas
E	=	expired gas
V	=	volume in litres
T	=	tidal

Lower-case letters are used to describe substances in the liquid phase.

a	=	arterial
v	=	venous
c	=	capillary

In a mixture of gases the *partial pressure* of a particular gas, is the pressure that gas would exert if it alone occupied the space available to it.

PO_2	=	partial pressure of oxygen.
PaO_2	=	partial pressure of oxygen in arterial blood.
$PaCO_2$	=	partial pressure of carbon dioxide in arterial blood.
FIO_2	=	fractional inspired content of oxygen. Air is about 21% oxygen, so breathing air the FIO_2 = 0.21
H^+	=	hydrogen ion.
$[H^+]$	=	hydrogen ion concentration.
pH	=	a non-linear scale for measuring hydrogen ion concentration.
FRC	=	functional residual capacity

UNITS

cm H_2O	=	centimetres of water pressure.
mmHg	=	millimetres of mercury pressure.
kPa	=	kilopascals of pressure. 7.60 mmHg = 1 kPa 1.36 mmHg = 10 cm H_2O

In the UK the kilopascal (kPa) is the preferred unit for measuring pressure.

DEFINITIONS

Apnoea is the complete absence of breathing.

Breathing is the mechanical act of moving air in and out of lungs.

Hypercarbia is an excess of carbon dioxide in the body.

Hypoxaemia occurs when the PaO_2 falls below 60 mmHg (7.89 kPa)

Hypoxia occurs when there is not enough oxygen to allow the cells carry out their normal function.

Hypoventilation is failure of lungs to eliminate carbon dioxide. It is measured by a rise in the partial pressure of carbon dioxide in the arterial blood.

Respiratory rate (RR) is the number of breaths taken each minute.

Tidal volume (TV) is the amount of air moved into or out of the lungs with each breath.

Minute volume (MV) is the volume of air moved into or out of the lungs in one minute. MV = RR x TV

Dyspnoea occurs when the patient feels he cannot get his breath.

Table 15.5

USEFUL NORMAL VALUES		
Arterial partial pressure of oxygen	PaO_2	100 mmHg 13.3 kPa
Arterial partial pressure of carbon dioxide	$PaCO_2$	40 mmHg 5.3 kPa
Alveolar partial pressure of carbon dioxide	$PACO_2$	40 mmHg 5.3 kPa
Respiratory rate	adult child neonate	12-15 breaths/min up to 20 breaths/min up to 60 breaths/min
Tidal volume	TV	7 ml/kg
Minute volume		65 ml/kg

ACID AND BASE BALANCE

Acids are substances that release hydrogen ions and *bases* are substances that accept or react with hydrogen ion. Although pH is widely used for measuring the hydrogen ion concentration in the body it is a convention rather than a useful concept. (pH is defined as the negative logarithm to base 10 of the hydrogen ion activity). If you remember that hydrogen ion is just an ion, as are sodium and potassium ions, then much of the mystery of acid base balance disappears.

Before describing how the body handles acids and bases, it is useful to have a perspective on very large numbers. You can fit about a million (10^6) peas in a big deep freeze unit (that is, a cubic metre). A thousand (10^3) deep freeze units would hold a billion (10^9) peas. A millimol (mmol) is one thousandth (10^{-3}) of a mol and a nanomol is one billionth (10^{-9}) of a mol.

Each day the mitochondria produce about 22 500 million nanomols of hydrogen ions If each nanomol of hydrogen ion were the size of a pea, this would be enough to fill up 22 500 deep freeze units. Lined up a metre apart this would be a line of 45 kilometres (just over 28 miles) of deep freezes, all filled with peas. Yet at any given instant there are only about 40 nanomols of hydrogen ion in each litre of extracellular fluid. This can be represented by about a third of a cupful of peas. You can now see that the body has an enormous ability to dispose of hydrogen ions because it holds this level almost constant despite the tidal wave of hydrogen ions continuously flowing through it.

The hydrogen ion (H^+), which is really a naked proton, is very reactive. Its powerful electric field attracts negative charges and repels positive charges. All proteins carry an uneven charge distribution around them, because electrons are more likely to be found around some parts of the molecule than other parts. As a hydrogen ion comes near a protein its positively charged field bends the protein out of shape, repelling the more positively charged parts of the molecule, and attracting the more negatively charged parts. Enzymes are complex proteins with specially shaped receptor sites. Too much (or too little) hydrogen ion in the vicinity of enzymes disrupts their shape and their function. The wrong amount of hydrogen ion in the cell causes metabolic chaos, because its biochemical reactions slow down, or sometimes, speed up. Take three deep breaths and you will feel dizzy. This occurs because your cerebral enzymes have been bent out of shape by the change in hydrogen ion concentration in your cerebrospinal fluid. Many drugs are carried on proteins in the blood stream. These too, alter shape and this affects their ability to bind the drugs, either increasing or decreasing the amount of free drug in the plasma.

Hydrogen ion is very potent, and just a few extra can cause metabolic havoc. In health there are about 40 nanomols of hydrogen ion per litre of extracellular fluid (pH 7.40). This means there are about 5 hydrogen ions for ever 100 million molecules of water. Just 3 more hydrogen ions added to those 100 million molecules of water (equivalent to distributing just 3 extra peas in 100 deep freeze units all full of peas) will make the body acidotic, increasing the hydrogen ion concentration to 64 nanomols per litre and giving a pH 7.20.

pH	Hydrogen ion concentration nanomol/litre	Effect
6.80–7.00	160–100	life threatening acidosis
7.00–7.20	100–64	severe acidosis
7.20–7.30	64–50	moderate acidosis
7.30–7.35	50–45	mild acidosis
7.35–7.42	54–38	normal limits
7.42–7.50	38–32	mild alkalosis
7.50–7.55	32–38	moderate alkalosis
7.55–7.65	28–22	severe alkalosis
7.65–7.80	22–16	life threatening alkalosis

A fundamental concept is that the body always compensates to attempt to maintain a normal hydrogen ion level. To do this it excretes or retains carbon dioxide through the lungs (the *respiratory component*). Hydrogen ion combines with oxygen in the mitochondria of the cells to form water. Carbon dioxide made in the process, is excreted by the lungs. Each water molecule is formed from two hydrogen ions and one oxygen ion making up the familiar molecule H_2O. To get rid of the 22 500 million nanomols of hydrogen ion each of us makes in a day we produce about 300 ml of water.

The kidneys also excrete or retain bicarbonate and hydrogen ions (the *metabolic component*). Hydrogen ion is also excreted as fixed acids These include tiny amounts of sulphuric acid, acetoacetic acid, and phosphoric acids formed from substances we have eaten.

The diagnosis of acid–base disorders involves not only an analysis of the blood gas results, but also a clinical appraisal of the patient.

The body always attempts to adjust
its hydrogen ion concentration to a normal level.

Acidaemia and Acidosis

The terms acidaemia and acidosis (alkalosis and alkalaemia) are used interchangeably by many anaesthetists, others make a lot fuss about the distinction. In practice it is probably not important as long as all the blood gas results are presented. To be pedantic the -aemias are what we measure in the blood, while the - oses are the effects in the tissues. The -aemias can be altered by compensatory mechanisms. Thus a man with severe chronic bronchitis and a chronically raised PaCO2, but a normal pH would have a chronic respiratory acidosis but no acidaemia.

THE HENDERSON EQUATION

$$[H^+] = \frac{24\ PCO_2}{[HCO3-]}$$

where: [H+] = hydrogen ion concentration in nanomols/litre.

PCO$_2$ = partial pressure of CO$_2$ in arterial blood measured in mmHg

[HCO3–] = actual or measure bicarbonate ion concentration in millimol/litre

Do not use the standard bicarbonate for this value, but get the actual bicarbonate ion concentration from a serum electrolyte analysis.

In essence this equation says that if you know two of the values, you can calculate the third. The often quoted Henderson–Hasselbach equation is derived by logarithmically converting the simple Henderson equation, but it is cumbersome and rarely used in a clinical situation.

Bicarbonate ion is one of the most important hydrogen ion buffers in the extracellular fluid. A *buffer* is a substance that soaks up hydrogen ions (like a sponge), or releases them to keep their concentration in the surrounding tissue fluid constant.

You can use the equation as a guide on how to use a ventilator to control PCO$_2$ and hence pH. It is also useful to work out the effects of various components of an acid–base disorder and the compensatory mechanisms.

STANDARD BICARBONATE
If you nominate the arterial PCO$_2$ as 40 mmHg, that is, you assume that the lungs are excreting a normal amount of carbon dioxide, then knowing the hydrogen ion concentration, you can calculate the bicarbonate concentration. This mathematical manipulation gives you the *standard bicarbonate*. The standard bicarbonate calculation assumes that any disturbances in bicarbonate level is not due to respiratory dysfunction, but is a measure of metabolic disturbance.

BASE EXCESS/DEFICIT
Sometimes the laboratory will give a value for base excess/deficit. This is an indicator of the amount of sodium bicarbonate needed to correct the acid base disorder and restore the pH to normal. It is seldom used these days, although some physicians still regard it important.

Respiratory causes of acid–base disturbances

Normally the pressure exerted by carbon dioxide in arterial blood is about 40 mmHg (5.3 kPa). Excess carbon dioxide dissolves in water to form hydrogen ion (a strong acid) and bicarbonate ion (a weak base). If a patient hypoventilates so that the excess carbon dioxide dissolves in the body water, hydrogen ion is released and the patient is said to have a respiratory acidosis. If the patient hyperventilates and carbon dioxide is blown off then there will insufficient hydrogen ion and the patient will be said to have a respiratory alkalosis.

Common causes of respiratory acidosis in the recovery room are, those that cause the patient to hypoventilate, such as:

- excess opioids;
- inadequate reversal of muscle relaxants;
- uncommonly drugs such as midazolam, or diazepam.

Respiratory alkalosis is uncommon, and is usually due to excessive hyperventilation during the anaesthetic. If a lot of carbon dioxide has been washed out of the body by excessive ventilation, it takes some time for the carbon dioxide to again build up in the tissues. Another cause of hypocarbia is interstitial pulmonary oedema. This may be due to fluid overload, cardiac failure, septicaemia, fat emboli, or early adult respiratory distress syndrome and reflex over-breathing. The patient feels breathless, his respiratory rate rises and his $PaCO_2$ falls.

Metabolic causes of acid–base disorders

If the liver fails to metabolize lactate, or the kidneys to excrete acids or alkalies, these are called metabolic disturbances. Causes of a metabolic acidosis are:

- hypoxia where lactic acid from anaerobic metabolism accumulates in the tissues faster than it can be metabolized by the liver;
- unstable diabetics where keto acids accumulate;
- serious sepsis where bacterial endotoxins have damaged the liver so it cannot metabolize organic acids;
- renal failure where the kidney cannot excrete acids.

Metabolic reasons for alkalosis are uncommon, and are usually due to severe preoperative potassium depletion, or the injudicious use of sodium bicarbonate. Occasionally following massive blood transfusion the liver metabolizes citrate to bicarbonate causing a metabolic alkalosis a few days later.

Acute or chronic disorder?

Disturbances can occur within minutes or hours, and these are known as *acute* disturbances, while others creep up slowly on the patient over days or weeks, and are known as *chronic* disturbances. Patients with acute disturbances either in the production or excretion of hydrogen ion tend to have an abnormal level of hydrogen ion (pH) in their plasma. Those with stable chronic disturbances have normal hydrogen ion concentrations.

Management of Acid–Base Disorder

Acidosis

Most acidaemia is caused by tissue hypoxia. The hypoxic cells switch of their mitochondria and revert to inefficient anaerobic metabolism with the production of lactic acid (sometimes simply called *lactate*). When the oxygen supply is resumed the liver and skeletal muscle rapidly metabolizes the lactic acid (re-paying the so called *oxygen debt*). Apart from being a sign of serious tissue hypoxia, in general, an acidosis is not a bad thing. The excess hydrogen ion alters the shape of haemoglobin so that oxygen is more readily released to the tissues. The body has buffer systems that soak up excessive hydrogen ions, and tissues such as the heart and kidney have a great tolerance for excess hydrogen ions. Tissue blood flow and cardiac output increases, and the body makes every effort to provide more oxygen to the tissues. Enzyme systems do not begin to fail until the hydrogen ion concentration exceeds about 80 nanomols per litre (pH 7.10).Do not treat an acidosis until the pH is less than 7.10 and there are signs of cardiac failure. In general, it is better to improve tissue oxygenation and allow the body to correct the problem for itself. Occasionally, particularly in severe diabetic ketoacidosis, or grave haemorrhagic shock you may need to give a small dose of bicarbonate slowly intravenously over 5–10 minutes. To prevent giving too much sodium ion dilute 100 ml of 8.4% sodium bicarbonate (that is 100 mmol) in 900 ml of 5% dextrose and start with a dose of 150 ml of this mixture in an adult.

Alkalosis

While acidosis is well tolerated and the hydrogen levels may rise to much more than 100 nanomols per litre before the heart starts to pump ineffectively, alkalosis is both dangerous and not well controlled by body buffers. Postoperatively alkalosis is usually iatrogenic, caused by excessive administration of sodium bicarbonate. Occasionally excessive vomiting, where hydrochloric acid is lost, can cause a metabolic alkalosis. Insufficient hydrogen ion causes haemoglobin to bind oxygen more firmly, so that it is not readily released in the tissues. Body enzyme systems are quickly disrupted and phosphate energy dependent pumps in the cells rapidly fail. Cardiac arrhythmias and increased binding of calcium by proteins cause problems. With an ongoing alkalosis, urinary potassium and chloride losses can quickly cause potentially fatal hypolkalaemia, so you will need to measure and replace these ions. Acetazolamide (Diamox®) can be used to prevent the kidney excreting hydrogen ion. Occasionally the alkalosis may need 0.1M hydrochloric acid infused into a central vein. Aim to increase the hydrogen ion concentration to 25–30 nanomols per litre very slowly over 2–3 hours.

INTERPRETATION OF ARTERIAL BLOOD GASES

Normal values

pH	7.35 7.42	[H+]	35-45 nanomols/litre
PaO_2	85–100 mmHg		(11.0–13.1 kPa) while breathing air
$PaCO_2$	37–42 mmHg		(4.9–5.5 kPa)
HCO3-	22–25 millimol/litre		

1. What is the hydrogen ion concentration (pH)?
If [H+] > 45 nanomols/l (pH< 7.35) the patient has an acidaemia
If [H+] < 35 nanomols/l (pH > 7.42) the patient has an alkalaemia

2. What is the arterial PaO_2?
If PaO_2 < 60 mmHg (7.9 kPa) then the patient is hypoxaemic.
If PaO_2 < 35 mmHg (4.6 kPa) then the patient is dying.
Whenever you quote the arterial PaO_2 you must state also what per cent oxygen the patient is breathing.

3. What is the arterial $PaCO_2$?
If $PaCO_2$ < 35 mmHg (4.6 kPa) then the patient is hyperventilating.
If $PaCO_2$ > 45 mmHg (5.5 kPa) then the patient is hypoventilating.

4. What is the 'actual' bicarbonate ?
If it is nearly normal then there is a respiratory component.
If it is abnormal then there is a metabolic component.

For example, where a woman is admitted to the recovery room after haemorrhaging on the operating table, present the results in the following form: This 35-year-old woman is acidaemic with a pH of 7.20, and hypoxaemic with a PaO_2 of 40 mmHg breathing 100% oxygen. She is hyperventilating with a $PaCO_2$ of 20 mmHg. The actual bicarbonate of 7.5 mmol/l suggests a severe metabolic acidosis.

---

1. McKenzie A. J. (1987). *Anaesthesia and Intensive Care*, 17: 412–17
2. Prohit D. M., Ellison R. C., *et al.* (1985). *Paediatrics*, 76: 399–44
3. Jackson R. M. (1985). *Chest*, 88: 900–5

16. RESPIRATORY PROBLEMS IN THE RECOVERY ROOM

Breathing Patterns

Dyspnoea

Dyspnoea occurs when the patient feels short of breath. This is sometimes called *respiratory distress,* because the patient's response ranges from being uncomfortable; to extreme panic, fighting for breath, and being unable to talk. On the other hand, a dyspnoeic patient need not necessarily have respiratory failure or be hypoxic, and respiratory failure can occur with, or without, dyspnoea.

Pleuritic pain

Pleuritic pain occurs postoperatively, if the pleura has been breached at surgery, or the patient has a pneumothorax. Characteristically an intense sharp pain limits inspiration. To avoid this the patient breathes in shallow pants, and stops abruptly with a grunt if he feels the pain.

Kussmaul's breathing

Kussmaul's breathing *(or air hunger)* is a sign of metabolic acidosis. The patient breathes deeply, and feels breathless. Be careful not to depress this compensatory hyperventilation with excessive opioid, because the acidosis will get worse.

Cheyne–Stokes breathing

Cheyne–Stokes breathing is an easily recognized pattern of breathing. The patient takes a series of breaths, and then stops (*the apnoeic phase*), only to start again. In infants, or the elderly, who are sedated, the respiratory centres in the brainstem do not respond as readily to a rising $PaCO_2$. The $PaCO_2$ has to rise sufficiently during the apnoeic phase to trigger the next breath.

Restrictive and obstructive lung disease

Restrictive lung disease limits the patient to short, rapid breaths. Compare this to obstructive lung disease where he takes longer, deeper breaths. If someone squeezes you tightly around the chest, you will breathe with a restrictive pattern. If you try to breathe through a drinking straw, you will adopt the pattern of obstructive lung disease.

See-saw breathing

Until the patient's airway is secure always watch both the chest and the abdomen, normally they will rise and fall together. See-saw breathing can be seen sometimes with life-threatening airway obstruction. In attempting to breathe, the severely obstructed patient's chest will be seen to fall, as the abdomen rises. This 'see-saw' breathing is known as *paradoxical breathing*. If the obstruction is severe, and the patient does vigorous forced valsalva manoeuvres against a closed glottis, he may develop pulmonary oedema[1]. This can happen rapidly if the patient is young and fit.

RESPIRATORY FAILURE (HYPOXIA AND HYPOVENTILATION)

Respiratory Failure

By definition respiratory failure occurs when either the PaO_2 falls below 60 mmHg (7.9 kPa); or the $PaCO_2$ rises above 50 mmHg (6.6 kPa).

Respiratory failure has two components. Hypoxia and hypoventilation. Assess and treat hypoxia and hypoventilation separately.

Table 16.1

DIFFERENCES BETWEEN HYPOXIA AND HYPOVENTILATION

Hypoxia	Hypoventilation
Low PaO_2	High $PaCO_2$
Lethal	Not lethal
• confusion	• drowsiness
• restlessness	• coma
• agitation, aggression	• bounding pulse
• coma	• vasodilation
Treat with oxygen	Treat by improving breathing

Hypoxia

Following an operation respiratory problems are the commonest cause of death and injury. At some time up to 64 per cent of patients in the recovery room have an oxygen desaturation below 90 per cent[2].

Signs of Hypoxia

Early signs of hypoxia are:

- confusion;
- restlessness, aggression, and agitation;
- deterioration in mental state;
- hypertension, tachycardia;
- cyanosis.

Late signs are:

- pallor;
- bradycardia and hypotension;
- convulsions;
- coma;
- cardiac arrest.

Confusion, agitation, aggression, restlessness and deterioration in mental state are signs of cerebral hypoxia indicating early neural dysfunction that can swiftly progress to fitting and coma.

Hypertension and tachycardia are responses of the sympathetic nervous system to the stimulus of hypoxia.

Cyanosis occurs when there are more than 3 grams of deoxygenated haemoglobin circulating. This corresponds to a PaO_2 of about 55 mmHg (6.6 kPa).

Pallor, hypertension and tachycardia are caused by the sympathetic nervous system responding to the hypoxic stress.

Bradycardia and hypotension are signs of a critically hypoxic heart, which if unrelieved, will stop in asystole.

Causes of Hypoxia[3]

Loss of lung function

Oxygen diffusion from the lung into the blood is reduced by pulmonary collapse, oedema, aspiration, surgical resection of lung tissue, pneumothorax, haemothorax, or fluid overload leading to pulmonary oedema.

Intraoperative pulmonary fat, or amniotic emboli cause severe hypoxia. Pre-existing diseases include obesity, and asthma. These problems cause respiratory distress. Patients with long standing lung disease, such as chronic bronchitis or emphysema, or chest wall deformities may, or may not have respiratory distress.

Acute complete or partial airway obstruction (see page 328)

High tissue oxygen demands

Shaking and shivering can increase muscle oxygen demands by up to seven fold. Anaemia or cardiac failure impair oxygen transport from the lungs to the tissues.

Hypoventilation

As already discussed (see page 306) physiology hypoventilation will cause hypoxia unless supplemental oxygen is given.

Signs of hypoventilation in a patient who is not hypoxic are:
- bounding rapid pulse;
- peripheral vasodilation;
- drowsiness;
- hypertension.

Causes of Hypoventilation

Depression of the respiratory centres

Opioids impair the normal stimulation of a rising $PaCO_2$, and reduce the desire to breathe. The patient is notably not distressed or dyspnoeic; he just does not feel like breathing. Morphine can depress ventilation for up to seven hours. Fentanyl can cause delayed respiratory depression which occurs some hours after the last dose of fentanyl. This is a hazard, particularly in the elderly. In contrast patients who are affected by residual anaesthetic drugs are usually still comatose in the recovery room.

Intraoperative hyperventilation causes the plasma PCO_2 to fall, removing the normal respiratory drive. It imitates the effects of opioids, but lasts for less than 10 minutes.

Failure of the respiratory muscles

Muscle relaxants may still be working making it difficult for the patient to take deep breaths. The patient will be distressed, struggling for breath and using his neck muscles to help him breathe.

After upper abdominal and thoracic surgery the diaphragm does not contract properly making breathing difficult. Neurological disease, such as multiple sclerosis, motor neurone disease, and Parkinson's disease weaken the respiratory muscle and make it difficult for the patients to cough.

Management of Hypoxia and Hypoventilation

1. Initially give 100% oxygen by mask, and attach a pulse oximeter.
2. Check the A,B,C,D,E of resuscitation (see page 146).

3. Call for help, and attach an ECG.

4. Examine the patient to ensure that there is no airway obstruction, and air entry is evenly distributed to both lungs. Exclude pneumothorax and signs of cardiac failure.

5. Is the patient's ventilation normal? Use a respirometer to check his tidal and minute volumes. The tidal volume should be greater than 5 ml/kg. If it is less then the patient is clinically hypoventilating and you will need to support his breathing with a bag and mask until you have found the reason.

6. Take arterial blood gases, check the haemoglobin levels, and order a chest X-ray.

7. Record the perfusion status of the patient (see page 236); monitor the blood pressure and pulse. Check the jugular venous pressure; if it is normal or high exclude cardiac failure, and pulmonary emboli, if it is low consider hypovolaemia.

8. Where a pulmonary shunt is involved, increasing the inspired oxygen concentration will only increase the PaO_2 a small amount. The worse the shunt, the smaller the rise in PaO_2. Further therapy could include intubation and the application of positive end expiratory pressure (PEEP) and the use of nitric oxide.

Hints:

• Monitor all patients in the recovery room with a pulse oximeter.

• Learn the limitations of a pulse oximeter (see page 388).

• Hypoxia is difficult to assess, it may give no signs, and the absence of cyanosis does not exclude it.

• Postoperative hypoxia contributes to postoperative confusion, and increases the risk of myocardial ischaemia, renal failure, and liver damage.

• Treat ALL restlessness, agitation, confusion or deterioration in mental state as hypoxia to start with. Give oxygen, support breathing and then find the cause.

• Hypoxia occurs during transfer of the patient from the operating theatre to the recovery room, so give oxygen during transport.

• Give at least 60% oxygen to all patients who are emerging from anaesthesia, during their transport from the operating theatre, and for at least 10 minutes in the recovery room.

• Use a mask giving 4–6 litres per minute. Nasal prongs do not give enough oxygen, and are useless if the patient breathes through his mouth.

- Treat persistent neuromuscular blockade by continuing to ventilate the patient; do not use repeated doses of neostigmine.
- Naloxone (Narcan®) works for about 35–50 minutes, and may wear off before the opioid. Giving it intramuscularly prolongs its action. Nalorphine (Lethidrone®) is a longer acting alternative opioid antagonist.
- Opioids used in the anaesthetic may cause respiratory depression for many hours, especially in the elderly. Send patients to the ward on oxygen, and continue it while the patient is still affected by opioids.

Hypoxia is treated with supplemental oxygen.
Hypoventilation is treated by improving breathing,
this may require a ventilator.

Postoperative hypoxia[4]

In the ward the major risks in the early postoperative period are opioid induced hypoventilation, and sputum retention leading to pneumonia.

Episodic hypoxia occurs for up to five days postoperatively in some patients. These patients may have no other clinical evidence of lung damage. At risk, are elderly patients, following hip surgery, and especially upper abdominal and thoracic surgery. Those with pre-existing cardiac or lung disease; and those receiving on-going opioid analgesia are even more at risk. It would seem logical that these patients receive continuous supplemental oxygen for this period, but in many hospitals this is not common practice.

Many recovery rooms do not give oxygen to children because they are so active and won't tolerate a mask over their face. Yet nearly half the children in recovery room have moderate to severe hypoxia at some stage[5].

Indications for Postoperative Ventilation

It is difficult to decide preoperatively if a patient should be mechanically ventilated postoperatively.

Preoperative risk factors are:
- pre-existing lung disease;
- abnormal preoperative blood gases;
- ineffective cough;
- obesity;

- smoking;
- elderly patients;
- anaemia;
- cardiac failure;
- neuromuscular disorders;
- patients from the intensive care unit.
    Operative risk factors include:
- upper abdominal surgery;
- thoracic surgery;
- surgery involving the diaphragm;
- aspiration of gastric contents.

Table 16.2

A ROUGH ESTIMATION OF POSTOPERATIVE REDUCTION IN RESPIRATORY FUNCTION.		
Site of incision	Preoperative FEV$_1$	Estimated postoperative FEV$_1$ as percentage of preoperative level.
Upper abdominal	100%	25–35%
Lower abdominal	100%	45–55%
Thoracic	100%	55–65%
Elsewhere	100%	10%

Airway Obstruction

Airway care is the most important skill required by recovery room. No staff should be left alone with unconscious patients until they are confident that they can maintain an airway, and cope with airway emergencies. Close and careful observation of the patient will enable problems to be detected early.

Noisy breathing is obstructed breathing,
but not all obstructed breathing is noisy.

In every recovery bay a high capacity sucker, laryngoscopes, Magill forceps, and airways, must be instantly available to remove foreign material from the airway. It is good practice to place the sucker under the right-hand side of the patient's pillow where it can be quickly found. Patients have died because the sucker was out of reach, or not turned on.

ESTIMATION OF POSTOPERATIVE RESPIRATORY FUNCTION

A useful, but rough guide can be obtained preoperatively by measuring the patient's forced expiratory volume over one second (FEV_1) with a spirometer. This is a dynamic test which is influenced by the amount of airway obstruction. Normally the FEV_1 should be at least 70–80% of the forced vital capacity (FVC). Using table 16.2 above, estimate the patient's postoperative FEV_1.

If predicted FEV_1 < 10 ml per kg ventilatory support likely to be needed.

If predicted FEV_1 10–15 ml per kg, then reassess in the recovery room.

If predicted FEV_1 > 15 ml per kg, then respiratory failure is unlikely.

Example case:

Consider a 60-year-old woman who smokes, weighs 60 kg, and is to have an open cholecystectomy.

Data: Weight   = 60 kg

Smoker 25% function

(a non-smoker would have 35% function)

Her preoperative FEV_1 = 3200 ml.

Estimated postoperative FEV_1 = 3200 x 25/100

= 800 ml

FEV_1 per kg   = 80/60

= 13 ml/kg

At a predicted postoperative FEV_1 of 13 ml/kg this woman will need reassessment in the recovery room. On admission to the recovery room she was stable, but within 30 minutes her respiratory rate rose to 28 breaths per minute and her oxygen saturation fell to 90%. Her pain was then managed with intercostal blocks, and she was encouraged to deep breath and cough. She improved rapidly, but was sent to a high dependency nursing ward for close observation for the next 36 hours.

Factors that predispose towards respiratory support are:

* a respiratory rate > 25 breaths per minute;
* an oxygen saturation < 92%;
* inability to take a deep breath and cough effectively;
* an alveolar–arterial oxygen gradient of greater than 250 mmHg when the patient is receiving 100% inspired oxygen.

If the predicted FEV_1 were to be much less than 10 ml/kg then consider keeping the patient intubated and ventilated, and reassessing them in the intensive care unit.

Wherever possible nurse comatose patients on their side in the coma, or *recovery position* (see page 11). Even conscious patients are safer like this. Drowsy patients lying on their backs are always at risk of airway obstruction postoperatively, and furthermore they are more likely to develop postoperative chest infections. Lay drowsy patients in the recovery position on the trolley when they are being transported back to their ward.

Signs of an Obstructed Airway

Partial obstruction

Partial obstruction of the airway causes the patient to make a snoring noise. This is called *stridor*. Stridor (including snoring) leads to hypoxia.

> *No patient can be allowed to snore*
> *in the recovery room.*

Complete obstruction

Complete obstruction is revealed by the absence of air coming and going from mouth and nose. Normally this tidal air exchange can be easily felt in the palm of the hand.

Cyanosis and falling oxygen saturation is a late and alarming sign of airway obstruction, and may be accompanied by ECG signs of ischaemia, such as sinus tachycardia, which will soon be followed, more ominously, by a nodal bradycardia. ST depression is a sign of severe myocardial ischaemia.

CONTENTS OF A DIFFICULT AIRWAY TROLLEY

Laryngoscope with Macintosh and Magill blades of different sizes;
Right-handed laryngoscopes
Endotracheal tubes, catheter mounts and tight fitting connections;
Stylets and gum elastic bougies;
Magill forceps;
Laryngeal masks;
Cricothyroidotomy kit;
Retrograde intubation kit;
Oral airways;
Nasopharyngeal airways;
Seldinger wires

Drugs:
- thiopentone;
- propofol;
- suxamethonium;
- adrenaline;
- ketamine;
- diazepam;
- atropine;
- salbutamol.

Causes of an Obstructed Airway[6]

Anatomical abnormalities

The commonest cause of airway obstruction in the recovery room is the tongue falling back into the pharynx to obstruct the airway. This is likely to occur if patients are lying on their backs.

Complete airway obstruction is silent,
and quickly and quietly will kill the patient.

Anticipate anatomically difficult airways in patients with:
• short or fat bull necks;
• stiff necks or previous cervical spinal surgery or injury;
• prominent protuberant upper teeth;
• underslung jaws or with receding chins;
• Down's syndrome;
• Turner's syndrome;
• atlanto-axial instability;
• patients who cannot open their mouths widely.

Patients with arthritis in the hands
often have stiff necks—be gentle.

MANAGEMENT
1. Inspect the patients airway with a laryngoscope.
2. Suck out any secretions or foreign bodies.
3. Give 100% oxygen by mask.
4. Firmly lift the patient's jaw forward by inserting the fingers behind the angle of the mandible and pulling firmly upwards; in general the ears should be lifted anterior to the clavicles.
5. Insert an oral Guedal or similar airway.
6. Sometimes a well lubricated nasopharyngeal airway can useful in maintaining a difficult airway.

Laryngospasm

Laryngospasm is a protective reflex where there is an occlusion of the glottis by the action of the intrinsic laryngeal muscles which prevents foreign material entering the tracheo-bronchial tree. This is a common and dangerous problem. The patient makes a harsh crowing noise when he attempts to breathe in. This is called 'inspiratory stridor'. Laryngospasm is often accompanied by violent coughing or breath holding for surprisingly long periods. It is a sign that something is irritating the upper airway or some foreign material is present.

Irritation induced laryngospasm follows extubation, (especially if there has been an earlier difficult or traumatic intubation), bronchoscopy, or pharyngeal or laryngeal surgery. It is particularly common in children after upper airway surgery occurring in about 20 per cent after tonsillectomy.

Foreign bodies include vomit or acid gastric contents which can be inhaled into the trachea and lower airways. Aspiration pneumonitis is a devastating complication and can cause fulminating and often fatal bronchopneumonia.

A foreign body can also be:

- a piece of tooth;
- a forgotten throat pack;
- a fragment of adenoid tissue;
- the coroner's clot.

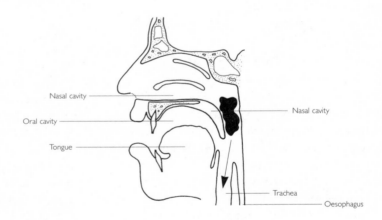

Fig 16.1 The coroner's clot

MANAGEMENT

1. Get help; you will need two assistants. The first assistant should attach an ECG, pulse oximeter and measure the pulse rate and blood pressure. Your second assistant should fetch the emergency trolley (cart), and prepare to draw up drugs.
2. Meanwhile inspect the patient's airway with a laryngoscope,

3. Suck out any secretions or foreign bodies.
4. Give 100% oxygen by mask.
5. Firmly lift the patient's jaw forward by inserting the fingers behind the angle of the mandible and pulling firmly upwards. In general the ears should be anterior to the clavicles.
6. Once you are sure the airway is clear, use a bag and mask to apply firm positive airway pressure in an attempt to relieve the spasm.

Further management if the above is unsuccessful:
1. Your assistants should prepare for urgent intubation.
2. Try lignocaine 1.5 ml/kg intravenously as a bolus. Often this will relieve laryngospasm [7,8].
3. Should this fail, intubate the patient to establish an airway.

Laryngeal or pharyngeal oedema

Laryngeal function is disturbed for at least four hours after tracheal extubation; even if the patients appear alert[9]. During this time the patient should remain under observation. This is especially important in child day cases who have been intubated.

Oedema in the upper airways occasionally follows extubation in children, and especially neonates and infants. A small amount of reactive oedema will intrude on the narrow lumen rapidly occluding it. Mild cases will respond to warmed humidified oxygen enriched gas mixtures. However, it may be necessary to use nebulized adrenaline. Take a 1 ml ampoule of 1 in 1000 adrenaline and make it up to 5 ml in normal saline. Give this by oxygen driven nebulizer at a 5 litre per minute flow to a face mask. The effect lasts about 2 hours. Although this sounds a big dose for a small child it has been found to be very effective[10].

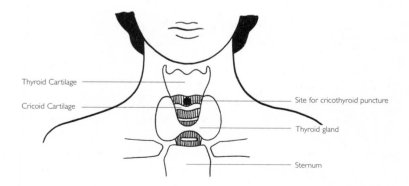

Fig 16.2 Location of cricothyroid puncture

In adults other causes are:

- Following thyroidectomy, carotid endarterectomy, or other operations on the neck;
- airway burns;
- trauma to the neck;
- subcutaneous surgical emphysema.

CRICOTHYROID PUNCTURE

There are a number of commercially available tracheostomy sets which are designed for quick and easy insertion. However, in an emergency situation, where the patient is becoming cyanosed, or his conscious state is deteriorating, you may not have time to organize this. You may have to perform an acute cricothyroid puncture. Take the largest bore intravenous cannula you have, (preferably 10 G or bigger) and insert it through the cricothyroid membrane into the trachea. Attach the barrel of a 2 ml syringe into the needle and then jam a No. 8 endotracheal 15 mm adaptor into the barrel of the syringe. It will now be possible to attach the cannula to a self-inflating bag or T-piece to support the patient's oxygenation until a tracheostomy or other means of establishing an airway can be achieved.

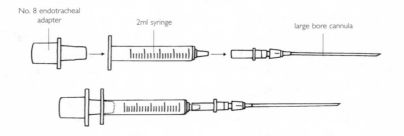

Fig 16.3 Improvised cricothyroid puncture set

Vocal cord paralysis

This is a rare complication, which may follow intubation, but is more common after thyroid surgery where the recurrent laryngeal nerve has been damaged.

Unilateral vocal cord paralysis is usually a benign condition which presents as hoarseness in the recovery room and resolves over several weeks. If the cords have been damaged the patient will be unable to say 'Eeeeee' in a high pitched voice.

Bilateral vocal cord paralysis is a more serious condition which presents as upper airway obstruction as soon as the patient is extubated. Laryngoscopy will show motionless vocal cords which lie adducted with a very narrow glottic aperture. Try ventilating with a mask and self-inflating bag but the patient will usually require reintubation and a tracheostomy. Bilateral vocal cord paralysis also has been described in patients with raised intracranial pressure who have been extubated.

Obstruction of an artificial airway

Patients awakening from anaesthesia often clench their jaws tightly. If they are still intubated they can bite hard on their endotracheal tube or laryngeal mask obstructing it. Prevent this by inserting a Guedal airway alongside the endotracheal tube.

Endotracheal tubes can become obstructed with mucus plugs, they can become kinked and the cuff may herniate over the distal end obstructing it. If there appears to be obstruction of the endotracheal tube then remove it.

Asthma[11]

Asthma is not usually a problem in the recovery room. Asthma is often diagnosed incorrectly, because not every patient who wheezes has asthma. Other causes of wheeze to consider are left ventricular failure, aspiration of foreign material into the bronchial tree, allergic responses to drugs and blood products, and acute pulmonary embolism. If the breathing is shallow the patient may not wheeze at all.

Signs are:
- dyspnoea;
- wheeze;
- use of sternomastoid and accessory muscles of respiration;
- distress;
- cyanosis (a dangerous and late sign in asthmatics).

Clinical assessment[12]
- If the wheeze is localized to one lung, or a segment of one lung, consider aspiration, of a foreign body in the lower airway, or pulmonary embolism.
- If the patient is using accessory muscles the bronchial obstruction is critical.

INITIAL MANAGEMENT
- Give oxygen at 6 litres per minute by mask;
- sit the patient up;

- attach an ECG monitor, pulse oximeter and automated blood pressure machine;
- inform the anaesthetist.

Wheeze?
Consider aspiration, allergy and cardiac failure.

Ongoing management includes:

1. If the patient is conscious give 5 ml 0.5% salbutamol in saline with a nebulizer.
2. If the patient is still anaesthetised give salbutamol (Ventolin®) 100 microgram intravenously, and repeat it at 3 minute intervals if necessary. Salbutamol will cause a tachycardia.
3. Ipratropium (Atrovent®), an anticholinergic agent is a useful to supplement salbutamol in the conscious patient. It can be given by nebulizer (250 micrograms/ml), or metered inhaler (20 micrograms/puff).
4. Check to see that the patient has not been receiving maintenance oral theophylline before considering using intravenous aminophylline. The gap between therapeutic and toxic blood levels of aminophylline is small. Aminophylline toxicity is hazardous and difficult to treat.
5. If the asthma is severe give a large dose of hydrocortisone hemisuccinate, at least 200 mg intravenously. This takes up to 8 hours to reach its peak effect.
6. Suspect aspiration, or an allergic response if a previously well patient becomes wheezy in the recovery room.
7. In a severe asthmatic consider the possibility of a pneumothorax, which may have occurred, unsuspected, during the anaesthetic.
8. Never sedate a restless asthmatic.

Aspiration Pneumonitis (see also page 229)

Aspiration pneumonia is one of the greatest risks of anaesthesia, and may occur, sometimes unrecognised, before the patient reaches the recovery room. It is often assumed that this calamity is due to some error, or negligence on behalf of the anaesthetist. This is not necessarily so.

The risk of aspiration cannot be predicted, although there are identifiable risk factors, such as obesity, hiatus hernia, pregnancy, bowel obstruction, trauma surgery, full stomach, and diabetes. Aspiration is a risk at any point while the patient is comatose, and for some time after regaining consciousness.

The mortality is quoted to be between 3 and 70 per cent. Aspiration of small amounts of fluid in the upper airway, not necessarily from the stomach, increase the incidence of postoperative respiratory infections. Aspiration of particulate matter causes more complications than aspiration of clear fluid. Aspiration in children is usually associated with some sort of airway abnormality.

Aspiration of gastric contents in pregnancy or in the puerperium causes a devastating form of aspiration pneumonitis called *Mendelson's syndrome*. This is often fatal, and it is essential to prevent this disaster.

Signs of aspiration are: rattling noise when breathing, especially if the patient has just vomited or regurgitated, dyspnoea, wheeze, cyanosis, use of sternomastoid and accessory muscles for breathing, distress and panic, hypertension.

INITIAL MANAGEMENT

1. Roll the patient into the coma position.
2. Give high flow 100% oxygen by mask.
3. Clear the airway with a sucker.
4. Call for assistance.
5. Attach an ECG, pulse oximeter, and automated blood pressure machine.
6. Prepare to take blood gases.

Further management includes:

1. Consider a bronchoscopy. This may be needed if there is suspicion that lumps of matter have been aspirated. If there is any doubt, perform a fibreoptic bronchoscopy to check. If you cannot hear breath sounds over a significant part of the lung, assume something is blocking a major airway. Bronchial lavage is contraindicated, and may spread infective material to unaffected parts of the lung.

2. Bronchodilators will help improve oxygenation and the treatment is essentially the same as for acute asthma.

3 Corticosteroids should not be used as they prevent localization of the inevitable infection, and impair the lungs defence mechanisms.

4. Broad spectrum antibiotics are not recommended at the early stage, because they select out resistant bacteria. The patient is bound to get a mixed flora bacterial pneumonia, including anaerobes. if possible take specimens of tracheal aspirate for culture. Most physicians would delay the use of antibiotics until the patient developed a fever and cough. Sputum cultures can be taken when this occurs and rational antibiotic therapy started.

5. If the patient has a PaO_2 less than 70 mmHg (9.2 kPa), transfer the patient to an ICU for monitoring. It may be necessary to ventilate these patients, but this should be avoided if at all possible because it abolishes the vital ability to deep breathe and cough.

6. A chest X-ray in the recovery room is not helpful. A characteristic blotchy picture, especially over the lower lung fields, will develop within a few hours.

Chronic Obstructive Airways Disease

In patients with chronic obstructive lung disease respiratory depression can occur with surprisingly low doses of opioids. Pain is best relieved with regional blockade. If the patient becomes drowsy in the recovery room, suspect that respiratory depression is causing carbon dioxide retention.

Encourage deep breathing and coughing. Sit the patient up and support his wounds. A heated humidifier, such as an Aquapack® or Conchapak® will help keep his sputum loose. Continue the chest physiotherapy and breathing exercises in the ward. Good analgesia is the key to success, because it is difficult to cough effectively if it hurts. These patients need thorough pre-operative physiotherapy, and explanations of how they are expected to co-operate in the immediate postoperative period. It is useless to start these explanations in the recovery room when the patient is confused and in pain.

If the patient can not cough tenacious, sticky sputum past his vocal cords, insert a cricothyroidotomy (such as a Minitrak®) in theatre before the patient comes to recovery room.

Do not be afraid to give oxygen to patients with chronic obstructive airway disease (COAD). Hypoxia kills. If the patient slows his breathing it can always be assisted while the problem is sorted out. Patients who depend on hypoxic respiratory drive nearly always have signs of cor-pulmonale; which is obvious preoperatively with dependent oedema and other signs of severe right heart failure.

Once a patient with COAD has become tired and drowsy, consider early ventilatory support in the intensive care unit. Respiratory stimulants will not help at this stage.

Pneumothorax

Pneumothorax occurs when air, which is normally confined to the lung, leaks into the pleural space and is trapped there. It may collect under tension and progressively distort the lungs, heart and major vessels. This can cause the patient to suddenly collapse in the recovery room. It may present with one or more of the following: sharp chest pain, tachycardia, cyanosis (particularly above the nipple line), hypotension, wheeze, or shortness of breath. Characteristically the patient pants and can't get his breath. The trachea is pushed away by the tension of the air in the pleural space. If you listen over the affected side with a stethoscope you hear no breath sounds. On percussion the chest sounds hollow—it is the same sound you hear when you percuss a pillow. The following are risk factors: recent insertion of a central line, brachial plexus and intercostal nerve blocks, upper abdominal (particularly kidney or hiatus hernia) surgery, thoracic, thyroid or cervical surgery, acute trauma, laparoscopy and any patient who has been intubated. In some tall thin young people they occur spontaneously. If the patient has collapsed, do not wait for a chest X-ray to confirm the diagnosis. You will need to arrange to insert a chest drain on the affected side.

Pulmonary embolism

During surgery blood clots can form in large veins, particularly in the pelvis and legs, and then break away sometime later to lodge in the pulmonary circulation. A range of events may occur from catastrophic circulatory collapse, shock and hypoxia causing death, to minimal symptoms such as chest pain from pleurisy, a minor cough or wheeze. They are sometimes symptomless. It is a useful rule to regard any patient who becomes abruptly short of breath in the recovery room to have had either, a pulmonary embolis, or a pneumothorax. Risk factors are obesity, pelvic surgery, or lower limb orthopaedic operations, application of an Esmarch bandage, legs in stirrups during the operation, woman on the oral contraceptive pill, and cardiac failure. Physical signs are often scarce. Sometimes a wheeze may be heard over the affected lung. You may be fortunate enough to detect a loud second sound in the pulmonary area, with a tapping heave on feeling the left second intercostal space in line with the centre of the clavicle, and a raised JVP, but this is unusual. The mainstay of treatment is heparin—but skilled advice will be needed if this is to be used in immediate postoperative period because of the danger of haemorrhage. If the situation is grave you may need to intubate, ventilate, and support the patient with ionotropes while a decision is made on further management. Formal open embolectomy may be an option.

1. Barin E. S., Stevenson I. F., et al. (1986). Anaesthesia and Intensive Care, 14: 54–7
2. Oh T. E. (1992). Recent Advances in Anaesthesia, 17: 103–15
3. Jones J. G., Saapsford D. J., et al. (1990). Anaesthesia, 457: 566–73
4. Aakerlund L. P., Rosenberg J. (1994). British Journal of Anaesthesia, 72: 286–90
5. Motoyama E. K., Glazner C H. (1986). Anesthesia and Analgesia, 65: 267–72
6. Hartley M., Vaughan R. S. (1993). British Journal of Anaesthesia, 71: 561–8
7. Bareka M. (1978). Anaesthesia and Analgesia, 57: 506–7
8. Gefke K., Andersen L. W., et al. (1983) ACTA Anaesthesiology of Scandinavia, 27: 111–12
9. Burgess G. E., Cooper J. R., et al. (1979). Anaesthesia, 51: 73–7
10. Child C. S. (1987). Anaesthesia, 42: 322
11. Cottam S., Eason J. (1991). Anaesthesia Review 8 (ed by Kaufman L.) p 71
12. Hirsman C. A. (1991). Canadian Journal of Anaesthesia, 38: 26–38
13. Chen C. T., Toung T. J. (1984). Anaesthesia and Analgesia, 63: 625–7

17. THE KIDNEY

Physiology

The kidney filters the blood, and reabsorbs most of its useful components back into the blood stream, excreting the unwanted wastes in the urine. Most of the wastes are protein break-down products from food and cellular metabolism, but the kidney also has an important role in excreting drugs. The kidney controls the volume, and composition of the of the extracellular fluid by regulating the balance of water, sodium, potassium, hydrogen ion and other water soluble substances in the body. It also produces hormones, erythropoietin, activated vitamin D, renin and prostaglandins.

The kidney receives 20–30 per cent of the cardiac output (about 1250–1500 ml per minute), which is far more than the amount needed to preserve its viability, but is important for its role as an excretory organ. If the extracellular fluid volume falls, the kidney will respond by diverting up to a litre per minute of its blood supply to boost the central circulation. It also retains sodium and water in an attempt to maintain the extracellular fluid volume. The kidney can survive for 30 minutes to an hour on a circulation as little as one tenth of its normal blood flow, but its ability to function becomes progressively impaired.

RENAL BLOOD FLOW

The *glomerulus* is a loose coil of blood vessels running into the upper end *(Bowman's capsule)* of the *nephron*. The glomerulus is rather like a hose with small holes in it. If the blood pressure inside the glomerulus is sufficient (>45 mmHg) then fluid will lead through the holes and flow down the nephron. Useful components of this *glomerular filtrate* are reabsorbed by the renal tubules and the waste flows on to be excreted as urine. It is important to understand that the blood first flows through the glomerulus, and then goes on to supply oxygen to the renal tubules. This blood flow is controlled by the systemic blood pressure, the activity of the sympathetic nervous system, and hormones such as adrenaline, vasopressin and angiotensin. Events which activate the sympathetic nervous system to cause renal vasoconstriction, and thus decrease renal blood flow, are haemorrhage, shock, pain, cardiac failure, hypoxia, and sepsis.

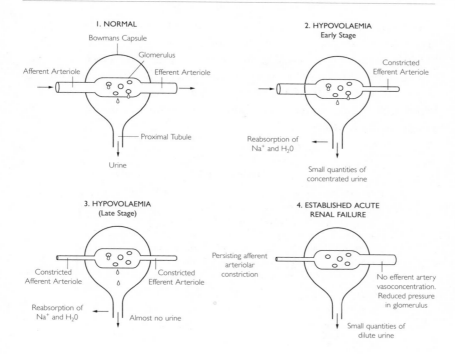

Fig 17.1 *Renal changes in hypovolaemia*

As shown in Fig 17.1, at first the sympathetic nervous activity restricts the outflow of blood from the glomerulus. This maintains the pressure sufficiently to force the plasma *filtrate* through into the nephron, but the blood supply to the renal tubules falls and they may become hypoxic. On the other hand, provided there is no renal vasoconstriction, blood may flow through the glomerulus and on to oxygenate the tubules, even though the pressure in the glomerulus is not high enough to form urine. This is the rationale for using a renal vasodilator such as dopamine to preserve renal oxygenation, and prevent hypoxia precipitating acute renal failure.

In the recovery room a kidney producing 0.5 – 1 ml/kg/hour of urine is not necessarily a sign of a properly oxygenated, healthy kidney. Nor can you be sure that because the urine output is low, or even absent, that the kidney is hypoxic and in danger of failing. The overall outcome depends on renal blood flow, and the activity of the sympathetic nervous system. A critical clinical sign is, that in early hypovolaemia, cold hands are a sign of a poorly perfused kidney.

To check the health of the kidney we need to look at the composition of the urine, especially its concentration and sodium content. A healthy kidney will respond to hypovolaemia by concentrating the urine, removing almost all the sodium and most of the water. The urine will be concentrated (high osmolarity), but with a low sodium concentration. If the kidney is hypoxic the tubules stop retaining sodium, and produce a dilute urine with a high sodium concentration.

DOPAMINE

It is controversial whether dopamine is an effective renal vasodilator, and what role it plays in improving renal perfusion in impending renal failure. At low doses of 3-5µg/kg/min it probably dilates the renal vascular bed. As the dose increases the effects are progressively due to increasing cardiac output, and raising renal perfusion pressure. It also has a direct diuretic effect on renal tubular function[5]. Clinically it is a useful drug in the preservation of renal blood flow, and the prevention of renal hypoxia.

CAUSES OF RENAL FAILURE

Oliguric Renal Failure

Without doubt the major cause of renal dysfunction in the recovery room is renal hypoperfusion with associated hypoxia, and the causes of this are in order: hypovolaemia, hypoxia, and hypotension. Hypovolaemia is the most likely cause of postoperative acute renal failure.

Renal hypoperfusion causing hypoxia
is the most important cause of acute renal failure.

In a fit young patient hypotension (mean BP down to 60 mmHg) is well tolerated, providing the patient is not also hypovolaemic.

Normovolaemic response

Hypotension induced by epidural anaesthesia, or deliberate vasodilation, may result in little urine being formed; but despite the lack of urine the kidney may not be hypoxic. This is because the kidney's autoregulation of blood flow ensures perfusion and oxygenation are maintained, even though the blood pressure in the glomerulus may not be enough to force fluid through the sieve to produce urine.

HYPOVOLAEMIA AND RENAL FAILURE

There is an ordered progression from hypovolaemia to renal failure. It starts with afferent arteriolar vasoconstriction, and cortical hypoxia; and progresses with impairment of autoregulation failure of efferent arteriolar constriction, with reduction in glomerular pressure; and finally neural and humoral effects on blood flowing to the kidney tubules. This progression is accelerated by renal vascular disease, diuretics and nephrotoxins such as gentamicin[1].

The fractional excretion of sodium (FeNa+) is a useful indicator of established acute renal failure.

$$FeNa+ = \frac{\left[\dfrac{Urine\ [Na^+]}{Plasma\ [Na^+]} \right]}{\left[\dfrac{Urine\ [Cr]}{Plasma\ [Cr]} \right]}$$

[Cr] = creatinine concentration   [Na+] = sodium ion concentration

Hypoxic injury   FeNa+ < 0.01

Acute renal failure   FeNa+ > 0.01

Hypovolaemic response

If the patient is hypovolaemic, or is in cardiac failure, his autonomic nervous system controls renal blood flow. The kidney is exquisitely sensitive to adrenaline and noradrenaline. It responds to hypovolaemia by progressively shutting down its blood flow.

Clinically we are warned of this renal hypoperfusion by the fact that the patient has cold hands, a poor perfusion status, a tachycardia and low blood pressure.

Cold bloodless hands = cold bloodless kidneys.

High Output Renal Failure

A second major cause of impaired renal function in the recovery room is drug toxicity. In this situation acute renal failure can occur when there is a good urine output. This is called *high output failure*.

Risk Factors

The hypoxic kidney is sensitive to toxins and many antibiotics, especially aminoglycosides such as gentamicin, some of the cephalosporins, and radiocontrast solutions used during angiography. Other toxins are frusemide, non-steroidal anti-inflammatory drugs (NSAIDs), especially ketorolac, and endotoxins from sepsis. Patients who, preoperatively, were taking angiotensin-converting enzyme (ACE) inhibitors are also at risk. The combination of frusemide, gentamicin, and hypovolaemia is well known for precipitating acute renal failure.

The combination of gentamicin and frusemide
are toxic to the underperfused kidney.

Other risk factors:
- Jaundiced patients undergoing operations on the liver and biliary tract are at risk from the hepato-renal syndrome. The renal damage is probably a combination of endotoxins, formation of granular pigment casts, and renal hypoxia. It is prevented by adequate fluid replacement, and encouraging a urine output with mannitol 0.5 g/kg.
- Patients having aortic or cardiac surgery, especially if the surgeon has had the aortic clamps on for more than 30 minutes.
- Adrenaline and noradrenaline infusions, that decrease tubular blood flow.
- Patients taking antihypertensive drugs.
- Diabetic patients.

Do not give frusemide to hypotensive patients.

Management of Oliguria

1. Identify the patients at risk.
2. As far as possible avoid the risk factors.
3. Give oxygen, and aim at a PaO_2 of at least 100 mmHg (13.3 kPa).
4. Monitor blood pressure, oxygenation and perfusion status.
5. Restore blood volume as quickly as possible.
6. Use low dose dopamine (3–5 micrograms/kg per minute) to maintain blood pressure. Aim at a mean blood pressure of 90–95 mmHg to compensate for impaired autoregulation of renal blood flow.
7. Use frusemide cautiously. Start with 0.5 mg/kg intravenously and repeat it every 20 minutes until a dose of 7.5 mg/kg has been reached. Doses beyond this are unlikely to be successful.
8. Consider mannitol, but high doses of mannitol can damage kidneys. Dose limits are less than 1 g/kg in healthy patients, and less than 0.5 g/kg in those with renal dysfunction. Mannitol is useful if there is a need to flush pigment through, such as occurs with myoglobinuria or haemoglobinuria.

9. Prevent non-oliguric renal failure from converting into oliguric renal failure. Non-oliguric renal failure is a milder disease, with a shorter duration, and a lower mortality. The commonest cause of non-oliguric renal failure is an aminoglycoside antibiotic.

If a patient has received gentamicin in theatre, make sure they do not become hypovolaemicwhile in the recovery room.

NEPHROTOXINS

GENTAMICIN[2]

Gentamicin is frequently used during urological surgery. Aminoglycosides are excreted exclusively by the kidney and are toxic to the renal tubules. Other factors that aggravate the renal toxicity (and ototoxicity) are hypoxia, hypovolaemia, diuretics, hypokalaemia, and hypomagnesaemia. This combination of factors is more likely to be encountered in the elderly. The loading dose for both normal patient, and patients with renal impairment is gentamicin 1–2 mg/kg. Gentamicin induced nephrotoxicity can be minimized by reducing the frequency of administration, and using peak and trough levels to guide therapy. Once daily dosing is the best way of giving gentamicin. The major site of damage is in the tubules, so the earliest signs of toxicity are impaired acid excretion, and depressed urine concentrating ability. A rising serum creatinine is a late sign.

ASPIRIN

Elderly patients often have heart failure, or atherosclerosis that decrease renal perfusion. They are also often taking aspirin for its prostaglandin mediated antiplatelet activity to prevent stroke and coronary ischaemia. Aspirin inhibits the cyclo-oxygenase, that is needed to maintain autoregulation of the kidney's perfusion. Aspirin stops the renal blood vessels dilating in response to early hypovolaemia or hypotension. Elderly patients are at high risk of acute renal failure if they become hypovolaemia, hypoxic, or hypotensive while they are taking this drug. Aspirin should be stopped about 7–10 days before surgery. Anti-platelet activity in patients with angina can be achieved with transdermal nitroglycerine[3].

NSAIDS

These drugs cause similar damage to aspirin, and no NSAID is exempt from this problem. Ideally NSAIDs should be withdrawn about 5 days before surgery. Paracetamol can be used as a substitute for pain relief.

RADIOCONTRAST MEDIA

Acute tubular damage by radiocontrast media used during vascular surgery in the elderly may be as high as 80–90%[4]. Hypovolaemia is the major avoidable risk factor. The problem is also exacerbated by co-existent diabetes, vascular disease, and age-related reduced renal function. The effects can be minimized in the recovery room by ensuring adequate hydration.

DIURETICS

To manage pulmonary oedema or renal failure in the recovery room, you will need to use one of the three powerful *loop diuretics*: frusemide, bumetanide, and ethacrynic acid. These drugs work by inhibiting the uptake of chloride in the ascending loop of Henle in the kidney, producing a brisk, and usually large diuresis even if the glomerular filtration rate is low. They all cause loss of sodium, potassium, and magnesium. They are all nephrotoxic. If given high doses, too fast intravenously they will cause ringing, or humming, in the ears (*tinnitus*); giddiness (*vertigo*) and irreversible hearing loss. This is much more likely if the patient is also receiving an aminoglycoside such as gentamicin or streptomycin. Cephalothin is another drug that increases their toxicity.

Frusemide (Lasix®) is the most commonly used of the three loop diuretics. It is called furosemide in the USA. Usefully, in pulmonary oedema, frusemide dilates the venous side of the circulation causing a decrease in the right heart filling pressure (preload). This vasodilation is a bonus, because it lowers the pressures in the pulmonary capillaries, so the patient gets quick relief from their dyspnoea. If a large dose is given rapidly intravenously, it will probably cause hypotension. It reaches its peak effect in 30 minutes, and a single dose will wear off in about 3 hours. After a dose of frusemide, the urine will contain 120 mmol/litre of sodium ion (or even more). The initial dose in pulmonary oedema or renal failure is 40 mg intravenously given at 5 mg per minute. If there is no effect after 20 minutes, then check the urinary catheter is not blocked, and then double the dose to 80 mg. If, after a further 20 minutes there is little or no diuresis then slowly give 120 mg. After a total dose of 240–250 mg it is unlikely that further frusemide will achieve an effect, and may have toxic effects. A dose of as little as 5 mg of frusemide in a young person with normal kidneys will produce a huge urine output of more than a 1000 ml in the first hour. Frusemide can be diluted in 0.9% saline, but is incompatible with glucose containing solutions.

Ethacrynic acid is sometimes used because it reaches its peak effect much faster, in about 5 minutes, and wears off in about 2 hours. It is considered more toxic than frusemide.

1. Badr K. F., Ichikawa I. (1988). *New England Journal of Medicine*, 319: 623–9
2. Walker R. (1994). *The New Zealand Medical Journal*, 107: 54–5
3. Lacost L. (1994). *American Journal of Cardiology*, 73: 1058–62
4. Thomson N. (1995). *The Medical Journal of Australia*, 62: 543–7
5. Duke D. J., Bersten A. D. (1992). *Anaesthesia and Intensive Care*, 20: 277–302

18. THE BLEEDING PATIENT

This chapter is divided into three parts. The first part describes blood transfusion, its risks and practical aspects The second part describes haemorrhage, its causes, investigation, and management; and the third part describes blood and blood products, and plasma expanders.

The recognition of HIV, and other diseases transmitted by blood transfusion have altered the way we use blood during, and after surgery. Anaesthetists are more reluctant to give blood intraoperatively, and patients are more afraid to receive it. Advances in understanding the physiology of tissue oxygenation have made it possible to reduce the amount of blood transfused. Keep the risks in perspective. Transfusion is a life-saving therapy, and when properly screened, is safe. When blood is needed to save a life, do not withhold it because of unrealistic fears of transfusion transmitted disease.

There are various alternatives to homologous blood (blood donated by another person) available. Autologous blood is the patient's own blood. It is collected several weeks before the operation, and is suitable for non-urgent surgery. Sometimes one or two units of blood are removed at the beginning of anaesthesia, and then re-infused at the end of the operation. Scavenged blood, which is washed and filtered, can also be returned to the patient. The equipment for this is expensive, and only practical in patients who are expected to lose more than 1500 ml of blood.

BLOOD TRANSFUSION

Haemorrhage becomes life threatening when tissues are deprived of their oxygen supply.

Therapeutic Principles[1]

1. Give blood to prevent tissue hypoxia. Do not use blood just to expand plasma volume, or in the absence of anticipated tissue hypoxia.
2. Avoid automatically giving a blood transfusion because the haemoglobin has fallen to less than 10 g/100 ml.
3. Try to avoid elective transfusion with homologous blood.
4. Give blood on a unit-by-unit basis. One unit of blood may be enough. Aim to keep blood pressure, and pulse within normal limits.

PHYSIOLOGY OF BLEEDING[2]

Neonates and infants are at risk after losing only 10 per cent of their blood volume (25 ml in a 2.5 kg baby). An haemorrhaging infant can neither increase his cardiac output, nor adequately vasoconstrict his circulation to maintain his blood pressure and tissue perfusion. On the other hand, healthy young adults can tolerate up to a 30 per cent loss of blood volume (about 1500 ml) before haemorrhage becomes life-threatening. In younger patients the blood pressure may actually rise in early haemorrhagic shock, because of a brisk neurohumoral response to the stress. Elderly patients drop their blood pressure earlier than younger patients, and have a lower pulse rate.

An adult responds to haemorrhage in two stages.

1. Arterial stretch receptors (baroreceptors) in the carotid and aortic arch detect a fall in arterial pulse pressure, and send messages to the hypothalamus and cardiovascular centres in the brainstem which, in turn, stimulate the secretion of adrenaline from the adrenal medulla, and noradrenaline from sympathetic nerve endings. These catecholamines cause vasoconstriction in the arterioles, especially in the gut, kidney, muscle and skin. They also cause the heart's rate and force of contraction to increase. The heart attempts to push blood against the constricted arterioles and the blood pressure rises, or is maintained, ensuring blood flow through the vital structures of the coronary arteries and the cerebral circulation.

2. When about 35 per cent of the blood volume is lost (about 1600 ml in an adult), the reflex sympathetic drive switches off. The blood pressure drops rapidly, the cardiac output falls, and blood bypasses oxygenated areas in the lungs. The supply of oxygen to the tissues starts to fail. Ischaemic gut and pancreas release *shock factors* into the circulation, that depress the heart, and damage capillaries. The results are a progressive circulatory collapse, with profound tissue hypoxia, leading to ischaemia of heart and brain, and then death.

Patients at risk from low oxygen carrying capacity include those with:
- myocardial ischaemia;
- coronary artery disease;
- congestive heart failure;
- haemodynamically significant valvular heart disease, such as, aortic stenosis;
- a history of transient ischaemic attacks, or suspected cerebral ischaemia;
- a history of previous thrombotic stroke.

To make sound clinical judgement you will need to understand the physiology of tissue hypoxia (see page 301). Most young fit adults can withstand a haemoglobin of 6–7 g/100 ml, providing they have no lung, or heart disease, and their vascular volume is normal.

Signs that blood transfusion may be needed are:

• continuing bleeding;
• persistent tachycardia;
• dyspnoea;
• postural hypotension, where the blood pressure falls when you sit the patient up;
• angina;
• deterioration in conscious state, associated with confusion or anxiety.

Table 18.1

CLINICAL SIGNS IN A 70 kg YOUNG ADULT MALE				
Severity of shock	Mild	Moderate	Severe	Critical
American College of Surgeons' Class[3]	Class 1	Class 2	Class 3	Class 4
Blood loss (ml)	< 750	750–1500	1500–2000	> 2000
Pulse rate	80–110	> 110	> 120	> 140
Blood pressure	Normal	Normal	Decreased	Decreased
Pulse pressure	Normal	Decreased	Decreased	Decreased
Respiratory rate	12–20	20–30	30–40	> 40 (gasping)
CVP (cm H_2O)	2 to 5	−2 to 2	−2 to −5	< −5
Urine output ml/hr	> 30	20–20	5–15	minimal
Perfusion	cool hands	pale hands	cold hands	sweating
Psychological status	anxious	agitated	confused	lethargic/coma

The blood pressure does not necessarily fall
early in haemorrhagic shock.

Management of Blood Loss

Continuing bleeding

Bleeding can be either concealed haemorrhage inside the thorax, abdomen or a limb where it is easily missed; or revealed haemorrhage which is obvious to all. Bleeding following tonsillectomy can be concealed if the patient has swallowed the blood, or revealed if the blood loss is obviously draining out of the mouth.

Then:

• lay the patient flat;

- raise his legs on two pillows, do not use a steep head down tilt;
- give oxygen at 6 litres per minute with a facemask;
- if possible, locate the site of bleeding;
- control bleeding by direct pressure using a pad and a gloved hand;
- call for help, notify the surgeon and anaesthetist;
- measure pulse rate and if possible, the blood pressure;
- attach ECG, pulse oximeter, and automated blood pressure cuff.

Blood loss with hypotension is an emergency.
Call for help!

Restore blood volume

Aim to replace the lost blood as quickly as possible. Give blood to replace the blood loss. If blood is not immediately available, do not wait for it to be cross-matched or come from elsewhere, use polygeline (Haemaccel®), pentastarch, or albumin solutions. If these are not available 0.9% saline or Hartmann's solution will suffice for a short time. The aim is to maintain renal perfusion, and prevent renal vasoconstriction. Titrate the volume until you can see the jugular venous pressure, or the central venous pressure is positive.

Transfuse whole blood

Blood is a living tissue transplant, and it starts to deteriorate as soon as it is taken from the refrigerator. Unless otherwise indicated give 2 ml per minute for the first 5 minutes, and during this time watch for untoward reactions (see page 353). Consider transfusing the remainder in less than 60 minutes. If possible transfuse a 400 ml pack of whole blood in no more than 2 hours.

Monitor progress

While the patient is haemodynamically unstable record the pulse and blood pressure at 5 minute intervals. The pulse rate rises long before the blood pressure starts to fall especially in young people. Do not rely on hypotension to confirm the diagnosis of haemorrhagic shock. Check the peripheral perfusion. Record the perfusion status in the patient's chart (see page 236).

If cardiovascular instability remains a problem then consider inserting a central venous catheter, and an arterial pressure line to monitor blood pressure, and to take samples for blood gas analysis. Repeat the recordings at 10 minute intervals to establish a trend.

Initially take blood to establish base-line haemoglobin, packed cell volume, and blood clotting status. As the bleeding continues, the circulating volume will contract. To start with, the haemoglobin levels remain steady; but once other fluids are given, the blood is diluted and the haemoglobin falls. As a rough rule in an adult, for each 500 ml of blood loss the packed cell volume falls by 5 per cent, and the haemoglobin drops by about one gram per 100 ml of blood.

Preserve renal function

Urine output is a sensitive index of tissue perfusion. Insert a urinary catheter. An output of less 30 ml an hour is a sign of poor tissue perfusion. Support renal perfusion with low dose dopamine infusion 3–5 micrograms/kg per minute, give oxygen, maintain blood pressure and consider using frusemide.

Prevent hypothermia

If you are giving more than two units of blood in a short time then use an in-line blood warmer to heat the blood to 37°C. Each unit of cold blood from the refrigerator will decrease the patient's core temperature by about 0.25°C. Rapid infusion of cold blood into peripheral veins is painful. Given quickly down a central venous line, cold blood can cause cardiac arrhythmias and reduce cardiac output. Some patients have cold agglutinins in their blood. These react with the cold transfused red cells causing them to clump and clog small vessels.

Warming transfused blood from 4° to 37°C decreases its viscosity 2.5 times, and dilates the patient's veins allowing the transfusion to run faster. It slows transfusions to run them through a standard blood warmer. To overcome this difficulty, there are two expensive systems available, the Level 1™ delivers 500 ml per minute, and Rapid Infusion System™ 1500ml/minute.

Never warm blood by heating the pack in warm or hot water. This causes rapid deterioration of the red cells, and may even cook the blood, rupturing the red cells. Never warm blood or blood products in a microwave oven.

Filter blood (see page 358)

Monitor hyperkalaemia

The concentration of extracellular potassium in stored blood rises by about one mmol per day, so that by its expiry date blood may contain up to 30 mmol/litre. This can cause cardiac problems especially in children, or patients with renal failure, acidosis and hypothermia. The ECG will initially show signs of peaked T waves. Consider giving 0.1 ml/kg calcium gluconate 10% slowly intravenously to counteract the effects of hyperkalaemia on the heart.

Do not automatically correct metabolic acidosis

Haemorrhagic shock causes a low PaO_2, usually a compensatory low $PaCO_2$, and a metabolic (lactic) acidosis. The acidosis will resolve in about an hour, providing tissue oxygenation is adequate, and the blood pressure and liver perfusion are restored. A moderate acidosis improves tissue oxygenation, so hesitate before using bicarbonate to correct it. Severe acidosis with pH less than 7.0 may need correction, but only if it is compromising myocardial contractility. Use slow increments of intravenous bicarbonate 0.2 mmol/kg into a central vein, and monitor the response. Use bicarbonate with extreme caution.

Massive Blood Transfusion

The normal blood volume is 70–80 ml/kg. A massive blood transfusion is defined as the patient's estimated blood volume replaced in a period of less than 24 hours.

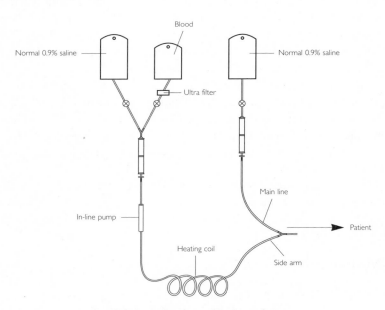

Fig 18.1 Set up for massive blood transfusion

After six units of blood have been given notify the haematologist-on-call.

Measure:
- haemoglobin;
- platelet count;
- partial thromboplastin time;
- prothrombin time.

Coagulation problems

Prophylactic administration of platelets or fresh frozen plasma is not useful in controlling haemorrhage during massive blood transfusion. The old philosophy of giving these components after 6 (or 8 or 10) units of blood should be abandoned. Wait for the onset of clinical coagulopathy, oozing from the operation site and around intravenous cannulas, before giving the appropriate components. The coagulation system shows great tolerance to a low platelet count, and clotting factor depletion.

Techniques of last resort

In cases of uncontrollable haemorrhage consider using fresh whole blood, and drugs that may reduce transfusion requirements such as aprotinin and desmopressin. Nearly fresh whole blood, less than 7 days old, is remarkably effective in all forms of coagulopathies and bleeding patients. We believe it is an under used resource.

RISKS WITH BLOOD TRANSFUSIONS[4]

Blood Transfusion Reactions

Severe transfusion reactions are rare[5] and include:
1. Acute haemolytic reactions transfusion reactions occur in about 1:6500 transfusions;
2. Febrile non-haemolytic reactions occurs in about 1–3 per cent of transfusions;
3. Anaphylaxis and anaphylactoid reactions occur in about 1:20000 transfusions.

Acute haemolytic transfusion reaction

Acute haemolytic transfusion reaction (HTR) is caused by red cell incompatibility. Reactions occur in about 1:6500 transfusions. They are characterised by fever, chills, hypotension, nausea, headache, dyspnoea, chest pains, back pains, shock, and uncontrolled bleeding; sometimes leading to death. The diagnosis is made on clinical signs, but can be confirmed later by: a blood film showing signs of abnormal red cells and haemolysis; with accompanying haemoglobinaemia, and haemoglobinuria. If renal failure occurs, then the mortality is high.

Initial management:
1. Turn off the transfusion, but do not remove the intravenous cannula.
2. Give oxygen at 10 litres per minute via face mask.
3. Change the drip set and continue the infusion with 0.9% saline.
4. Monitor with pulse oximeter and ECG.
5. Re-identify patient and blood pack.
6. Inform the blood bank and return unused blood and pack.

Further management:
1. If there has been major fall in blood pressure, associated with dyspnoea, treat for anaphylaxis (see page 142).
2. Treat wheeze with nebulized salbutamol, and hypotension with a plasma expander. Take care as patients may be allergic to the plasma expanders too.
3. If haematuria occurs, or urine output falls below 0.5 ml/kg/minute, give mannitol 1.5 g/kg IV to promote a diuresis. Mannitol works within minutes and lasts for about 3–4 hours. Commence a dopamine infusion through a central line at 3–5 micrograms/kg per minute.
4. Be prepared to manage disseminated intravascular coagulopathy (see page 362).

DRUGS DECREASING TRANSFUSION REQUIREMENTS

Desmopressin (DDAVP®) induces the release of von Willebrand's factor and procoagulant components of factor VIII and may be useful in bleeding due to platelet abnormalities occurring with uraemia. It is sometimes used during operations where large blood losses are expected such as the insertion of Harrington's rods.

Antifibrinolytics. Tranexamic acid and epsilon-aminocaproic acid (Amicar®) stabilize existing clots, and prevent primary fibrinolysis. These drugs inhibit the conversion of plasminogen to plasmin, so preventing fibrin breakdown. Aprotinin (Trasylol®) inhibits fibrinolysis,and also inhibits kallikrein-induced activation of the coagulation cascade. It appears to diminish postoperative blood loss. Antifibrinolytics occasionally promote pathological thrombosis.

Febrile non-haemolytic reactions (FNH)

Febrile non-haemolytic reactions are caused by sensitivity to donor granulocytes. They occur in about 5–7 per cent of transfusions, and are characterized by febrile, non-haemolytic reactions. Usually fever begins within 30–60 minutes of starting the transfusion, but may occur at any time up to two hours after the transfusion has started. These reactions are seldom dangerous, and are treated by stopping the transfusion. Only one patient in eight who has an FNH reaction will have a similar reaction to the next blood transfusion. Use leucocyte-poor blood if the patient has had two previous FNH reactions.

Urticarial reactions

Urticarial reactions are usually caused by antibodies to the donor plasma proteins. They occur in 1–3 per cent of transfusions. An urticarial reaction is characterized by local erythema, urticaria (hives) itching, but seldom fever. Treat it by stopping the transfusion. The urticaria will resolve in a few hours.

Anaphylaxis can be fatal

It is rare, and the incidence is estimated to be about 1 in 20 000 transfusions. Its usual cause is an antibody reaction to donor IgA. Suspect anaphylaxis if features occur after only a few millilitres of blood have been transfused. Coughing is usually the first sign, followed by acute wheezing, respiratory distress, hypotension, abdominal cramps, vomiting, diarrhoea, shock and collapse. (See page 142 for treatment.)

Other Problems with Blood Transfusions

Non-cardiogenic pulmonary oedema. This is sometimes known as transfusion-related acute lung injury (TRALI). It is more common than previously suspected. The usual cause is passive infusion of antibody to leucocytes inducing complement activation. The patient becomes dyspnoeic after a small volume of blood has been received. It may be accompanied by fever, chills, cyanosis, and hypotension. A chest X-ray will reveal interstitial pulmonary oedema.

Circulatory overload

Pulmonary oedema from too rapid infusion will present with a wheeze, dyspnoea, coughing, cyanosis, tachycardia, added heart sounds and raised jugular venous pressure. Neonates, infants, and patients with heart disease are at greater risk.

Infected blood

Blood can be contaminated during collection from the donor. Some bacteria, particularly coliform and pseudomonas species, will grow in a blood pack in the refrigerator. Contaminated blood is often a chocolate brown colour with bubbles in it, and the pack may be distended with gas. Do not even think of opening the pack, return it to the laboratory or blood bank. Contaminated blood, if transfused, can kill a patient almost instantly, or cause high fever, shock, haemoglobinuria, intravascular coagulation, renal failure, abdominal cramps, and generalized muscle pain.

Blood transfusions and blood products can transmit many diseases from the donor to the recipient which include:

- Hepatitis B, C, and D;
- human retroviruses: HIV (AIDS), HLTV-1 and 2,
- cytomegalovirus;
- toxoplasma;
- hepatitis A, and E, (oro-faecal hepatitis);
- herpes virus 6;
- Epstein–Barr virus, malaria, trypanosoma, brucellosis, Lyme disease, syphilis, babesiosis, Chagas disease, Creutzfeldt–Jakob agent, and many others.

Dilutional coagulopathy

Depletion of coagulation factors and particularly platelets is a complication of massive blood transfusion. If bleeding becomes a problem, initially treat it as a platelet deficiency, because coagulation factor depletion occurs later.

Immunosuppression

Although immunosuppression is not an immediate concern in the recovery room, it can become a problem to the patient later. It is probable that in cancer patients blood transfusions are associated with a greater risk of tumour recurrence, than in non-transfused patients. Blood transfusion is associated with a very real risk of wound or chest bacterial infection following surgery. Transfusion poses a greater risk than other factors such as wound contamination, shock, or duration of surgery. Whole blood seems to suppress the immune response, more than packed cells; and fresh frozen plasma is the worst offender[6].

PRACTICAL ASPECTS OF BLOOD TRANSFUSION

Checking blood

Every hospital has a routine procedure for checking blood before infusing it into a patient. Know your hospital's routine. Human error is responsible for nearly all deaths due to incompatible blood transfusion. Be absolutely sure the patient's identification exactly matches the one on the blood pack, and the cross matching form.

Transfusing blood?
—watch for transfusion reactions.

To prevent errors, two trained staff at the bedside should independently check the patient's identification: hospital number, name and initials with those on the blood pack and the laboratory's cross-matching form.

Cross-matching

The blood bank *types* (or groups) donor and recipient blood in the *ABO and Rh(rhesus) systems*, and then screens for other antibodies to red cell antigens. During the cross-match procedure the patient's serum is mixed directly with donor's red cells to make sure that undetected antibodies in the serum don't haemolyse the red cells.

If further blood is needed for cross-matching, do not to take the blood sample from a vein above the site where a drip is running, because the blood will be diluted with the contents of the drip, and furthermore the puncture wound will ooze.

Blood for cross-matching?
—send 8 ml of blood in a plain tube.

Take and process blood for cross-matching from one patient at a time. Be especially careful if there are two patients booked on the day's operating lists with the same surname.

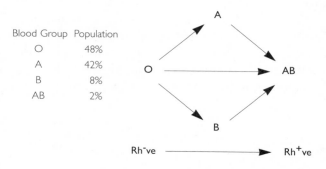

Blood Group	Population
O	48%
A	42%
B	8%
AB	2%

This diagram is NOT valid for transfusions of fresh frozen plasma.

Fig 18.2 Blood or platelet groups theoretically safe to give

Cross-matching usually takes 20–60 minutes. It can take longer if the patient has been receiving dextran 70, or the antihypertensive drug methyldopa. Tell the laboratory about these drugs.

In an emergency you can give type-specific, but uncross-matched blood. The chance of a severe reaction, although still possible, is less than one per cent.

Type O red cells lack both A and B antigens and consequently cannot be haemolysed by anti-A or anti-B antibodies in the recipient's plasma. Many operating theatres keep a few units of low plasma antibody titre type O negative blood. Use packed cells rather than whole blood. This is because type O plasma may contain anti-A or anti-β antibodies, which could cause haemolysis in an A, B, or AB patient. In desperate circumstances type O positive blood can be used in males, or post-menopausal females where Rh sensitization can never cause a threat to a fetus. If more than two or three units of uncross-matched blood has been used without signs of an adverse reaction, then continue transfusing the same blood rather than switching to properly cross-matched blood. This precaution is necessary because the already transfused uncross-matched blood may contain antibodies to any properly cross-matched blood.

Drip sets

When starting a blood transfusion use a set with a 170–260 micron filter incorporated in the drip chamber to remove lumps of debris.

Filters

Stored blood contains microaggregates, and the longer it has been stored, the more there are. A 40 micron filter will remove most of the microaggregates. These microaggregates contribute to the development of adult respiratory distress syndrome, non-haemolytic febrile reactions and cause a thrombocytopaenia in some patients[7]. It is advisable to use a filter if you anticipate that you will be infusing more than two units of blood, because donor white cells cause major depression in the recipients immune system[8].

Do not prime blood lines with
calcium containing solutions.

Packed cells will run more quickly through these filters if they have been re-expanded with saline. Use a Y-infusion set with the blood on one arm and the saline on the other. Run the saline into the blood bag. (See illustration on page 352.)

Compatibility

Use 0.9% saline to prime the drip set. Do not prime the line with electrolyte solutions containing calcium (such as Hartmann's solution, or Haemaccel®), because the calcium will neutralize the citrate anticoagulant, and clots will form. The only fluids compatible with blood are 0.9% saline, or blood products (5% normal serum albumin (NSA) and fresh frozen plasma). Once all the blood has run through put up a new drip set. Do not follow blood with 5% dextrose, polygeline, Hartmann's solution, parenteral nutrition fluids, or any other fluid apart from 0.9% saline, because the residual blood will clump in the drip tubing.

Never add, or infuse any drug with blood.

Do not vent plastic blood containers. Be careful not to put your finger on the needle introducer of the giving set in such a way that it carries your skin flora into the bag.

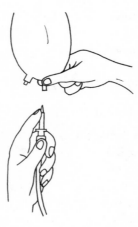

A common mistake when setting up a drip. Note the forefinger contaminating the sterile needle as it is being inserted into the bag of intravenous fluid.

Fig 18.3 Introduction of skin flora into bag of blood

Cannulas

The best cannula size for blood is either a 14 G or 16 G cannula. Blood can be infused through smaller cannulas, but only slowly. Cannulas as large as 10 G are available. For a rapidly running drip use a short, wide bore cannula and a high drip stand. If you cannot find a vein consider cannulating the femoral vein using a Seldinger wire technique and a 8.5 F sheath. To increase the rate further use an in-line pump, or an inflator bag.

Sterility

Be careful to maintain sterility if you are connecting a new drip set to a cannula that is already in the patient. Wear sterile gloves, swab the drip cannula and site with poviodine (Betadine®), and give it 90 seconds to work.

Wear gloves when handling blood.

HAEMORRHAGE

Causes of on-going bleeding, in order of frequency, are:
1. Inadequate surgical haemostasis;
2. Drug therapy such as warfarin, heparin or aspirin;
3. Platelet deficiencies;
4. Venous congestion particularly in head and neck operations;
5. Plasma clotting factors deficiency;
6. Disseminated intravascular coagulation;
7. Citrate toxicity;
8. Hypofibrinogenaemia;
9. Fibrinolysis;
10. Blood transfusion reactions.

1. Inadequate Surgical Haemostasis

As the patient's blood pressure rises in the recovery room, bleeding from the surgical incisions may occur. Watch wounds and especially drain bottles. If they drain blood at more than 200 ml per hour inform the surgeon. Bleeding can usually be controlled by direct pressure on the bleeding site. Put on a pair of gloves, pad the site and press firmly. Pressure dressings are not effective, and cause venous congestion aggravating the problem.

2. Drugs

Heparin

Some patients are given heparin in theatre, especially during vascular surgery. Heparin interferes with the function of factors II and X in the clotting pathway. It normally has a clinical life of about 50 minutes, but this is prolonged after blood loss or hypothermia. Check whether the heparin has been reversed with protamine before the patient came to the recovery room. An additional dose of protamine is sometimes needed. Protamine 1 mg will reverse the effects of about 100 units of heparin. Give the protamine slowly intravenously, no faster than 5 mg per minute, because it is a potent cause of hypotension, and pulmonary vasoconstriction. Excessive protamine can aggravate bleeding by depressing platelet function. If the patient is allergic to protamine (derived from fish testes), use polybrene (derived from whale testes) instead.

Oral anticoagulants

Some patients are taking warfarin for the long term treatment of deep vein thrombosis, atrial fibrillation, or because they have a prosthetic heart valve. Warfarin interferes with the ability of vitamin K to activate factors II, VII, IX, and X of the clotting pathway (see Fig. 18.4). Warfarin is usually stopped about 72 hours before surgery, and the prothrombin ratio (or INR) is checked on the day of surgery to make sure it is within acceptable limits. The residual effects of warfarin can be reversed with fresh frozen plasma. Vitamin K, or its analogues, take 4–8 hours to work and make it difficult to restabilize the patient on their oral anticoagulant regime after surgery. If you need to give them use vitamin K, infuse 25 mg over 30 minutes.

Non-steroidal anti-inflammatory drugs (NSAIDs)

This group of drugs (see page 202), all inhibit clotting, and patients who have taken them preoperatively are more likely to bleed in the recovery room.

3. Platelet Deficiency

Aspirin in particular, has an anti-platelet effect which lasts for up to 10 days after the patient's last dose. Patients sometimes neglect to mention they are taking aspirin and may bleed excessively following surgery, particularly after a hip or knee replacement. The bleeding tendency can only be reversed by a platelet transfusion.

Platelet deficiency is the most probable cause of bleeding during a massive blood transfusion (see page 352). Platelets can be deficient in numbers or in quality. Bleeding time increases if the level is less than $100000/mm^3$. Surgical bleeding may be hard to control if the level is below $40000–60000/mm^3$. Life-threatening spontaneous haemorrhage can occur if the level is below $20000/mm^3$. A platelet transfusion of 100 ml will raise the platelet count by about $10000/mm^3$. If platelet deficiency is the cause of bleeding give 6 units of platelets, and reassess the situation.

4. Clotting Factor Deficiency

After about a week in storage blood is deficient in platelets, factors V and VIII. Fresh frozen factor contains factor V (labile factor), and factor VIII (antihaemophilic globulin). Occasionally dilutional coagulopathy occurs after about 10 units of whole blood or packed cells have been infused, but most bleeding in massive blood transfusion is due to platelet deficiency.

5. Venous Congestion

Venous congestion will cause bleeding. The most common causes are tight bandages or plasters. Typically the blood is dark, and the skin is purple. Notify the surgeon.

6. Disseminated Intravascular Coagulation (DIC)

DIC is a hypercoaguable state where fibrin plaques out along vessel walls. So many of the clotting factors and proteins are consumed in the process, that if bleeding occurs there are not enough left to ensure proper clotting.

This condition has a mortality exceeding 50 per cent. It is caused by many things including:
• head injury;
• multiple trauma;
• severe sepsis;
• massive tissue damage;
• incompatible blood transfusion;
• any severe illness;
• a dead foetus.

The signs are the same as for a coagulation defect and include:
• uncontrollable bleeding from wound edges;
• excessive blood draining from the operating site;
• oozing occurs from old venipuncture sites and drip sites;
• blood stained urine;
• bleeding mucosal surfaces;
• a sudden fall in urine output.

Prevention includes early stabilization of fractures and debridement of wounds, early adequate resuscitation, and early use of antibiotics to control infection, urgent delivery after death in utero.

Laboratory confirmation of the clinical diagnosis of DIC includes:
• falling platelet count;
• elevated fibrin degradation products;
• falling fibrinogen;
• prolonged prothrombin ratio;
• prolonged partial thromboplastin time;
• a blood film that shows microangiopathic haemoglobinaemia.

Management of disseminated intravascular coagulation:
- replace blood loss;
- replace clotting factors with platelets and fresh frozen plasma;
- seek expert help.

7. Citrate Toxicity

Citrate toxicity is rare. Citrate phosphate dextrose (CPD) is the anticoagulant in packs of stored blood. It is readily metabolized by the liver, however if the patient is hypothermic, or receiving more than a litre of blood every ten minutes, then blood levels of citrate rise to form complexes with free calcium ions. Citrate acts as anticoagulant, because it binds calcium ions and interferes with many parts of the clotting pathway. Citrate may cause hypocalcaemia with hypotension and continued bleeding. Awake patients may complain of tingling around the mouth and muscle twitches. The ECG may show a prolonged QT interval, and cardiac arrhythmias. Serum calcium levels will not help with the diagnosis because they do not distinguish between free calcium ion and bound calcium. Treat hypocalcaemia with 10 ml of calcium gluconate 10% and then a further 2 ml with each successive 500 ml unit of blood. The standard serum calcium blood test does not distinguish the ionized from the complexed fractions. Each mol of citrate is eventually metabolized in the liver to 3 mols of bicarbonate, which explains the metabolic alkalosis seen a day or so after massive blood transfusion.

8. Hypofibrinogenaemia

Hypofibrinogenaemia (fibrinogen less than 100 mg per cent) occurs as a complication of:
- haemorrhage;
- abortion;
- intrauterine fetal death;
- amniotic embolism;
- hydatiform mole;

Treat it with fresh frozen plasma, or more specifically 10–20 units of cryoprecipitate.

9. Fibrinolysis

Fibrinolysis may complicate prostatectomy where the patient continues to bleed from the prostatic bed. Use tranexamic acid, which inhibits plasminogen activation. Give 0.5–3 grams slowly intravenously. EACA (*epsilon aminocaproic acid*) is sometimes used as an alternative.

10. Blood Transfusion Reactions (see page 353)

PROBLEMS WITH BLOOD CLOTTING

Clotting Studies

Clotting studies enable you to work out the cause of bleeding and the adequacy of the clotting mechanisms. Order clotting studies in the bleeding patient after major surgery. If possible collect the blood from an established arterial line, take 5 ml of blood and discard it before collecting your sample. Be sure there is no heparin, or other contamination, in your sample. If taking venous blood, collect it with a fine needle, or you may not be able to stop the bleeding from the venipuncture site. Do not take blood samples from veins in which a drip is flowing.

Table 18.2

USE THE RIGHT TUBE FOR CLOTTING STUDIES		
Test	**Abbreviation**	**Laboratory tube**
Cross match	X-match	8 ml in plain tube
Haemoglobin	Hb	5 ml in heparin tube
Platelets	Plat	5 ml in EDTA tube
Activated partial Prothrombin time	aPTT	5 ml in citrate tube
also called INR	PT INR	5 ml in citrated tube
Fibrin degradation products	FDP	5 ml in special FDP tube
Fibrin D-dimer	XDP	5 ml in EDTA tube

Interpretation Of Clotting Studies

To understand the process of clotting and how it can fail Fig. 18.4 will be helpful.

Whole blood coagulation time

Normal range is 3–12 minutes. If it is abnormal further tests are needed to identify cause. You will need the help of a haematologist.

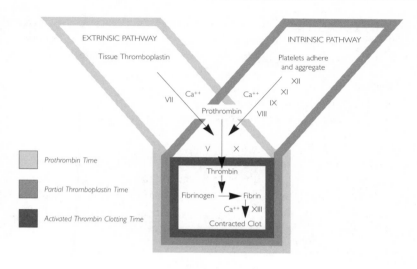

Fig 18.4 Clotting diagram

Haemoglobin (Hb)

During acute haemorrhage the venous capacitance vessels contract around the diminishing blood volume. This is the reason haemoglobin levels do not fall in early haemorrhage.

Platelets

The normal range of platelets is 150 000–400 000/mm^3. Deficits are treated with platelet infusion (see page 368).

Activated partial thromboplastin time (aPTT)

The normal range is 25–37 seconds, but some laboratories use different standards and the normal values may range widely. Check the local standard with your laboratory. Bleeding is unlikely to occur with ratios less than 1.5 of normal.

Prothrombin time (PT)

The normal value is 13–17 seconds. Some laboratories report it as the prothrombin ratio which is normally not greater than 1.5. Recently this test has been renamed as INR (International Normalized Ratio), which has a normal value of 1.0. Deficits are corrected initially with fresh frozen plasma.

Fibrin degradation products (FDP)

The normal values are under 40 micrograms/ml but check your local standards as the normal range varies between laboratories. Elevated concentrations indicate fibrinolysis usually secondary to disseminated intravascular coagulopathy, but it also occurs after massive crush injury.

Fibrinogen levels

The normal range is 1.6–5 g/litre (160–500 mg per cent). Less than 1.6 g/litre (160 mg per cent) indicates a coagulopathy.

Fibrin D-dimer levels

Fibrin D-dimer levels are a measure of fibrinolysis, This can be secondary to disseminated intravascular coagulation (DIC) or a primary event. Primary fibrinolysis is rare but can occur after amniotic embolism, resection of carcinoma of the prostate, in cirrhosis of the liver and after cardiopulmonary bypass. It is treated with tranexamic acid.

BLOOD CLOTTING

Blood clotting is a complex series of biochemical reactions involving clotting factors, platelets, calcium ions and the microvasculature. Once triggered it progresses like the chain reaction that occurs when you knock over a row of dominoes. Prothrombin and coagulation factors VII, IX, and X are made in the liver with the help of vitamin K. The coagulation factors circulate in an inactive form in the blood ready to help form a clot.

When a blood vessels is breached, the circulating *platelets* (little plates) come into contact with exposed collagen, either in the vessel wall, or in nearby tissue. The platelets *adhere* to the exposed collagen. They then change to a burr-seed shape, and become sticky. Other platelets became tangled (or *aggregated*) with them. A long stringy plasma protein called *fibrinogen* also gets stuck to the platelets as it floats by. The aggregated platelets then release a number of factors (such as adenosine diphosphate, prostaglandins, and 5-HT) that are needed for the chain reaction known as the coagulation cascade. In the presence of calcium ions the coagulation factors then convert circulating prothrombin into thrombin. The thrombin causes the fibrinogen, (already stuck to the platelets) to turn into a loose *fibrin* mesh. This fibrin mesh snares passing platelets, red cells, and white cells. Factor XIII then shrinks the mesh, to form a tight fibrin plug that blocks the hole in the blood vessel.

Fortunately blood does not clot unless it needs to. Factors preventing this are

- a good blood flow through vessels;
- rapid removal of activated clotting factors by the liver;
- a special circulating enzyme called plasmin that dissolves clots.

This fibrinolytic system involves a precusor called plasminogen which is activated into plasmin in the vicinity of clots. Plasmin breaks down fibrin into fibrin split products, and prevents the fibrin mesh being formed.

Hess' test for capillary fragility

Draw a circle 2.5 cm in diameter on the flexor surface of the forearm, and note any purple dots (*petechiae*). Apply a blood pressure cuff to the upper arm and inflate to 80 mmHg for 5 minutes. Count the number of petechiae inside the circle. If there are more than 10, capillary fragility is greater than normal, or the platelet count is low. Look for petechiae under the blood pressure cuff. If you see them, inform the anaesthetist.

BLOOD, BLOOD PRODUCTS AND PLASMA EXPANDERS

Blood and Blood Products

Blood issued by a blood bank is different from blood in the body. Unlike normal red cells, banked blood is deficient in 2,3 diphosphoglycerate (2,3 DPG). These banked red cells pick up oxygen readily, but in the absence of 2,3 DPG are bound strongly to the haemoglobin, and not released to the tissues. The banked red cells are rigid, and circulate in clumps like stacks of plates. They do not easily deform, to flow through the microcirculation. It takes about 18–24 hours for the banked red cells to regain their normal function. Potassium leaks out of the banked blood cells, and may cause hyperkalaemia, so be sure that a transfused patient maintains a good urine output.

Whole blood

Whole blood contains red blood cells, and plasma components. It comes as a 450 ml pack of blood from one donor. It is only indicated for patients who are likely to get symptoms from insufficient oxygen carrying capacity. Use whole blood in a bleeding, or traumatized, volume depleted patient.

Blood will keep for about 35 days in a special refrigerator held between 2–6°C. Components of the blood deteriorate at different rates. Platelets deteriorate more rapidly than plasma clotting factors and platelet counts around 100 000/mm^3 can still be found in whole blood after proper storage at 4°C for 5–7 days[9]. Clotting factors and immunocytes deteriorate more slowly than previously thought. The levels of factor V and VIII exceed 50 per cent of normal after 5–7 days, and factor III exceeds 70 per cent for some 2–3 weeks. This means that fresh whole blood, which has been stored for less than 7 days, can help greatly in the management of some coagulopathies especially during massive blood transfusion.

Try to use Rh negative blood for the 15 per cent of the population who are Rh negative. This is important if the patient has had a previous transfusion, or is a female of child bearing age. If you give Rh positive blood to an Rh negative woman in the child bearing years, give anti-Rh antiglobulin to prevent maternal antibodies damaging future babies.

Rh negative blood can be given to Rh positive patients provided the ABO blood group is compatible; but Rh positive blood cannot be given to Rh negative people.

BLOOD STORAGE

Do not store blood in a normal refrigerator, especially in the freezing compartment. Frozen blood cells are dead. If thawed and then given to a patient the cells will haemolyse releasing haemoglobin that will clog the kidneys causing renal failure. Blood should be dripping into a patient or stored correctly at 4°C. Do not leave packs of blood lying around at room temperature.

Packed cells

Units of packed cells contain 350 ml of red cell concentrate, but little plasma, and no clotting factors. Packed cells can be reconstituted with 0.9% saline and used when whole blood is not available. Packed cells are also useful where it is necessary to increase the oxygen carrying capacity of blood and there is a risk of fluid overload.

Platelets

Platelets comes in packs of 70–100 ml at room temperature. They are issued in O, A and B blood groups only. The normal range of platelets is 150 000–400 000 mm^3. One unit of platelets raises the platelet count by about 10 000/mm^3. If Rh positive platelets are given to an Rh negative women, then give anti-D immunoglobulin. Platelets are damaged if they are sucked up into a syringe and injected through a fine needle. If you are keeping them for more than two hours before use they should be gently agitated on a special shaker. Store platelets at room temperature, and not in the refrigerator. Since they are stored at room temperature, platelets are more likely to incubate bacteria than other blood products. Diseases can be transmitted by platelet transfusion in the same way as blood. The effects of giving platelets with bacterial contamination are similar to a transfusion of contaminated whole blood; they may cause massive cardiovascular collapse.

Indications for platelet transfusion do not rest solely on the platelet count. Not only do drugs such as aspirin, NSAIDs, calcium channel blockers, β blockers, and local anaesthetics inhibit platelet function, but peristaltic blood pumps, used during cardiac surgery also damage the platelets. In these circumstances the platelet count may still be normal, but the platelets are not working. Consider platelet transfusion after neurosurgery, or operations on the eye or ear, because slight bleeding, or even ooze, can cause serious damage.

Do not filter platelets
—use a special giving set with no filter.

Use platelets before fresh frozen plasma in surgical induced bleeding. Bleeding is unlikely to occur until the platelet count have been diluted to less than 40 000/mm³.[10] Because pooled platelet concentrates expose the patient to many donors, try to use single donor packs where available.

Preferably give type (group) specific platelets. If you cannot get the appropriate type, then in an emergency, patients can be given type O positive platelets. If the recipient is a pre-menopausal Rh negative female then they will need to be simultaneously given *anti-rhesus* antibody to prevent damage to a fetus during future pregnancies. The situation is outlined in Fig. 18.2.

Fresh frozen plasma (FFP)
Fresh frozen plasma comes as packs of 180 ml of beige ice for adults, and 60 ml packs for infants. It contains all the clotting factors, including Factor V, Factor VIII and fibrinogen; and can transmit HIV and hepatitis. It is stored at $-18°C$, and deteriorates at warmer temperatures, so it is often delivered packed in dry ice. Many hospital blood banks will thaw it for you. Otherwise place the pack of fresh frozen plasma in a watertight protective bag, and thaw it under running cold water. This takes about 20 minutes. Never thaw it in a microwave oven. Microwave or hot water will cook it, destroying its enzymes. Use it within six hours of thawing.

Preferably give type (group) specific fresh frozen plasma. If you cannot get the appropriate type, then in an emergency, patients of type O blood can be given type A, B, or AB fresh frozen plasma. This is the reverse of the situation outlined in Fig. 18.2. If possible use Rh negative fresh frozen plasma, but if you have to Rh positive, then in Rh negative women, who may bear children, you will have to give an antibody.

When giving fresh frozen plasma
—administer the appropriate ABO blood group.

Indications for the use of fresh frozen plasma include :
- correction of a coagulopathy in a bleeding patient;
- reversal of the effects of warfarin.
- if the patient has a damaged liver, or has disseminated intravascular coagulopathy.

In these cases the prothrombin time (or INR), or activated partial thromboplastin time should be greater the 50 per cent above normal before fresh frozen plasma is given.

Table 18.3

INDICATIONS FOR THE USE OF FRESH FROZEN PLASMA				
Test	Range	Mean	Abnormal	50% prolonged
Prothrombin time (PT)	13–17 sec	15 sec	20 sec	22 sec
INR		1.0	1.5	1.5
Activated partial thromboplastin time (aPTT)	25–37 sec	31 sec	40 sec	44 sec (a ratio of 1.5)

If platelet concentrates do not stop the bleeding,
then try fresh frozen plasma.

5% Normal Serum Albumin (NSA)

5% Normal serum albumin is similar to HPPD (Human Purified Protein Derivative) and PPF (Plasma Protein Fraction). Useful facts about this colloid are:
- it comes bottles of 500 ml amber-coloured clear solution;
- store it at 5°C;
- it is stable for about 6 months at room temperature and many years at 4°C;
- the plasma half life is about 16 hours;
- it has been heated to 60°C for 10 hours and so it carries no risk of hepatitis or HIV;
- chills and fever occur in about 1:150 recipients.

It can be used to support blood pressure in a bleeding patient while waiting for blood to be cross-matched. It is usually reserved for patients who are specifically deficient in serum albumin.

Blood Substitutes and Plasma Expanders

Colloid solutions are used to expand plasma volume in cases where blood is, either not available, or not needed. They do not contain any clotting factors.

Polygeline

The polygelines are suspensions of gelatin in saline (Haemaccel®, Gelofusin®).

Useful facts are:
- it comes in 500 ml plastic bottle of clear solution of polymerized gelatin;
- it is a useful substitute for plasma proteins and much cheaper;
- it is cleared from the circulation in 8–12 hours, the half life is about 5 hours;
- allergic reactions occur in about 1 in 1500 patients;
- use it with care in atopic patients such as those with asthma;
- do not infuse polygeline with blood because the calcium ions will cause the blood to clot;
- it does not interfere with haemostasis or cross-matching.

Esterified starches

Hetastarch ('Hespan®'), and pentastarch ('Pentaspan®') are esterified amylopectin solutions. Hetastarch causes allergic reactions in about 1 in 1200 patients. Pentastarch is better than hetastarch, because it does not interfere with clotting, is cleared from the plasma in half the time (12 hours), and is completely degraded by circulating amylase. Pentastarch has a higher colloid osmotic pressure, and produces an initial plasma volume expansion of 1.5 times the administered volume.

Dextran 40 (Reomacrodex®)

Useful facts about dextran 40:
- it is a clear solution of polymerized dextran;
- it is sometimes used to improve tissue flow;
- do not use it in the treatment of shock, because it can damage kidneys.

Dextran 70 (Macrodex®)

Useful facts about dextran 70:
- it is a clear solution of polymerized dextran;
- it can be used for plasma expansion in the case of hypovolaemia;
- It lowers the incidence of deep vein thrombosis but is not as effective as low dose heparin;
- can cause allergies in about 1/1400 patients. Allergic reactions can be

blocked by pre-treatment with small dextran fragments; this is called *hapten inhibition*[11]. Use 20 ml of 'dextran 1' (Promit®);

• do not use dextran 70 in pregnancy[12];
• it may interfere with blood cross matching. Take blood for typing and cross matching before infusing any dextran 70 solution.

1. Audet A., Goodnough L. T. (1992). *Annals of Internal Medicine,* 116: 403–6
2. Van Leeuwin A. F., Evans R. G., *et al.* (1989). *Anaesthesia and Intensive Care,* 17; 312–19
3. American College of Surgeons' Committee on Trauma. *Shock in Advanced Trauma Life Support Program.* Chicago. (1989). 57–73
4. McClelland D. B., (1992). *Clinical Anaesthesiology,* Vol 6, No. 3 pp. 539–60 (1992), published by Ballière, London.
5. Duffy B. L, Harding J. N., *et al.* (1994). *Anaesthesia and Intensive Care,* 22: 90–2
6. Blumberg N, Heal J. M. (1992). *Australian Anaesthesia 1992,* pp. 159–163, published by Australian and New Zealand College of Anaesthetists, Melbourne.
7. Bareford D., Chandler S. (1987). *Journal of Haemotology,* 66: 574–6
8. Blumberg N, Heal J. M. (1992). *Australian Anaesthesia 1992,* pp. 159–163, published by Australian and New Zealand College of Anaesthetists, Melbourne.
9. McNamara J. J. (1978). *Surgery, Gynacology and Obstetrics,* 147: 505–9
10. Phillips T. F. (1987). *Journal of Trauma,* 27: 903–6
11. Ljungström K. G. (1988). *Acta Scandinavia Chirugae,* S43: 26–30
12. Berg E. M., Fasting S., *et al.* (1991). *Anaesthesia,* 46: 1033–3

19. MONITORING

Monitoring is not a substitute
for patient observation.

On emerging from anaesthesia, and for some time afterwards, the patient is in an unstable physiological state, and many things can go wrong. In the operating theatre the anaesthetist gives the patient his full attention and deals with problems as soon as they arise; in the recovery room, if monitoring is not so close, events may progress further before being effectively dealt with[1]. The monitors will warn you of approaching problems, but they are not a substitute for carefully observing the patient.

The most useful electronic monitor in the recovery room is the pulse oximeter. For an infant, a debilitated, sick, hypothermic, or elderly patient, you will need an ECG and other monitoring equipment.

Much modern equipment is complex, and can confuse even the most competent staff. All personnel in the recovery room need to know how to use the monitors, and especially to understand what can go wrong with them. This requires a continuing education programme for new staff, and to refresh the memory of more experienced staff. If you are worried about the readings from a monitor, (and before assuming the monitor is faulty) go to the patient, and check the fundamentals.

BLOOD GASES

Arterial blood gases (ABG) are best taken from an arterial cannula, or failing that the radial or femoral artery. You can use the brachial or dorsalis pedis arteries, but do not use them in diabetics or patients with peripheral vascular disease. Occlusion of these end-arteries can cause gangrene. Before sticking a needle into the radial artery, use a modified *Allen's test* to check patency of the collateral ulnar artery.

Reasonably cheap commercial kits are available for collection of blood gases. If you do not have these, use a 23 gauge needle, and a 5 ml glass syringe which has the lining lubricated with heparin. Make sure no heparin drops are left in the syringe, and no air enters the syringe. Air bubbles cause errors in the estimations. Once taken, the blood should be stored in melting ice and quickly sent to the laboratory. The results will be unreliable if more than 10 minutes elapse between taking the blood and processing it. The laboratory will also need to know the patient's temperature, and his inspired oxygen concentration.

ALLEN'S TEST

Get an assistant to curl the patient's hand into a fist. Compress both the ulnar and radial arteries. Release the ulnar artery first, and note if the hand flushes. If there is adequate collateral flow, the hand will flush within 15 seconds. If there is inadequate flow the hand will remain pale. It is unwise to puncture or cannulate the radial artery if there is not enough flow in the ulnar artery to supply the hand.

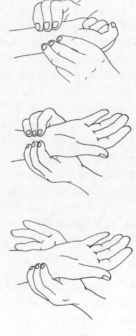

Fig 19.1 Allen's test

To prevent painful haematomas, use a pad to press firmly on the puncture site. After a measured 3 minutes, remove the pad to check if bleeding has stopped. Re-apply the pressure if necessary. Do not just tape a cotton-wool swab over the site, or the artery may continue to bleed.

Assess and treat any abnormal result quickly.

Acid–base balance in a hypothermic patient

Physiological pH and PCO_2 alter with the patient's temperature. Traditionally, arterial blood gases (ABGs) are measured in the laboratory at 37°C and then corrected back to the patient's temperature (pH-stat). Maintain the blood gases to achieve levels of pH = 7.40 and a PCO_2 = 40 mmHg when the blood is at 37°C. If the hypothermic patient's ABGs are correct at 37°C, then they will be physiologically correct at whatever they might be in the hypothermic or hyperthermic patient. For instance, if the blood gases are normal at 37°C, and read pH = 7.52 and a PCO_2 = 25 at 28°C, then this is the value at which the patient's physiology is optimal for that temperature; so don't attempt to correct it.

Table 19.1

QUICK GUIDE TO INTERPRETATION OF BLOOD GAS RESULTS				
	pH	PaO$_2$ mmHg (kPa)	PaCO$_2$ mmHg (kPa)	Standard HCO$_3$ mmol/l
Normal*	7.35–7.42	90–100 (11.8–13. 2)	35–42 (4.6–5.5)	22–26
Danger	< 7.25	< 60 (< 7.9)	> 45 (> 5.9)	< 16
Critical (moribund)	< 7.121	< 35 (< 4.6)	> 60 (> 7.9)	< 12

*For a normal patient when breathing air.

BLOOD PRESSURE

Errors can occur when measuring blood pressure with a manual blood pressure cuff. To prevent these errors you will need to:
• Explain to the patient what is about to happen.
• Check that the pulse is regular.
• Quickly inflate the cuff to above the expected arterial pressure.
• Estimate the blood pressure by feeling the return of the pulse with your finger on the radial artery.
• Quickly re-inflate the cuff to 30 mmHg above the arterial pressure.
• With the stethoscope over the brachial artery in the cubital fossa, let the cuff deflate no faster than 5 mmHg per second. To be accurate some authorities maintain this should be 2 mmHg per second[2]. however, this is uncomfortable for the patient.

- Listen at the point where the first sound is heard, this is the systolic
  blood pressure. The diastolic pressure is the point at which the sounds
  disappear completely; not where the sounds become muffled.

     Also make sure to:
- use the correct sized cuff;
- keep the mercury manometer at eye level to prevent parallax errors;
- check the blood pressure in both arms if the patient has vascular disease
  or diabetes;
- not allow the mercury column to fall too swiftly as you may pass the
  correct blood pressure between beats.

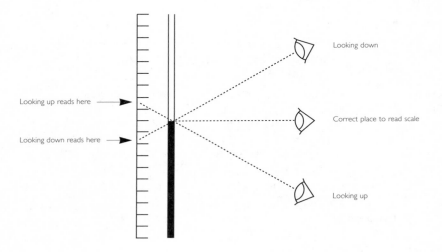

Looking down

Correct place to read scale

Looking up

Looking up reads here

Looking down reads here

How you position a mercury blood pressure machine may cause errors in the readings.

Fig 19.2 Diagram of parallax effect

     False readings occur because:
- the cuff is too narrow or too wide for limb;
- the cuff deflation is either too slow, or too fast;
- the mercury manometer is not at eye level.

     If you are making your own cloth blood pressure cuff covers, then the
bladder length should be at least 80 per cent, and the width at least 40 per
cent, of the circumference of the upper arm.

     In elderly patients, *pseudo-hypertension* may deceive you. The cuff
cannot compress the rigid calcified arterial walls to occlude the blood flow,

so you can still feel the pulse even though the cuff pressure is above the real systolic pressure. Many arteriosclerotic patients have different blood pressures in each arm.

Non-invasive blood pressure

Non-invasive blood pressure using an automated oscillometric monitor, usually called a NBP monitor; which is an abbreviation for non-invasive blood pressure. These are accurate if you are aware of the following points:

- Use the correct cuff size. If it is too large the device will under-read the blood pressure; and if the cuff is too small it will over-read.
- They tend to over-read at low blood pressures, and under-read at high blood pressures.
- They are inaccurate if the pulse is irregular, as with atrial fibrillation, or multiple ventricular ectopic beats.
- If the blood pressure is low they are slow to read and constantly re-cycle.

Invasive-blood pressure

Invasive-blood pressure uses an intra-arterial cannula attached to a transducer. To accurately measure the blood pressure ensure the transducer is level with the isophlebotic point (see page 381). These are commonly thought to be an absolutely accurate measure of continuous blood pressure. However, if the fluid dynamics of the system are not correct errors of 70 per cent, or more, can occur. The catheters must be matched to the transducer and must not be too stiff, too pliant, or too long; so use reputable makes. Check the first few readings with a manual blood pressure machine. Other problems that occur are loss of power supply, incorrect calibration, broken or faulty transducers, failure to correctly level the transducer relative to the patient, or air bubbles in the system.

Do not disturb the dressings around the arterial cannula. If the cannula is accidentally disconnected, put a syringe in the cannula and prepare to set up a new sterile line. If the cannula falls out and you cannot control the bleeding, immediately apply pressure to the site with your gloved hand. If you still cannot control the bleeding then inflate a pressure cuff on the arm to 250 mmHg to act as a tourniquet until help arrives.

If the arterial line crosses the wrist or elbow joint, splint the arm to prevent the cannula kinking.

The incidence of radial artery thrombosis is 2–25 per cent. Factors increasing the risk are[3]:

- large or long cannulas;
- the length of time the cannula is left in the artery;

- prolonged hypotension;
- the use of vasoconstrictor agents;
- accidental injection of drugs into an arterial line.

Accidental arterial injection

Accidental injection of a substance into an artery usually occurs when intravenous injections are attempted in the antecubital fossa, but may occur anywhere, even on the back of the hand. After inserting any needle check to see that bright red blood does not pulse back. If something harmful has been injected down the line the patient will complain of severe pain. In which case do not withdraw the needle, remove the syringe and replace it with a fresh syringe containing normal saline. Flush and then inject procaine 0.2 ml/kg. If the hand or arm turns white; phentolamine 1 mg made up to 10 ml in normal saline may be injected slowly to vasodilate the limb. This can be repeated, and the option of a continuous arterial infusion considered. It may be necessary to perform a brachial plexus, or stellate ganglion block although the results of these manoeuvres are disappointing. Consult a vascular surgeon and for medico-legal reasons keep careful notes of what has happened, and what has been done, and by whom.

CAPNOGRAPHY

Capnographs measure carbon dioxide concentration in the airways by shining infra-red light through samples of expired air, and calculating how much light is absorbed. A microprocessor looks for the highest reading at the end of a breath. It is assumed that this is the concentration of carbon dioxide in the alveoli, hence the other name for these devices; *end tidal CO_2 monitors*. The commonest reason for malfunction is water entering the sampling line.

Although frequently used during anaesthesia, capnography is not routinely used on extubated patients because it is difficult to obtain an undiluted sample of expired air. Capnography swiftly detects some emergencies:
- disconnection from, or malfunction of, a ventilator;
- obstruction of an endotracheal tube;
- a rapid fall in expired PCO_2 due to a fall in cardiac output, or a pulmonary or an air embolism;
- a rapid rise in CO_2 production associated with malignant hyperthermia.

CARDIOPULMONARY CATHETERS (SWAN GANZ CATHETERS®)

Swan Ganz® catheters are balloon tipped catheters used for measuring *pulmonary artery* (PAP), and *pulmonary artery wedge pressures* (PAWP). When the balloon is inflated, the tip floats forward and wedges in a small pulmonary artery blocking the flow of blood. The pressure in this still column of blood in the pulmonary capillaries is measured. This gives valuable information about the filling pressures of the left atrium, and performance of the left heart. They are often used in specialized units in patients with cardiovascular disease, or those having open heart or vascular surgery. Some catheters have a heat detecting thermistor at the tip, which is connected to a computer. If cold saline is injected up stream, the speed at which this saline reaches the tip can be used to calculate the cardiac output.

They measure the following parameters:
• central venous pressure;
• pulmonary artery pressure;
• pulmonary artery wedge pressure, which is an indicator of left ventricular function;

They can also be used to:
• measure cardiac output;
• infuse drugs and fluids;
• determine core temperature;
• sample mixed venous blood;
• derive systemic vascular resistance, cardiac index, and tissue oxygen delivery, and oxygen consumption;
• in newer modifications, continuously sample oxygen, carbon dioxide, and other substances.

Cardiac output

Perfusion status reflects cardiac output. As people come in different sizes, cardiac output is often standardized by calculating the *cardiac index*.

$$\text{Cardiac index} = \frac{\text{cardiac output}}{\text{body surface area}} = \frac{5.0}{1.34} = 3.73 \text{ litre/m}^2$$

Most monitors that measure cardiac output will have the facility to calculate the body surface area from the patient's weight and height.

Pulmonary oedema

Pulmonary oedema is likely to occur in healthy lungs if the wedge pressure is greater than 20–25 mmHg. Pulmonary oedema can occur at normal or lower pressures if the patient is septic, has adult respiratory distress syndrome (ARDS), or very severe hypoproteinaemia.

Problems that may arise during insertion of a Swan Ganz® catheter and appear in the recovery room are:

• carotid or sub clavian artery puncture and haematoma of the neck;
• pneumo- or haemo-thorax;
• catheter kinking, and occasionally intravascular knotting;
• balloon ruptures;
• inappropriate inflation of the balloon can rupture the pulmonary artery;
• cardiac arrhythmias;
• valvular damage or incompetence.

Table 19.2

NORMAL VALUES OF CARDIAC PRESSURES	
Central venous pressure	0–7 mmHg
Pulmonary artery pressures	14–32 mmHg systolic
	4–13 mmHg diastolic
	8–19 mmHg mean
Wedge pressure	6–12 mmHg
Cardiac output	70–100 ml/kg
Cardiac index	2.5–3.6 litres/min/m^2
Pulmonary vascular resistance	700–1500 dyne-sec/cm5
	77–150 kPa-sec/cm5
Systemic vascular resistance	20–120 dyne-sec/cm5
	2–12 kPa-sec/cm5
Oxygen consumption	3.5 ml/kg/min

CENTRAL VENOUS LINES

If you anticipate problems of fluid balance, or the need for potent ionotropes, consider inserting a central venous line. A catheter in the superior vena cava measures right heart filling pressures. In normal patients there is a correlation between right heart and left heart filling pressures, but in cardiac failure this correlation is lost, and there is no correlation whatsoever between the two. To monitor pulmonary artery pressures and left heart performance a Swan Ganz® catheter is needed.

Indications for a central venous line include:

• when peripheral venous access is difficult;

- to guide fluid replacement in trauma or haemorrhagic shock;
- to infuse drugs especially concentrated ionotropes or vasodilators;
- for parenteral nutrition following gastrointestinal surgery;
- in paediatric surgery where accurate fluid replacement is important;
- to monitor the right heart filling pressures, when the cardiovascular system is unstable, such as, after burns or removal of phaeochromocytomas.

The normal value for central venous pressure (CVP) is 0–5 cm of water. Unlike blood pressure which is measured in millimetres of mercury (mmHg), the CVP is recorded in centimetres of water. This is because the traditional way of measuring a CVP is a water column, although special transducers are used in many teaching centres. You need to know the position of the patient's right atrium to measure the CVP. The right atrium is at the level of the isophlebotic line; that is, the mid-axillary line.

How to measure a CVP

The principle involved is to balance the column of water in the manometer tubing with the pressure in the great veins (central venous pressure). To achieve this there must be a continuous column of fluid between the great veins and the manometer.

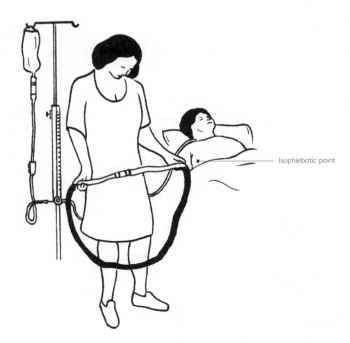

Isophlebotic point

Fig 19.3 How to measure central pressure with reference to the isophlebotic point

Fix the manometer to the central venous catheter and attach it to a drip stand. If you have positioned it correctly the fluid in the manometer should swing freely as the patient breathes. To get the zero point on the manometer level with the patient's isophlebotic line you can either use a carpenter's spirit level, or a closed loop U-tube filled with coloured fluid.

Three way taps can cause confusion:

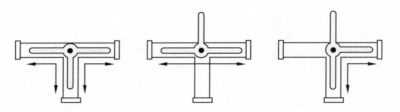

Fig 19.4 Flow with three -way taps

MANAGEMENT
- Pressure recordings as ordered by medical staff.
- Order an erect chest X-ray after insertion to check position, and ensure there is no pneumothorax.
- Monitor blood pressure, pulse and respiratory rate.
- Ensure the zero pressure reference point is at the specified place, usually the mid-axillary line (isophlebotic point). Frequently check the readings with a spirit level, or a loop of tubing partially filled with coloured fluid.
- Keep the line free of air bubbles.
- Have a continuous flowing infusion to ensure the line remains patent.
- Lock all connections to prevent accidental disconnection.

Fig 19.5 Luer® lock

- Maintain strict aseptic care of ports and infusions. Clean the puncture wound with poviodine (Betadine®), dry and dress it with a clear plastic dressing.
- Before you take any reading make sure the fluid in the manometer is swinging normally with the patient's breathing. If it is not swinging, then

the catheter is, either blocked, or in the wrong place. If there are large pressure swings, the catheter tip is probably in the right ventricle; so pull it back a bit.

• Securely fasten the lines to the skin so that they are not accidentally pulled out.

• Warn the patient to notify the nursing staff immediately if the line becomes disconnected.

• Sometimes a wide bore 10 gauge sheath is inserted into a central vein, to give blood at a fast rate.

Use of CVP in a bleeding patient

The CVP is a useful guide to fluid replacement in a bleeding, or traumatized patient. Normally about 3 litres of the blood volume are stored in the floppy walled great veins. There is a further one litre in the arteries, and another litre in the heart and lungs. When a patient bleeds, his blood volume falls. To start with, most of this blood comes from the veins, which gently contract to maintain the pressure inside them.

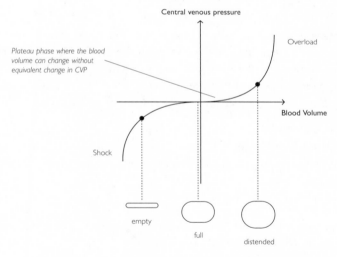

Cross-sectional shape of great veins as they follow the blood volume

Fig 19.6 Diagram of how central venous pressure follows blood volume

The first sign of a low blood volume is a gently falling central venous pressure. After a blood loss of about 500 ml the pulse rate starts to rise, and by the time 800 ml is lost the CVP starts to fall rapidly, this is followed later by a fall in the arterial blood pressure.

As the diagram shows, the CVP does not change as much as the blood volume changes between 0–5 cm H_2O where the graph line is almost flat. In other words you cannot tell whether the veins are almost full or almost empty. So, in a bleeding patient, it is better to aim to raise the patient's CVP to 5 cm H_2O. You may be surprised by how much fluid is needed, but you are unlikely to give too much fluid if the CVP does not go over 10 cm H_2O.

Interpretation of results: This is a rough guide.

1. CVP low and blood pressure low:
   • hypovolaemia;
   • shock.
2. CVP high and blood pressure low:
   • cardiac failure;
   • cardiac tamponade;
   • venous obstruction, such as pulmonary embolism.
3. CVP high and blood pressure high:
   • fluid overload.

Complications of Central Line Insertion

Pneumothorax

Pneumothorax occurs in 2–5 per cent of subclavian insertions, and in less than 1 per cent if the line is inserted through the internal jugular vein. If a chest x-ray shows that the lung has collapsed with greater than 3 cm between the lung and the chest wall, or the patient is short of breath, you will need to insert an underwater thoracic drain (see page 31).

Arterial puncture

If this occurs press firmly on the site for 10 minutes. Monitor the patient's blood pressure, pulse and breathing. Watch for signs of continuing haemorrhage.

Air embolism

Air embolism occurs if the lines become disconnected. The incidence is under 0.5 per cent; but can be fatal (see page 140).

If you find a collapsed patient with a disconnected central venous catheter, assume the patient has an air embolism.

Other problems are catheter sepsis, thromboembolism, brachial plexus injuries, damage to the thoracic duct, catheter kinking (or even knotting), pericardial tamponade, and cardiac arrhythmias.

ELECTROCARDIOGRAPHY (See also Chapter 14)

About half the arrhythmias detected in the recovery room are 'human detected' and the other half are 'monitor detected'. The ECG does not detect serious physiological changes, such as hypoxia, hypercarbia, and hypotension. Indeed a normal ECG in a dangerous situation may lead to unwarranted complacency[4].

A normal resting ECG does not exclude coronary artery disease, but is reassuring as adverse cardiac events occur in only 2 per cent of patients with a normal preoperative ECG; compared with 23 per cent if the pre-operative ECG is abnormal[5].

Studies have found that myocardial ischaemia and cardiac arrhythmias are common in the recovery room particularly if the patient has pre-existing factors[6]. We monitor patients over the age of 50 years. A good rule is to monitor if in doubt.

Guidelines to select those at risk could include
1. Patient factors:
   * known or suspected cardiac disease;
   * patient on drugs affecting the heart, such as digoxin;
   * hypertension, or systolic blood pressures greater than 160 mmHg;
   * age over 50 years;
   * peripheral vascular disease;
   * major intercurrent medical illness, such as diabetes;
   * pulse greater than 100 beats per minute or less than 60 beats per minute;
   * smokers over the age of 35 years;
   * lung disease;
   * oximeter reading of arterial saturation of 95 per cent or less;
   * abnormal perfusion status;
   * anaemia;
   * electrolyte imbalance;
   * obese patients.
2. Surgical factors:
   * thoracic operations;
   * emergency major surgery;
   * head injuries and neurosurgery;
   * patients with burns.
3. Anaesthetic factors:
   * arrhythmias during the anaesthetic;
   * severe pain in patients over the age of 45 years;
   * hypothermia;

- patients from intensive care unit;
- large blood transfusion;
- improperly reversed muscle relaxation.
  Practical hints about ECG monitoring
1. Post a diagram on the notice board so that every one knows exactly where to place the sticky ECG electrodes. Particularly lead V5, which is often positioned in an exotic location.
2. If serious arrhythmias, or signs of ischaemia, occur then do a 12-lead ECG so the trace can be kept and analysed later.
3. The commonest reasons for a poor quality ECG trace are:
   - The electrode has poor contact with skin. Shave and clean the skin with an alcohol swab. Re-apply an electrode.
   - The patient is moving, or shivering;
   - The leads are faulty;
   - The leads are picking up interference; usually because they are lying across power cables, or other metal objects. This can be seen as 50 cycle AC hum making the trace blurred or smudged. If you look at the trace closely you will see a tight sine wave pattern. Solve the problem by moving the leads away from the source of interference. Coiling the lead may also help.
4. Make sure your screen and print-outs are properly calibrated.
   On the vertical axis 1 cm = 1 millivolt; and on the horizontal axis 1 large square = 0.2 seconds.
5. To reliably detect ST changes, use the monitor in diagnostic rather than monitor mode.

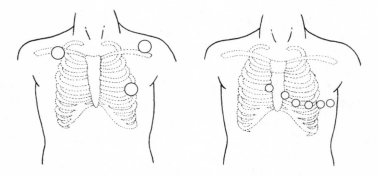

Modified CM5 position for the ECG electrodes   Position of ECG electrodes for a 12 lead trace

Fig 19.7 Placement of electrodes

Ischaemia

To detect ischaemic ST changes the modified CM5 lead is the most useful. Place the left arm electrode over the fifth left intercostal space in the mid axillary line, and turn the 'lead select' switch to Lead I.

Rhythm lead

Lead II is the best lead to detect changes in rhythm, and to view the P wave.

NEUROMUSCULAR BLOCKADE

NERVE STIMULATORS

Put two skin electrodes over the ulnar nerve near the wrist joint. Place the negative electrode distally. Look for a twitch of the thumb as the nerve is stimulated. It should jerk toward the palm of the hand as flexor pollicis brevis is stimulated. Ignore movement in the other fingers because the current directly stimulates the muscles so they will curl even if the nerve itself is not stimulated.

Two stimuli are given, a *train-of-four* twitches or a *tetanic stimulus* with a whole run of stimuli close together.

Using a train-of-four in the unparalysed patient causes the thumb to twitch equally all four times. The ratio of the fourth response of a train-of-four to the first response is a measure of recovery from neuromuscular blockade. The fourth twitch disappears when there is about 75% neuromuscular blockade still present. The third when there is about 80%, the second when there is 90% paralysis. Absence of all four corresponds to complete paralysis. Neostigmine and atropine will not adequately reverse neuromuscular blockade if two twitches or less are seen in a train of four. Three or four twitches need to be seen before the patient is safe to be reversed with neostigmine and atropine.

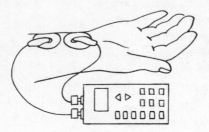

Fig 19.8 Where to place electrodes

Frequent use of a nerve stimulator during an operation may cause post-operative paraesthesia with a feeling of 'pins-and-needles' around the little finger and down the ulnar side of the hand. This resolves within a few hours.

If a patient is still unconcious and you suspect incomplete reversal of their muscle relaxing drugs, such as vecuronium or suxamethonium, a nerve stimulator can be used to gauge residual neuromuscular blockade.

Do not use a nerve stimulator on a conscious patient because it is painful. The best test of proper reversal of muscle relaxants is to ask the patient to lift his head from the pillow. Patients must be able to sustain a 15 second head lift before they are discharged from the recovery room. Other tests of muscle power are straight leg lift, coughing, and hand grip. To test hand grip offer only two of your fingers, otherwise you may be hurt.

PULSE OXIMETERS[7]

Pulse oximeters are the most important monitors to be developed in the last ten years. They should be available in every recovery room.

PULSE OXIMETER

Pulse oximeters measure the differential absorption of red, and infrared light, by oxygenated and deoxygenated haemoglobin. A light emitting diode located in a finger tip, or ear lobe probe sends light waves through the test site, and monitors the reflected wavelengths coming back as the blood passes through the capillaries. During systole, the extra surge of arterial blood absorbs additional light, and the reflected intensity falls. In this way the pulse can be detected. The difference in intensities is sensed by a photodetector in the probe, and the signal is fed into a microprocessor, that calculates the saturation, and pulse rate, and displays the reading on a screen.

Providing a patient is well perfused the measurements are accurate. Use a pulse oximeter on all patients until their protective reflexes return, and they have oxygen saturations greater than 96 per cent when breathing room air.

Causes of erroneous readings[8]:
• long fingernails and nail polish;
• poor peripheral perfusion with hypothermia, shock or vasoconstrictor drugs;
• ambient light (particularly infra-red lamps used to warm infants) entering a poorly fitting probe;
• bilirubin in heavily jaundiced patients;
• movement;
• iodine containing skin preparation;
• carboxyhaemoglobin gives a false high reading;
• methaemoglobin caused by prilocaine or nitroglycerine causes a trend toward 80 per cent saturation irrespective of the true haemoglobin saturation;

• dyes, such as methylene blue give a false low reading.

Some pulse oximeters run on rechargeable batteries which last about 10 hours. Remember to charge them every night for use the next day.

A useful way to protect the delicate sensory probe, is to encase it in plastic foam. This also excludes ambient light, which is a cause erroneous readings.

The saturation of haemoglobin can be used to calculate the patient's arterial PaO_2. The relationship between haemoglobin saturation and PaO_2 is described by the oxygen saturation curve (see page 309).

Pitfalls occur in use of the oximeter, because there is a false belief that a saturation is greater than 90% means the patient is not hypoxic. As the table below shows the PaO_2 depends on the pH of the blood.

Table 19.3

THE SATURATION METER AND ITS CORRELATION WITH PaO_2			
Oxygen saturation	PaO_2 at pH 7.25	PaO_2 at pH 7.40	PaO_2 at pH 7.55
60	36 < critical level	31	24
70	44	37 < critical level	28
80	53	45	34
81	55	46	35
82	56	48	36 < critical level
83	58	49	37
84	59	50	38
85	61 < danger level	52	39
86	63	53	40
87	65	55	41
88	67	57	43
89	69	59	45
90	72	61 < danger level	47
91	75	64	49
92	79	67	51
93	83	70	54
94	88	75	57
95	94	80	61 < danger level
96	102	87	66
97	113	96	73
98	129	109	83
99	157	134	101
100	241	204	155

Figures are calculated from Kelman modification of the Hill Equation for the oxygen dissociation curve[9].

In summary
Once the saturation falls to 90% the symptoms of hypoxia accelerate. A PaO$_2$ less than 60 mmHg (7.9 kPa) is dangerous, and a PaO$_2$ less than 35 mmHg (4.6 kPa) is potentially lethal in an otherwise well patient.

RESPIRATION MONITORS

Some monitors measure respiratory rate from changes in the voltages of the ECG.

There are also sensory pads on which neonates and young children lay to detect apnoeic periods. These should be used postoperatively, on any infant under the age of 12 months who was born prematurely.

TEMPERATURE

Infra-red tympanic thermometers[10]
Infra-red tympanic thermometers are the best and easiest way to accurately measure a patient's temperature. They respond rapidly, and measure the core temperature, because the tympanic membrane shares the same blood supply as the hypothalamus, which is where the body's thermoregulatory control centre is located.

Thermocouples
Another way of measuring patient body temperature is with an electronic thermocouple. These are cheap, robust, re-useable and reliable. Rectal probes are the most convenient. Never put thermocouple probes into patients' ears as it is easy to traumatize the delicate aural canal or tympanic membrane.

Thermometers
The normal clinical mercury thermometer is of little use in the recovery room, because they break easily, and do not measure temperatures below about 36°C. Axillary temperatures are totally useless in postoperative patients. Keep a special low reading rectal thermometer available for detecting hypothermia.

Should the patient's temperature rise above normal, exclude malignant hyperthermia. It has a high mortality unless quickly treated (see page 174). Other causes include thyroid crises, blood transfusion reactions and pre-existing febrile states.

VENTILATORY VOLUMES

The patient's tidal air exchange can be measured by a respirometer, (sometimes called an anemometer). To prevent expired air escaping it needs a tightly fitting mask, laryngeal airway or endotracheal tube to get accurate results. The two types available are Wright's Respirometer™ and the Drager Volumeter™.

VOLUME METERS

WRIGHT'S RESPIROMETER®

In this device gas passes over a two-bladed rotor which spins to measure the flow passing through it. These instruments, are very accurate, but are also very fragile. Look down the inlet port and you will see the paper-thin metal aerofoil blades. These aerofoils are easily torn by a moderate blast of air. If someone blows hard into this type of respirometer, the blades will shear off and the tiny cogs will be stripped. They are very expensive to repair or replace. To test a Wright's respirometer, wave it through the air, the dial will indicate an airflow.

DRAGER VOLUMETER®

This device is much more robust, a bit more bulky, but not quite so accurate. Two lightweight meshing rotors measure the volume of air passing over them. It has a useful timing device which stops measurement after one minute has elapsed, making it easy to get consistent readings. If necessary this device may be autoclaved.

Both instruments tend to under read at low flow rates and over read at high flow rates.

X-RAY

Portable X-ray may be needed for the following:
• respiratory distress;
• pneumothorax;
• following central venous line insertion;
• heart failure;
• suspected aspiration;
• following nephrectomy where there is a chance the pleural space has been entered.

1. Holland R. (1993). *Anaesthesia and Intensive Care,* 21: 501
2. 'The Management of Hypertension—A consensus statement' *Medical Journal of Australia,* (1994) supp. 160: S1–S16

3. Bright E., Baines D. B. (1993). *Anaesthesia and Intensive Care,* 21: 351–3
4. Ludbrook G. L., Russell W. J., *et al.* (1993). *Anaesthesia and Intensive Care,* 21: 558–64
5. Carliner N. H., Fisher M. L., *et al.* (1985). *American Journal of Cardiology,* 56: 51–8
6. Hollenberg M., Managano D. T., *et al.* (1992).
   Journal of American Medical Association, 268: 205–9
7, 8. Alexander C. M., Teller L. E. (1989). *Anaesthesia and Analgesia,* 68: 368–76
9. Kenny GNC. (1979). *British Journal of Anaesthesia,* 51: 793–96
10. Edge G., Morgan M. (1993). *Anaesthesia,* 48: 604–7

20. EQUIPMENT IN THE RECOVERY ROOM

(arranged in alphabetical order)

Airways - Nasopharyngeal (see page 404)

Airways - Oropharyngeal

Guedal airways are made either of clear plastic or black rubber with a metal flange inserted in the mouth piece to stop the patient clenching his teeth and obstructing the airflow. The black rubber airways are better and longer lasting. The plastic ones tend to deform after a while.

Size 4   for huge men.
Size 3   for adult men.
Size 2   for women, and men without teeth, and for children down to the age of 18 months.
Size 1   for children under the age of 18 months.
Size 0   small for neonates.
Size 00   tiny.

In the elderly, especially if they have no teeth, try using a smaller rather than a larger size to maintain the airway.

Batteries

Laryngoscopes, torches, and clocks use disposable alkaline batteries. Alkaline 1.5-volt batteries come in four sizes AA, A, C, and D. Some apparatus uses 9-volt batteries. Have a ready supply of batteries on hand. Store them in a dry airtight container in a cool place.

Rechargeable batteries. Some apparatus, such as a defibrillator, use rechargeable batteries. To make sure they are in good working order, charge them to the recommended levels, and for the recommended times. Do not overcharge these batteries.

To extend their life, some types of rechargeable batteries periodically need to be completely discharged, and then slightly overcharged. Properly maintained they will give service for 3 to 5 years, or more than 1000 charges. Include this procedure on your regular maintenance program.

Blood Pressure Monitors

Mercury sphygmomanometers with solid mountings are more reliable, robust and easier to repair than anaeroid devices. Choose ones with a bright (preferably yellow) scale, that is easy to see from a distance. Mount them at eye level to prevent parallax errors when reading the scale.

Anaeroid ones have a clock-face type dial. These are easier to read, but to remain accurate need recalibrating every 3 months. In humid areas the mechanism rusts quickly.

In addition to standard cuffs, you will need a broader cuff for obese adults, and a narrower cuff for children and thin adults. Wrap around cuffs are more durable than Velcro® or hook ones, and a local tailor can make you spares. In the tropics the rubber bladders perish quickly. Keep a supply of spares in an airtight container in cool dry place.

Non-invasive blood pressure monitors (NBP) are popular because they release staff to attend to other matters while monitoring the blood pressure at regular intervals, and give warnings if the blood pressure rises or falls beyond set limits. Well known makes are reliable and robust.

Invasive blood pressure measurement involves inserting a small cannula into an artery (usually the radial artery), and connecting it to a pressure transducer with plastic catheters. The signal is processed; and systolic, diastolic, and mean blood pressures along with the pulse wave form are displayed on a screen. Catheters can be either too soft or too hard; this interferes with the fluid dynamics of the system. With incorrectly matched catheters, fluid dynamic errors may be as much as 80 per cent. In other words the monitor may show a systolic blood pressure of 240 mmHg when the correct blood pressure is only 160 mmHg. Make sure that your lines and cannulas conform to the manufacturer's recommendations.

Blood Warmers

Blood warmers help prevent hypothermia.

Water-bath blood warmers heat the blood by passing it through a coil immersed in water maintained at a constant temperature. The temperature of the water bath must never exceed 40°C. Their major disadvantages are that water slops out if the bath is knocked or tilted, and the coil slows the rate of transfusions.

Dry heat blood warmers warm the blood by passing it close to a heated plate or cylinder. Recently the Atom™ Blood Warmer (BW385L), has been introduced. It is the first of a new generation of blood warmers that do not require dedicated disposables and, the makers claim, will accept any giving set.

It is difficult to run a rapid transfusion through a standard blood warmer. To overcome this problem there are two expensive systems available, the Level 1™ delivers 500 ml/min, and Rapid Infusion System™ 1500 ml/min.

Make sure your blood warmer has some means of indicating the temperature, a thermostat control, and preferably an alarm.

Bronchoscopes

Keep a sterile bronchoscopy tray with both adult and paediatric bronchoscopes available in the theatre suite. Make sure that the light source, cables, oxygen supply, suction devices and grasping forceps are all compatible, and in working order. Check this on your regular maintenance program.

Fibreoptic bronchoscopes require special care and are not as useful for retrieving foreign objects from the lower airways as a rigid bronchoscope.

Central Venous Lines

Central venous catheters should be radio-opaque. Do not buy the ones that are introduced through needles, because the needles can cut the cannula leaving the cut end in the vein. The best types are inserted using a vein dilator and a Seldinger wire. Manometers for central venous pressure measurement are disposable. An improvised manometer mounting board can be made with a half metre ruler.

Clocks

A clock with a clear-sweep second hand should be visible from all over the recovery room. These are cheap, readily available and run on batteries. Include battery replacement as part of your routine maintenance program. Use the 24-hour clock routinely for noting times on charts or records.

For example

midnight	=	00.00 hr
10. 20 am	=	10.20 hr
Noon	=	12.00 hr
8 pm	=	20.30 hr

Defibrillator

The defibrillator is an essential piece of equipment to treat cardiac arrest and some arrhythmias. In a small hospital share one defibrillator with the whole theatre block. Keep it with the resuscitation trolley in the recovery room. There are many types, but the most useful are portable and light weight, run on mains power or rechargeable batteries, and have their own internal ECG monitor. Include the care of the defibrillator on your regular maintenance program.

Since defibrillators put out as much as 7000 volts at 400 joules they are dangerous if not handled properly. Staff have been electrocuted while demonstrating its use on each other. Practice using the defibrillator but not while it is charged up. Defibrillators need special conductive jelly or conductive pads. Make sure they are available. In hot climates slightly moisten the pads with saline if they are dry. Do not allow the saline to leave the area of the pad or a short circuit may result. Do not use a non-conductive jelly (such as KY Jelly®) or water because it will cause deep burns during cardioversion.

As well as treating cardiac arrest, defibrillators are used to restore sinus rhythm in a patient with atrial fibrillation, and some supraventricular tachycardias. Reversion of these rhythms uses low-energy pulses. The shock pulse from the defibrillator needs to reach the heart at the peak of the R wave on the ECG. Most defibrillators have the facility to detect the peak of the R wave, and will deliver the shock pulse at the right time regardless of when the paddles are discharged. To use this facility switch the defibrillator to *synchronized mode*.

ECG and Patient Physiological Monitors

There are many ECG monitors on the market. It is wise to order them from the same manufacturer who supplies other monitoring apparatus to the hospital. This gives you greater bargaining power, and eases servicing and maintenance. Desirable features include a clear display, which can be read from 2 to 3 metres away, audible pulse monitoring, and pulse rate display, a cascade mechanism to view up to the last 30 seconds of trace, and a screen freeze function to allow analysis of a trace pattern. It is also helpful to have a paper trace readout to record arrhythmias for later analysis. This is an expensive option, and is not essential if your budget is tight.

Monitors are becoming increasingly sophisticated, and many have multiple functions enabling ECG, oximeters, non-invasive blood pressure and various other parameters to be measured and displayed. Some have menu driven displays and colours to show different parameters on the screen.

Ordering electronic equipment for humid climates?
Make sure that the components are sealed against moisture and mould.

Keep spare cables and sensors in stock. Be careful not to bend the cables, particularly near their sockets. When they are not in use coil them loosely and store them carefully.

The ECG is not a good monitor for hypoxia, and it is not a substitute for a pulse oximeter. By the time hypoxic damage is evident on the ECG, much damage will have occurred.

Mobile phones have been reported to interfere with monitoring equipment, and some hospitals have banned their use within the hospital precincts. This is excessively cautious, in fact, analogue phones are unlikely to cause any problems. The more powerful digital phones cause interference if used within 2 metres of a monitor[1].

Emergency Trolley

In the USA these are called *emergency carts* or *crash carts*. Recovery rooms must have a well designed and equipped emergency trolley ready for immediate use. They should carry all the drugs and equipment needed for the resuscitation of any collapsed patient. Keep a laminated plastic sheet, listing all the required items, tied to the trolley. Restock immediately after use. Discourage lazy staff from using this trolley as a source of stock for routine procedures. It is wise to leave drugs in their boxes until they are needed. Many mistakes have been made in selecting an emergency drug by inaccurate recognition of an ampoule's shape and colour. Drugs should be stored in alphabetical order of their generic names. Keep a list of their trade names and generic names with them.

Endotracheal Tubes

Clear plastic endotracheal tubes are preferable. You will need a range of sizes for different ages. Sizes are measured on their internal diameter. Children under the age of ten usually do not require cuffed tubes, however above this age cuffs are needed for a good gas seal, and to prevent fluid entering the lower airways.

The distance from the teeth to the midpoint of the trachea[2]

$$= \frac{\text{height (cm)}}{10} + 2$$

add 3 cm to allow space to tie or fix the tube.

Table 20.1

ENDOTRACHEAL TUBE SIZES	
NEONATES	
< I kg	2. 5 mm
I–3. 5 kg	3. 0 mm
3. 5– 6. 5 kg	3. 5 mm
INFANTS	
10 kg	4. 0 mm
12 kg	4. 5 mm
CHILDREN TO 16 YEARS OF AGE	
$\dfrac{age}{4} + 4$ = size of tube	
ADULTS	
60 kg	8. 0 mm
70 kg	9. 0 mm

In the larger tubes a 'Murphy eye', which is a second hole near the distal end of the tube, prevents occlusion if the tip becomes obstructed.

Check the tubes you buy are non-irritant. They should have either 'IT' or 'Z 79' printed on the side of the tube. If you are still using rubber endotracheal tubes, periodically check them to see that they are not perished. Throw away the old metal connectors and use well-made tight-fitting plastic 15 mm connectors.

Face masks (see page 407)

Keep a full range of anaesthetic face masks on the emergency trolley. Everyone working in the recovery room must be able to bag and mask a patient until help arrives.

Glucose Meters

Glucose meters are small electronic devices that accurately measure blood glucose using a drop of blood from a finger or heel prick. Some machines are simpler to use than others. Keep the instructions on how to use the device with the meter. They use special reagent strips; store them in a cool dry place. Do not take blood from the toes or feet of diabetics, or patients with peripheral vascular disease because they are likely to get infected. Serious ulcers can cause the patient to lose a limb.

Haemoglobinometers

These compact, cheap and accurate electronic devices read the level of haemoglobin on a reagent strip. Most of them are easy to use. Microcuvettes used in some makes are damaged by humidity giving inaccurate results[3].

Humidifiers

Humidity is a measure of the amount of water vapour present in a gas. Humidifiers increase the amount of water vapour in the inhaled gases, helping prevent the tracheobroncheal mucosa from drying out, and preserving the action of surfactant in lowering surface tension within the alveolus. Humidification is especially important in those with acute or chronic respiratory disorders, especially smokers.

Condenser humidifiers (such as the Humid Vent®) are disposable and weigh about 40 grams. They provide effective heat and moisture exchange, and help prevent the bronchial mucosa from drying out. They are attached to the upper end of an endotracheal tube and are often used during anaesthetics. As the patient breathes out, the expired water vapour collects in the baffles of the humidifier.

When the patient breathes in, the dry air rushes past the moisture-laden baffles and partially saturates with water vapour. These devices are only useful if the patient is receiving ventilatory support. Do not leave them on a patient who is spontaneously breathing through an endotracheal tube or laryngeal mask because they easily become blocked with sputum and may totally obstruct the patient's breathing.

Special condenser humidifiers are available for tracheostomies. If their baffles become clogged with sputum the end blows off so that the airway cannot obstruct.

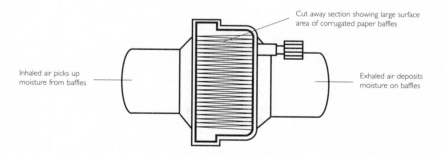

Cut away section showing large surface area of corrugated paper baffles

Inhaled air picks up moisture from baffles

Exhaled air deposits moisture on baffles

Fig 20.2 Condenser humidifier

Heated humidifiers are useful to warm hypothermic patients who are being ventilated. They deliver gas at 37–40°C at a relative humidity of 100 per cent. By humidifying gas in the trachea they prevent drying of the mucosa, preserve ciliary function, and keep the mucus fluid. The ones designed for ventilated patients are expensive. Fill them with sterile water because tap water may contain pathogens such as Legionella.

Temperatures greater than 42°C will cause tracheal burns, so most humidifiers have sensors near the patient's airway to warn of overheating.

Heated humidifiers require a lot of nursing attention. Make sure you have a service guarantee, proper instructions, and a service book with exploded diagrams showing all the parts, and how they fit together.

Cheap, compact heated humidifiers are available for the spontaneously breathing patient.

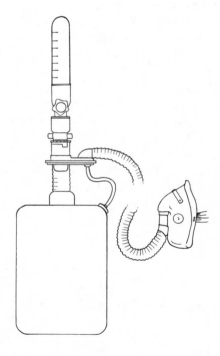

Fig 20.3 Aquapack®

Bubble-through humidifiers, where gas is passed through cold water, are barely effective. Use only sterile water. Tap water is a good source of aerosol infection especially in warmer climates.

Infusion Sets

Special infusion sets are available for blood transfusions with 120 micron filters. There are several variations in the giving sets available. A useful type has a squeeze pump incorporated into the line for rapid transfusion. A Y-giving set for blood or platelet transfusion is available. These sets have an internal diameter of 3.2 mm. Large-bore trauma sets 5.72 mm internal diameter are available for rapid transfusion.

Infusion Pumps, Syringe Drivers, and Drip Set Regulators.

Syringe drivers (such as the Atom®, Graseby®, Ohmeda® and Terumo®) use the turn of a screw to deliver small accurate volumes of fluid from a syringe. They are useful for giving precise amounts of concentrated drug. At flow rates under 10 ml per hour most have a slow start up time, and it may be as long as 10 minutes before the pump is delivering a steady flow. Inadvertant drug delivery is a risk from gravitational syphoning and also if an obstructed line is suddenly released.[4] Obtain a sturdy pump, adaptable to different syringes. Try to use the syringe recommended by the makers.

Fatal mistakes have been made because syringe drivers have been set at the wrong flow rate. The most frequent error is wrongly setting the decimal point. A good syringe driver has clearly marked figures. Two trained personnel should independently check the drugs, dilutions and the pump settings.

Infusion pumps (such as the Imed®) are drip rate regulators. These deliver a set number of drips, or millilitres per hour, through an intravenous line. Infusion pumps need a dedicated intravenous line. If anything else is to run through that line, a one way valve must be inserted to prevent back-flow. Multilumen central venous catheters are useful for running up to three separate infusions through a single intravenous catheter. Problems with infusion pumps include unintentional delivery if they are not set up correctly.[5]

A useful alternative to an infusion pump is a Dial-a-Flow®. These cheap, disposable, small drip set regulators are ideal for those recovery rooms who only occasionally need a precisely controlled infusions rates. Plug one into an intravenous infusion set, follow the instructions and you will find they are accurate enough for most infusions.

Laryngeal Masks

Laryngeal masks were introduced into general anaesthetic practice in 1989 and are justifiably popular. It is far easier to maintain an airway with a laryngeal mask than with a normal rubber face mask. They are inserted through the mouth and fit like a hood over the larynx. A cuff is then inflated to achieve a loose seal in the pharynx.

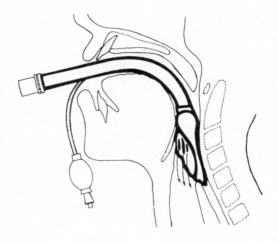

Fig 20.4 Laryngeal mask in situ

Advantages are that they:
• maintain a good airway;
• are easy to use;
• are atraumatic and do not irritate the upper airway;
• can be used with a CO_2 analyser;
• can be used in patients who are difficult to intubate;
• do not require muscle relaxants to insert;
• are less likely to cause sore throats, coughing or bucking than an endotracheal tube;
• are reusable after sterilization.
    Disadvantages are that they:
• require constant skilled supervision;
• do not protect the airway against vomiting or regurgitation of stomach contents;
• are expensive;
• with attempted ventilation they may fill the stomach with gas under tension;
• are unsuitable for fat patients who frequently have hiatus hernias, and may regurgitate gastric contents.

The laryngeal mask does not prevent regurgitation
and must only be used in fasted patients.

Hints for their use[6]
- Use a 20 ml syringe for inflating and deflating the cuff.
- A patient emerging from anaesthesia is likely to clamp his jaws shut, bite the airway and obstruct it. Fold a piece of gauze and use it to prevent the patient biting down on the tube. There is not enough room for both a laryngeal mask and a Guedal airway in most patients.
- The laryngeal mask can be left in place while the patient is being transferred to the recovery room.
- Where possible recover patients lying on either side in the coma position.
- To give oxygen attach a light T-piece made out of corrugated plastic tubing to the mask (see Fig. 20.8).
- Wait for the patient to take out his own laryngeal mask. If he coughs or gags on the mask remove it for him. Check to see no fluid is in the pharynx or mouth that could be aspirated.
- Be careful not to rip the laryngeal mask past the teeth, or you may tear it.
- Laryngeal masks can be used to intubate patients who have difficult airways. Insert either a small endotracheal tube, or a fibre optic bronchoscope down the lumen of the mask and through the larynx.

LARYNGEAL MASKS		
Sizes		**cuff inflation**
size 1	neonate	2–4 ml
size 2	small child	10 ml
size 2.5	large child	15 ml
size 3	small adult	20 ml
size 4	large adult	30 ml

Laryngeal masks sometimes do not sit very well in babies, probably because they have short fat necks, and not much room in their pharnyx. Do not persist if the mask keeps riding up, take it out and replace it with a Guedal airway.

Cleaning and sterilization
- Put the dirty laryngeal mask straight into a bowl or jug of water. Dried secretions are difficult to wash off.

- Soak the mask thoroughly in soapy water and use a bottle brush to gently clean the lumen. Rinse it thoroughly in clean water.
- Do not use glutaraldehyde (Cidex®), formaldehyde or ethylene oxide. Laryngeal masks may be autoclaved at low pressures and temperatures. Do not use the high-pressure high-temperature autoclave. To prevent the cuff from bursting as it is heated, deflate the mask almost completely before autoclaving.

Laryngoscopes

Many companies sell laryngoscopes, but unfortunately there is no standardization in design so that parts of one make of laryngoscope are not interchangeable with other models. There are dozens of shapes, sizes and designs, some made of plastic, and others of metal. When you are buying laryngoscopes for your recovery room, buy the same make and model as the rest of the hospital. This means parts can be interchanged.

Choose a type with a detachable blade that can be easily washed and autoclaved if necessary. Do not autoclave blades if they have a fibreoptic light cable because it will be destroyed. Handles rust easily so do not autoclave them; just remove the batteries, wash the outside and dry it carefully. Sometimes the electrical contact between the blade and the contact on the handle becomes corroded. Clean it with a piece of steel wool until the brass just shines. The strike strip from a box of matches is another useful abrasive to clean the contacts.

Check each day that the light is bright and white. If the light is dim or yellow check that the contacts are clean and shiny and that the batteries are fresh. A dim light is not due to a faulty bulb; they either work or they do not. Keep a good supply of spare bulbs on hand because they blow out easily; especially if the laryngoscope is knocked or dropped.

Most useful of the blades are:
- The Mackintosh curved blade. It comes in three sizes child, standard, and large and is the most commonly used blade for adult use. The standard sized (medium) blade is satisfactory for most needs, but have at least one of each of the other blades available.
- Kessel blade for fat patients with short necks. Have at least one of these available.
- Paediatric blades for infants are straight. Choose one with the light near the tip such as the Warne™ or Weston™ blade.
- To complete the range it is useful to have a right handed blade available.

Nasopharyngeal Airways[7]

It is worthwhile having a range of these available. They are useful in those adults whose airways are difficult to maintain. Size 5, 6 and 7 will cover most needs. Commercially available nasopharyngeal airways are made of soft plastic with a flange to prevent them slipping in too far. They can, however, be made by cutting a 15 cm length of an old soft silastic endotracheal tube. Push a safety pin through the outer end so that the tube cannot disappear into the nose. Lubricate well and insert by pushing them gently straight back, parallel with the floor of the nose. Do not push them upwards.

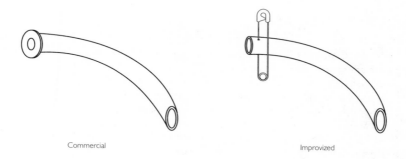

Commercial   Improvized

Fig 20.5 Nasopharyngeal airways

Nerve Stimulator

Nerve stimulators are useful to assess the degree and type of neuromuscular block in patients who remain paralysed after the end of an anaesthetic. (Nerve Stimulators, page 387.)

Non-reflux Valves

These should be fitted to the side part of infusion sets (drips) so that drugs can be given intravenously without the need to use a needle. This will reduce the chance of needlestick injury.

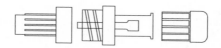

Fig 20.6 Non-reflux valve

Oxygen Concentrators

In regions where bottled oxygen is expensive or difficult to obtain *oxygen concentrators* can provide an economical supply of nearly pure oxygen from air. If you are working in an isolated hospital, oxygen concentrators are a most worthwhile proposition.

A small unit suitable for the recovery room will produce 3 to 5 litres at about 5 PSI of more than 90% pure oxygen per minute. The compressors in these units run on mains electric current but in emergencies they will run on the output from a small generator.

OXYGEN CONCENTRATORS

Air is basically a mixture of two gases: 21% oxygen and 79% nitrogen. A small compressor blows air at about 1000 kPa (20 pounds per square inch (PSI)) through a canister of artificial zeolite (a form of aluminium silicate) which acts as a molecular sieve. The nitrogen molecules are trapped on its surface and oxygen passes on to a storage tank. After about 20 seconds the zeolite sieve becomes saturated with nitrogen, and the supply of compressed air is automatically diverted to a second canister where the process is repeated. This gives a constant output of oxygen. While the pressure in the second canister is at 20 PSI the pressure in the first is reduced to zero. The nitrogen then comes off the zeolite, and is released to the atmosphere.

The World Health Organization has set down minimum standards of performance for oxygen concentrators under extreme conditions of heat, humidity, vibration and atmospheric pollution. The Puritan Bennett 'Companion' (Model 492 A), the Healthdyne (Model BX 5000), and the DeVilbiss (Model DeVO/MC44) are the first three oxygen concentrators to successfully meet all these standards. These concentrators are easy to use; the controls are simply an on/off switch and a flow meter. There is a pressure alarm which sounds when the unit is first turned on. If it sounds during use it usually means the filters need changing.

Oxygen Cylinders

There are four sizes of oxygen cylinders normally available:
G cylinder contains 7000 litres = 7 cubic metres (200–260 cubic feet);
E cylinder contains 3500 litres = 3.5 cubic metres (100–130 cubic feet);
D cylinder contains 1400 litres = 1.4 cubic metres (40–50 cubic feet);
C cylinder contains 400 litres = 0.4 cubic metres (12–15 cubic feet);

The gas in the cylinders is at extremely high pressure (120000 kPa or 2000 lb per square inch). Handle the cylinders carefully, Do not drop them, they have been known to explode with devastating effects similar to a bomb. Chain large cylinders upright so they cannot fall over. Store them in a cool place well away from direct sunlight. Do not accept delivery if they show signs of rust or the neck is damaged.

Make sure you have the right key to turn them on and off. Keep a supply of spare keys available. Cylinders need to be cracked before use. To crack a cylinder turn it on gently for an instant before connecting to the apparatus. This blows any dust or grit out of the neck of the cylinder that could otherwise damage the apparatus. Do not crack cylinders near inflammable or explosive gases. Oxygen is neither explosive nor flammable, but it vigorously supports combustion.

Oxygen Delivery Devices

Fixed oxygen delivery masks (Hudson®, McGraw®, Airlife®) deliver an oxygen air mixture. The masks are designed to give fixed percentages of oxygen. Oxygen flows through a small hole, called a venturi, entraining air. The concentration remains roughly fixed.

The standard oxygen mask gives about:
• 35% oxygen at a flow rate of 4 litres a minute;
• 50% oxygen at a flow rate of 6 litres a minute;
• 60% oxygen at a flow rate of 10 litres per minute.

At flow rates less than 4.5 litres per minute some re-breathing occurs. The masks do not deliver the intended oxygen concentration if the patient is taking deep breaths. For over-breathing patients increase the oxygen flow rate to 10–14 litres per minute. A tight fit is not necessary because the high flow rate constantly replenishes the oxygen supply.

Masks should be made of clear plastic so you can see the colour of the patient's lips. Do not purchase coloured masks because these obscure cyanosis. Masks can be washed, thoroughly cleaned and used again. Do not autoclave them because they melt.

Nasal prongs may be used to administer oxygen. They are not effective if the patient is breathing through his mouth. They give 25–28 per cent oxygen at flow rates of 2–3 litres per minute.

Nasal catheters are inserted straight back along the floor of the nose. Do not try to pass them upwards. Oxygen is delivered into the nasopharynx at concentrations of 25–40% at flows of 2–4 litres per minute.

Tracheostomy masks fit over a tracheostomy tube. They raise the oxygen content of the inspired air by a variable amount depending on how deeply the patient is breathing.

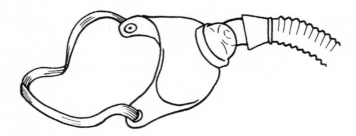

Fig 20.7 Tracheostomy mask

T-pieces are attached directly to an endotracheal tube, laryngeal mask, or tracheostomy tube. Usually made of wide-bore plastic corrugated tube, their advantage is that they are non-rebreathing with low resistance to gas flow, and do not increase the effort of breathing. Humidified gas is delivered at 6–8 litres per minute through one limb of the T, while expired air is washed out of the system by the fresh gas flow. The expiratory limb should not have a volume exceeding 2 ml/kg ml in an adult. The volume of the expiratory limb in children should not exceed 0.5 ml/kg body weight. Never attach the fresh gas flow to a high-pressure gas source, and preferably attach it to a heated blow over humidifier.

T-pieces are simply made and effective. They are ideal for weaning patients before extubation, and for giving oxygen to patients in the recovery room who have, either a tracheostomy, or laryngeal mask in place.

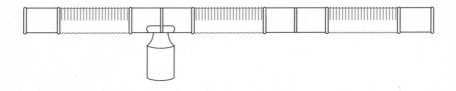

Fig 20.8 T-piece

Head boxes and incubators are only useful for infants. Head boxes require high flow rates, and it is necessary to monitor the oxygen concentration close to the child's face. Incubators and humidicribs at 3–8 litres per minute give up to 40 per cent oxygen.

Patient Controlled Analgesia Devices (PCA)

There are many pumps suitable for patient controlled analgesia. When purchasing one for your unit make sure:

- it has battery backup;
- disposable items are readily available;
- it is easy to use;
- it is tamper proof;
- it indicates the number of times the patient has pressed the button;
- it has internal safeguards that shut the machine down if any malfunction is detected;
- maintenance and servicing is readily available.

PATIENT CONTROLLED ANALGESIA

Postoperative pain control is a major problem. In 1968 it was found that a small intravenous dose of opioid given by a nurse, whenever the patient asked for it resulted in much better pain relief, with smaller total doses of drugs. This led to the development of devices allowing the patient to control his pain by pressing a button to give a small dose of intravenous opioid. A small computer (called a microprocessor) prevented further doses being given until a prescribed lock-out interval had elapsed. The lockout interval is chosen to allow time for the drug to work, and to prevent overdosage. Overdoses are unlikely because a drowsy patient will not press the button.

Pressure Infusion Bags

Pressure infusion bags are used to squeeze plastic bags containing intravenous fluids. Many are poorly designed and made. Check the one you buy has a clearly marked pressure gauge, and is constructed of strong woven material that will not burst or tear. The bulb used to inflate them should be large enough to rapidly and easily inflate the device.

A PRESSURE INFUSION BAG

A temporary device can easily be made. Carefully cut open the ends of a tough outer plastic bag in which many litre bags of intravenous fluid are delivered. Reinforce this with non-stretchable cloth surgical adhesive dressing (such as sticky zinc oxide tape) or Sleek® so that it can withstand pressure. Then attach a blood pressure cuff inflation bulb to an empty plastic litre bag. Slip the litre bag inside the reinforced outer bag to act as a bladder. A bag of blood attached to its giving set can then be compressed between the reinforced outer case and the inflatable inner bladder.

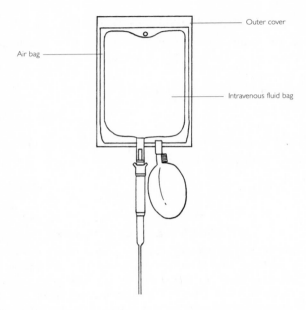

Fig 20.9 Improvized pressure infusion bag

Pulse Oximeters[8]

Pulse oximeters give an early warning of hypoxia. They are the single most useful electronic device for monitoring in the recovery room. Every recovery room bay should have a pulse oximeter. Well known makes are accurate if the patient is warm. They measure the oxygen saturation of haemoglobin as blood passes through the capillaries of the skin. Points to check before purchase are:

• size, weight and portability;
• ability to run on mains current and internal rechargeable batteries;
• display easily seen from all angles and in all light conditions;
• alarms easy to set;
• probes robust, easy to repair or cheap to replace;

Probes come in a suitable range of sizes to suit different patients. Ear or nose probes are useful for patients who have cold hands or poor circulation.

When testing a pulse oximeter check the display when the probe is exposed to the ambient light. Do not purchase a unit that shows a saturation reading when the probe is off the patient. Some makes are confused by flickering fluorescent or incandescent electric bulbs, where ambient light enters the sensor causing interference. This can be overcome by making a small light proof bag or sleeve to fit over the probe and finger to exclude light.

Probes are the items that cause the most problems. They can be very expensive to replace. Some probes can be repaired especially if the electrical connections have worked loose from repeated bending of the wire running to the sensor. An unmatched probe, which if not designed for your particular oximeter, can burn the patient's finger.

Respirometers (Anemometers)

The **Wright's respirometer**® is a fragile instrument. It has delicate vanes that rotate to turn a series of fine cogs. These move a needle on a dial to register the volume of gas passing through the instrument. Respirometers are easily damaged if dropped. If someone blows into them hard it will tear the vanes and shred the cogs.

Don't blow hard into a Wright's respirometer,
they are easy to damage, and expensive to replace.

The **Drager Volumeter**® is bulky and more robust. It has a useful timing device which stops the measurement after one minute, making it easy to standardize measurements. This device may be autoclaved and is a better choice for a remote hospital.

Resuscitation Bags

The two commonly used *self-inflating* types are the Ambu bag® and the Laerdal bag®. These bags are useful for transporting a patient when you are away from a compressed gas supply, because their shape automatically restores itself after it has been squeezed. The bags have a volume of about 1600 ml. Air is entrained through a one-way valve, and oxygen can be added if necessary. To enrich the inspired oxygen a reservoir bag must be attached to the Laerdal bag to act as an oxygen store.

Resuscitation bags are not easy to use. They require practice under supervision until you feel competent.

A **Mapleson C circuit**, sometimes known as the Magill circuit, is useful in recovery room.

It is easy to use in the resuscitation of a non-breathing patient. It has a major disadvantage; if it is attached to a spontaneously breathing patient he will rapidly become hypercarbic.

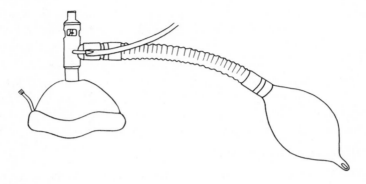

Fig 20.11 Magill circuit

To make this circuit safe for a spontaneously breathing patient remove the bag from the end and turn the fresh gas flow up to at least 10 litres per minute. This will convert it into a T-piece where carbon dioxide cannot accumulate.

Do not use a Mapleson C circuit
on a spontaneously breathing patient.

Space Blankets

Space blankets are thin shiny metallic-like sheets made from Mylar®. This is an exceptionally strong plastic material which has a layer of silver, a few molecules thick, adsorbed on to it. Mylar® sheets are hard to break, but tear easily. Put the silver side next to the patient. They are excellent for minimizing radiant heat loss; however, as they conduct heat readily they need to be separated from the patient's skin by a sheet or blankets to seal a layer of insulation around them. They also conduct electricity so keep them away from electrical apparatus. They are highly inflammable, and quickly burn with intense heat to form a shrunken, molten ball of red hot plastic.

A cheap and probably better alternative is bubble plastic used for packing fragile items for posting. This can be wrapped around the patient, cut to size and stapled with an ordinary office stapling machine. It is especially useful for keeping infants or neonates warm.

Spirit Level

Spirit levels are used for levelling transducers or central venous measuring lines with the isophlebotic point on the body. One can easily be made from a six foot (1.8 metre) length of plastic tubing that has its ends joined to make a loop. Half fill the tubing with coloured water (stained with methylene blue or ink). Join the ends together, seal the join with water proof tape, and label it so it is not discarded (see page 381).

Stethoscopes

People borrow stethescopes and do not return them. Buy easily identifiable coloured ones. Most disposable stethoscopes are not suitable for recovery room use.

Suckers

Y-catheters are used for either tracheal suction where they are passed down an endotracheal tube, or for pharyngeal suction where they are passed through the nose or mouth, to remove fluids collecting in the pharynx. Use only sterile catheters for tracheal suction.

Y-catheters are soft and flexible; they should be transparent, with a single hole at the tip. They must be long enough to pass beyond the end of an unshortened endotracheal tube. Their outer diameter (OD) should clearly labelled in millimetres. Since 1993, Charriere size (known as French gauge) has been dropped as the international standard.

Do not buy the type with an additional side hole or eye near the tip of the catheter. If the end hole becomes blocked by secretions the side hole sucks on to the mucosa and damages it. Argyle Aeroflo® catheters are cleverly designed to prevent this sort of damage. For endotracheal tubes, size 5 or less, select an appropriate sucker for every tube. The sucker must never be more than half the width of the internal diameter of the endotracheal tube.

Rigid suckers are made out of metal or plastic. They are sometimes called Yankeur, or dental suckers. Make sure their tips are firmly in place because they might come loose and be either swallowed or inhaled. If buying reusable suckers, check they are easily cleaned and sterilized.

Suction

The most important piece of equipment in the recovery room is a high-capacity, high-flow suction. This may come from a wall-outlet or an electrical pump. Foot pumps, and other devices are occasionally used. Whatever suction unit you use must run perfectly, and be strong enough to suck up the most viscid mucus or vomit. Each suction point must be capable of permitting a free flow of air of not less than 80 litres a minute and achieve an occluded suction of not less than 460 mmHg (60 kPa).

To prevent the suction inlet becoming blocked, have a fluid trap (usually a three litre glass or plastic container) between the sucker and the pump. This trap collects the secretions, blood and other fluids and prevents the pump becoming clogged with muck. Most suction pumps have a sintered brass filter at the wall inlet. These frequently become clogged which lowers the suction pressure. Establish a maintenance routine to clean, and replace these filters every few days. Change the tubing between patients, replace the collection bottles every shift, and get the hospital engineers to check the pressures and flows at the start of every day.

Temperature

Every recovery room needs a device for measuring low temperatures, because some patients will be hypothermic when they arrive in the recovery room. Normal clinical thermometers do not register below 35.5°C. Recently developed infra-red tympanic thermometers[9] accurately measure the patient's temperature. Devices such as *The Genius*™ (Model 3000A) and the *The Cyclops 33*™ are accurate, respond rapidly and are easy to use. The hypothalamus, where the thermoregulatory control centre is located, and the tympanic membrane share the same blood supply. They give the best estimate of temperature.

Cheap, accurate and reliable thermistor tipped catheters can be placed in the rectum or oesophagus. Do not put these devices in the ear, because you risk damaging the delicate tympanic membrane and auditory canal. Swan Ganz® catheters, too can give an accurate core temperature because they measure the temperature of the blood in the pulmonary artery.

Torches

Keep torches where they can easily be found in the dark if the lights fail. Have one torch available for every two beds. Each needs spare bulbs and batteries. Torches are also used for testing pupillary reflexes. To do this use the standard 100 W incandescent bulb held 60 cm (2 feet) from the patient's face.

Trolleys

Tables and sets of drawers on wheels are known as *carts* in the USA and Canada, and *trolleys* in the UK and elsewhere. These are designed to be taken to the patient's bedside for various procedures; for example, arrest trolleys (crash carts). The best ones have strong, large sprung castor wheels, and are made of stainless steel. Painted, or coated trolleys tend to chip and this makes them difficult to clean. Make sure the drawers cannot fall out and have stout runners to withstand heavy use.

Patient trolleys suitable for the recovery room have a specific standard dedicated to their design. Purchase those that conform to your local standard.

• Quickly tilted head or foot down at least 25° from the horizontal.
• The patient should be able to sit up with support.
• An adjustable foot rest or bed-end to stop the patient sliding down.
• A firm base and mattress.
• Trolley sides or rails are necessary to prevent the patient rolling off. They must be easily retracted or removable.
• Removable poles to carry intravenous fluids.
• Holders for drainage bottles and bags and urine bags.
• Large castor wheels for easy manoeuvrability.
• Easily applied brakes.
• Portable oxygen and suction easily available. This will require a cylinder, regulator, a flow device and a suction device on each trolley. This can be provided with a Twin-O-Vac® or similar device.
• A tray for carrying small articles such as the patient's history, false teeth and belongings.

Ventilators

Ventilators that have been inappropriately purchased or donated often become an embarrassing and expensive mistake. There are many makes and models and one is sure to fit your requirements. Seek expert advice. Make sure that the one you get will work in your recovery room. If you have a restricted supply of compressed gas, do not purchase a gas driven ventilator that is going to use many litres a minute to run; the Bird® ventilator and the Campbell® ventilator require between 11 litres and 25 litres of compressed gas a minute to power them.

If you have an unreliable electrical supply make sure that your auxiliary generators can cope with the load. Your ventilator should have an alarm to warn you if the patient has become disconnected. In case of ventilator malfunction, have a self-inflating bag near by so that you can use to ventilate the patient. Make sure all the connections can be attached to an endotracheal tube. Always have a clean ventilator ready. You may need it in a hurry.

The Manley Multivent® is a simple, reliable ventilator developed for anaesthesia in the geographically isolated hospital. It can be powered either by compressed gas from a standard cylinder or electricity. It cannot, however, be triggered by the patient, which limits its use to the paralysed or deeply sedated patient.

Warming Blankets (see Space blankets page 412)

Forced air warming devices blow warm air into a light plastic envelope which is laid around the patient. They are highly effective in preventing further heat loss, and help re-warm the patient in the recovery room. One of the most widely used is the Bair Hugger™; which when set on high, can increase body temperature by about 1.5°C/hr[10].

1. Australian and New Zealand Intensive Care Society Circular Sep 1994. ANZICS, College of Surgeons, Melbourne, Australia.
2. Eagle C. C. (1992). *Anaesthesia and Intensive Care*, 20: 156–60
3. Henderon M. A., Irwin M. G. (1995). *Anaesthesia and Intensive Care*, 23: 407
4. Rooke G. A., Bowdle T. A. (1994). *Anaesthesia and Analgesia*, 78: 150–6
5. Cook R. I., Woods D. O., *et al.* (1992). *Journal of Cardiothoracic and Vascular Anaesthesia*, 6: 238–44
6. Brimacombe J., Berry A. (1993). *Anaesthesia*, 48: 670–1
7. Stoneham H. D. (1993). *Anaesthesia*, 48: 575–580
8. Clayton R. K., Webb A. C. (1991). *Anaesthesia*, 46: 3–10
9. Edge G., Morgan M. (1993). *Anaesthesia*, 48: 604–7
10. Sessier A. I., Moayeri A. (1990). *Anesthesiology*, 70: 424–7

21. PURCHASING
EQUIPMENT AND SAFETY

When setting up a recovery room one of the most challenging tasks is to decide what equipment is needed, what is available, reliable and good value for money. Make sure any electrical equipment you buy conforms to the international safety standard for electromedical equipment (IEC 601–1). Do not approach supply companies until everyone agrees on the decisions.

When buying equipment keep in mind the KISS criteria. KISS stands for Keep It Simple and Safe. Equipment must be easy to operate, preferably so easy that just by looking at it you can work out what it does, and how to use it, without referring to an instruction book. Important functions, such as alarm settings, should be obvious. Remember many staff will use it and some may not have been trained in its use. Simplicity is important. Do not buy complicated equipment. Try to use the same equipment as the rest of the hospital; this means bits and pieces can be borrowed from, or shared with, other departments. It also helps the purchasing officer to buy and stock spare parts, and to negotiate on cheaper bulk purchases of disposables. Check with other recovery units in nearby hospitals about the reliability, and ease of servicing of the equipment you intend to buy.

Special Problems for the Isolated Hospital

Nominate one member of your department to be in charge of the purchase, care, and maintenance of equipment. This is an important and time consuming job.

Work out why you need the equipment in the first place.

- Will it improve patient safety; such as a pulse oximeter?
- Will it help staff work more efficiently by doing a routine chore better; such as a non-invasive blood pressure machine?
- Can it do something that was impossible before; such as an oxygen concentrator?
- Does it need a special power source? A gas powered ventilator is useless unless there is a reliable and cheap source of compressed gas to run it. Many isolated hospitals have to work with an erratic and unreliable power supply.

Equipment must be robust and reliable. Fragile equipment is useless if it constantly needs maintenance, or has to be sent a long distance for repairs. Reliability is essential. Before purchasing any piece of equipment, find out how often it breaks down. In engineering terms this is known as the MTBF (mean time between failures). For instance, for the best of the oxygen concentrators, this is about 6000 hours of operating time. Find out what happens when it does break down. Does it break down in a safe way? If in doubt about the reliability of the equipment, or its suitability for the task, telephone your nearest university teaching hospital and consult either the Biomedical Engineering Department or the Department of Anaesthesia. They should be able to give you helpful and unbiased advice.

HOW TO FIND OUT WHAT IS AVAILABLE

In the UK, the Department of Health periodically publishes evaluations of available equipment in Health Equipment Information In Australasia there is a master reference manual published annually by MIMS (Medical International Statistics) called Hospital Equipment and Supplies. This thick book gives comprehensive details on almost everything that is commercially available in the region. Included are such data as catalogue numbers, addresses and telephone numbers of suppliers. Unfortunately there is no attempt to evaluate the equipment. These catalogues are expensive, but if you write to MIMS Publishing in your official capacity they may send your hospital a free copy. In Australasia the address is MIMS, 49 Albany Street, Crows Nest, New South Wales, 2065, Australia. The World Health Organisation is collecting data on reliable, robust and economical equipment for use in the isolated hospital.

When buying expensive equipment, such as electronic monitors or ventilators; involve the engineering staff in the planning phase. Consider their advice on technical matters about the choice of equipment, and what sort of training they need; and particularly, the manufacturer's ability to provide support, such as manuals, maintenance contracts, spare parts, and training films or familiarity courses.

Do not buy equipment unless the company is willing to release circuit diagrams, and detailed workshop manuals of the equipment. Servicing is almost impossible if these diagrams are not available. Get at least two copies of the operator's manual and the maintenance manual; one for the hospital's biomedical engineers, and one to keep in the department. Check that they are complete and relevant to your piece of equipment. These manuals are an essential part of the equipment. They must be easy to understand, and have clear diagrams so that you can teach others. Poorly written, poorly translated, or incomplete manuals make equipment difficult to use, maintain and repair. Poor instruction manuals may also indicate that the equipment has not been carefully designed in the first place and may be unreliable. Sending equipment away for repairs or servicing can take many months and is very expensive. Often a local technician can do the work if he has access to the workshop manuals.

Where do spare parts come from? Getting spare parts from another country can take months. Make sure there is an *after sales service,* with a reliable supply of spare parts. It is a good idea to order spare parts when the equipment is purchased. Even with normal wear and tear some pieces will begin to break down almost immediately; for example the rubber suction bulbs, or rubber straps of an electrocardiograph, and blood pressure cuff bladders. This is especially true in tropical climates where rubber perishes quickly.

Servicing (with Special Reference to the Isolated Hospital)

Of all the areas in which the isolated hospital has problems servicing causes the most difficulty. Lying around departments of most isolated hospitals is broken down or unusable equipment. Thoughtful planning avoids such waste. Most equipment requires simple servicing by the people who use it. Establish a regular programme of checking the equipment with clear orders on what to is to be done, and enforce them or else it may not happen! Every time a service is carried out, enter it in a book kept with the equipment. This includes:

• daily or pre-use checks;
• routine calibration;
• daily or pre-use cleaning and the reporting of faults;
• ensuring accessories are serviceable and complete;
• consumerable items are available.

Regular checks should be done by the biomedical engineers. To make things proceed smoothly the following questions need to be considered:

• what is to be maintained?
• how it is to be maintained?
• when is it to be maintained?
• is the maintenance effective?

To answer the first question draw up an inventory or register of equipment that needs maintenance. Before putting equipment into use it needs to be *commissioned.* This involves setting up a maintenance programme and training staff to use and care for the equipment. The regular maintenance schedule must balance the manufacturer's recommendations with how often the equipment is used. Obviously the more often the equipment is used, the more frequently it should be checked.

Documentation is crucial, and card index systems are best in a smaller hospital. We hesitate to recommend computer based systems in an isolated hospital because they require expert staff to run them. If the computer breaks down (and proper back-ups have not been made) all your data can be lost.

Some items of biomedical equipment, such as blood gas machines require periodic calibration by an outside agency. Try as far as possible to calibrate the apparatus on the spot to avoid long periods without the equipment, and the risk of damage during transport. Bring the technician to the machine, try not to send the machine to the technician.

If servicing and maintenance is beyond the resources of your biomedical engineers it is possible for regions, or even countries, to co-operate and share a technician at regular intervals. This reduces costs, and increases efficiency.

If it cannot be repaired, condemn broken biomedical equipment. Do not leave it in your department. Ask your Supply department to organise its disposal, and attend to the proper inventory and accounting procedures. Consider modifying the equipment to extend its useful life, or use parts of it for other things.

Disposables

It is tempting to buy disposable items, because they release staff from the chores of cleaning and sterilization. Disposables save wages, and time, and reduce the chance of cross infection. However, they are expensive, and need lots of storage space. If you are working in a isolated hospital think carefully before you discard, or stop using reusable items such stainless steel dishes, glass syringes, metal suckers and linen drapes. Circumstances can make disposables unobtainable. Once the routines for cleaning and sterilising reusable items is abandoned, it is hard to start again.

An inventory system is needed to automatically re-order disposables. Delegate this clerical function to the pharmacy, or the supply office.

Re-using disposable items is a controversial issue. Many disposable items, which have not been exposed to blood, or body fluids, can be washed, and then sterilized and safely reused. In many countries medico-legal problems make re-use impracticable.

Budgets

Most hospitals require every service area, such as the recovery room to have their own budget with the freedom, within set limits, to purchase and maintain their equipment. Until you are familiar with budgets it is worthwhile sitting down with a hospital administrator to check through the figures to see how the department is managing financially.

Safety in the Recovery Room

Electrical Safety

Make sure that all equipment has been checked by an accredited technician before it is put into service, such as an electrician, or an electrical engineer from your hospital's biophysics department.

Report anything you suspect is faulty, such as :
- kinks in wires;
- plugs not fitting their sockets properly;
- worn or frayed electric leads;
- damaged outer coats on power cables;
- instances where someone has felt tingling, or has received a minor shock;
- spillage of liquid into electrical equipment.

Disconnect the suspect equipment, put a large 'Unsafe—Do not use' label on it, and report it.

Also:
- keep electric leads as short as practicable;
- keep electrical leads off hot surface, pipes or taps;
- do not use extension cords, because of the danger of fluid entering the junction;
- do not stand on a wet floor when operating or plugging in electrical equipment;
- do not stand on electric leads, or run trolleys over them.

(Electrical safety in the design of the recovery room, see page 427.)

Fire Safety

All staff should have lectures about what to do in the case of a fire, and attend a fire drill at least twice a year.

Put up notices in conspicuous places giving clear, simple instructions about what to do in the case of fire. You will need to **RACE** to prevent tragedy.

Rescue	Remove patients to a safe place.
Alarm	Sound alarm.
Contain	Close windows and doors to isolate the fire.
Extinguish	Only attempt to put out the fire if you are certain of what you are doing.

Put Anglia® or similar evacuation sheets under each mattress on the trolleys. These tough sheets have handles, straps and buckles and use the mattress to wrap the patient in a protective shell. It is easy to drag this shell along the floor, and even down stairs, if necessary.

The best type of fire extinguisher for recovery room is one that uses carbon dioxide. This copes with fires involving wood and paper, flammable liquids, live electrical equipment, and oil. Ensure fire extinguishers, fire hoses and fire blankets are installed in prominent places. Get the advice of your local fire department on this matter. Be sure to include a review of your fire equipment on your routine maintenance programme.

22. DESIGN OF THE RECOVERY ROOM

SITE OF THE RECOVERY ROOM

Shortly after the first anaesthetic was given in 1846, Florence Nightingale recognized the need for a special area, and special nursing care of patients recovering from ether anaesthesia. She wrote in her book *Notes on Hospitals* that the patient should be placed in a small room near to the ward, with clean fresh sand on the floor, clean bedclothes, and windows to admit the sunlight and fresh air.[1]

The recovery room is normally part of the operating suite, located close to where the anaesthetic was given, but readily accessible to medical staff who are in their street clothes. Staff tea rooms should be nearby so that the doctors, having a break at the end of a case, can have quick access to the patients if needed. Preferably, have the intensive care unit on the same level, and close to the recovery room. In hospitals with fewer than 200 beds it may be useful to have the intensive care unit next to the operating theatre. The recovery room can then be a functional part of the intensive care unit, but remain a separate area, away from the normal intensive care beds. Such an arrangement means that staff, facilities, and equipment can be shared between the two areas. A further advantage is that after hours, when there are less staff on the wards, patients can be recovered overnight in the intensive care unit. The big disadvantage is the risk of transferring infection from the intensive care patients to the surgical patient. Staff will need education, and discipline to prevent this *nosocomial infection.* Hand washing, and the wearing protective gowns are crucial parts of this program.

PLAN FOR THE RECOVERY ROOM

The following section is an overview of the major features of a well-designed recovery room.

Square recovery rooms are more efficient than rectangular ones. Arrange the trolley bays around three walls, with a nurses' station, and open storage space on the fourth wall. The number of bed or trolley spaces should be sufficient for expected peak loads. You will need about 3 recovery room trolley bays for each operating theatre. Make sure there is easy access to the patient's head, and an adequate working area around the patient. Allow about 12 square metres of space for support utilities. Modular cupboards can be expanded to meet the future requirements. Each trolley bay needs at least 1 cubic metre (9 cubic feet) of storage space within the room, and at least 3 square metres (28 square feet) of shelving and storage nearby.

STANDARDS

There are many things to consider when planning, and building a recovery room. Fortunately architects, and engineers have access to help in the form of *standards*. Standards are sets of specifications that cover almost everything to do with the construction, design, safety, and purchase of buildings, and equipment used in hospitals. Many countries including Australia, United Kingdom, and the European community, and USA have their own standards that specify such things as the design of buildings, the supply of piped gases, the quality of lighting, the fittings for anaesthetic apparatus, the formulation of drugs, electrical safety, hospital signs, medical records, and so on.

The International Organization of Standardization (ISO) based in Switzerland is struggling to get agreement between the various national standardization bodies, and is slowly bringing them into line. This means that apparatus designed, and used in one country, can be used equally safely in another; and the various fittings, pipes and colour codes, are uniform. In the European Community the Commité Européen de Normalisation has made rapid progress towards standardization, and their determinations were made mandatory in 1992.

Make sure that anything you design, builds, or buy complies with the accepted standards in your area. We have drawn freely on various standards to list ideas that may help you to design, and manage your recovery room. Our emphasis is on the needs of geographically isolated hospital.

Too much storage space
is better than too little.

Plan an open, and uncluttered recovery room, with no structures obstructing your view. Every trolley bay should be visible from anywhere within the room.

If the recovery room is designed as part of the intensive care unit, consider building an *isolation room* for managing patients with infections, contaminated wounds, and those who are immunosupressed. This room should have both negative, and positive air conditioning.

Make sure the patient trolleys can move easily around the room, with a minimum number of corners to negotiate. Have two wide doors for access; one from the operating theatre, and one to the wards. Ideally these should be at opposite ends of the recovery room.

All the recovery room bays should be identical with the same things in the same place. Do not design bays that are mirror images of each other, a confusing technique favoured by many architects.

RECOVERY ROOM BAYS

Utilities

Each patient trolley bay needs its own service utilities mounted on the wall at the head of the patient trolley.

Ideally there should be:

- two high-pressure oxygen outlets equipped with flow meters and nipples;
- two high-vacuum, high-flow suction outlets, including receiver, tubing, rigid hand piece, and a range of suction catheters;
- two high-pressure medical air outlets;
- six electric (general) power outlets;
- one mobile examination lamp, that can be swung to provide light to any point on the patient;
- at least two shelves with slightly raised edges to prevent things falling on the floor;
- appropriate facilities for mounting monitoring equipment;
- somewhere to keep the patient's chart;
- storage space for items, and the patient's belongings.

Equipment

Provide each recovery room bay with:

- a sphygmomanometer attached to the wall at eye height;
- a good stethoscope;
- over head runners similar to curtain rails are preferable to drip stands;
- a place to keep the patient's chart;
- suction equipment, sterile suction catheters;
- oropharyngeal airways, and nasopharyngeal airways;
- a range of needles, syringes, and skin cleaning preparation;
- sterile disposable gloves;
- a pressure infusion bag for giving intravenous fluids rapidly;
- clear plastic masks so you can see the patient's mouth and lips;
- oxygen tubing with connectors;

- T-pieces for delivering oxygen to intubated patients, or those returning with a laryngeal mask still in place;
- self-inflating bag for inflating the lungs with oxygen;
- a pulse oximeter;
- bowls, and kidney dishes;
- small hand towels;
- paper tissues;
- scissors;
- containers for haematology, and pathology specimens;
- blood gas syringes;
- sealable plastic bags for transport of potentially infected fluids.

RECOVERY ROOM FACILITIES

Air-conditioning should maintain the temperature of the recovery room at between 21°C and 24°C with the capability of increasing it to 26°C, and with a relative humidity of between 40 and 60 per cent under all conditions with at least 6 air changes each hour. Anaesthetic gas pollution can be high in the recovery room, because patients continue to exhale the gases for some time after leaving the operating theatre.

Emergency power

Emergency power is essential in case the mains supply fails. This should automatically switch on if there is mains power failure. To avoid the recovery room being plunged into total darkness install one or more emergency, battery powered lights, that automatically switch on when the mains power supply fails.

Electrical safety

Macroshock causes electrocution, with the heart going into ventricular fibrillation. *Microshock* occurs when a tiny current of a few millivolts passes through an electrolyte infusion or pacemaker wire to cause ventricular fibrillation. Isolation transformers or core balance earth leakage devices protect against macroshock.

Emergency station

Establish an emergency station where the defibrillator, and trolleys *(crash carts)* for managing a cardiac arrest, and other emergencies are kept. Keep this easily accessible. The emergency station needs its own power outlets to keep the portable equipment's batteries charged.

ELECTRICAL PROTECTION DEVICES

Ordinary wiring used in domestic houses has its electrical protection (*Class A*) limited to fuses, and an earth wire in the cord. The recovery room should be a *Body Protected Area* (*Class B*) giving protection from macroshock in event of an accident. Macroshock protection is provided by either isolation transformers or core balance earth leakage devices. *Isolation transformers* may be fitted to the main electricity supply. These prevent a person being electrocuted if they touch the electrically live (or active) wire of the power supply while in contact with an earth. They are designed so that current cannot flow through a person or other electrical conductor to the earth. They are expensive, and need regular maintenance. A far cheaper alternative is a *core balance earth leakage device*. It detects a current flowing to earth, and automatically cuts off the power supply before it causes harm. For most recovery rooms this device is sufficient to minimize the risk of electrocution. To ensure they work properly all earth points in the ward need a common heavy copper grounding cable. The engineering specifications for these areas are set out in special safety standards. *Cardiac-protected areas* (*Class Z*) are similar to Class B areas but include special wiring to ensure no exposed surfaces of the plumbing, electrical equipment monitors etc, in the vicinity of the patient can create an electrical gradient sufficient to cause microelectrocution.

Flooring

Lay a non-slip floor, with a non-absorbent surface of uniform colour that can be easily cleaned. Patterned or speckled flooring hides dirt, and makes it difficult to find small objects that have fallen on the floor.

Hand washing

A hand basin with hot and cold running water, liquid-soap dispenser, paper towels, and a waste bin. To prevent cross contamination do not use linen towels. Avoid installing hot-air hand dryers, because they are noisy, and spray germs, and skin squames all over the room.

Imprest system

A drug and disposables *Imprest system* makes restocking easier. This is a system for holding commonly used items in the recovery room. It is the duty of the pharmacist, and supply officer to check, and restock them as they are used. Recovery rooms use a wide range of drugs. Store them lockable drug cupboard. A set of recessed shelves with a door that is rolled down at the end of the day is ideal. Organize the drug cupboard in such a way that drugs can be quickly found. Post an alphabetical list of available drug under both their generic and trade names. It is a good idea to have a third list with the drugs classified under their pharmacological actions; for example, a list of antibiotics, and cardiac drugs.

Library

Install an unlocked bookcase for a small library of reference books.

Lighting

If natural daylight is not available, light the room with special colour-corrected fluorescent tubes. Do not use blue-light fluorescent tubes, or incandescent light bulbs, because they make it difficult to judge the patient's colour, and delay the recognition of cyanosis. The lights should provide 100 candela for every 10 square metres of floor space. Effectively, this is enough light to read the printing on a drug ampoule at arm's length with one eye covered. For most purposes two 25 watt fluorescent tubes would be enough to cover 10 square metres.

Linen and laundry

Make provision for the collection of soiled linen, and other contaminated waste. Plan for the orderly disposal of paper, and clean plastic. Have a meeting to decide what can be safely be recycled, then make the process easy with clearly labelled containers.

Notice board

A notice board and a white board with erasable pens for teaching, and planning patient management.

Painting

Paint walls, and ceilings light, neutral colours. Avoid colours such as blues, reds, greens or yellows, because they reflect misleadingly on the patient's skin.

Piped gases

Fit all *piped gases* with failure alarms that are easily identified by both a sound and a light. Install these in a conspicuous place. Frame a set of instructions on what to do if the alarm sounds, and screw them to the wall next to the warning light. Supplies of oxygen, and suction for emergencies are best kept under every trolley bay.

Plumbing

Share toilets and space for equipment cleaning with the operating theatres.

Telephones

Consider installing telephones to make outgoing calls only. Noisy telephones disturb patients, and demand to be answered. Furthermore, nursing staff are tempted to leave their patient to answer the phone. Trivial in-coming calls are a nuisance, and best handled by the theatre receptionist or secretary.

Utility cables

The desk, and nurses' station, will need power points. Install a utility cable duct to carry cables for telephones, intercoms, computers, and paging systems. Make these ducts easily accessible to allow you to lay more cables in the future.

X-ray machines

Install a suitable power outlet for the portable x-ray machine used in your hospital.

X-ray viewing screens

Attach X-ray viewing screens, and a bright light for examining films on the wall near the nurses' desk.

EQUIPMENT FOR THE RECOVERY ROOM

Blood warmers

In-line blood warmers to reduce transfusion pain, help prevent hypothermia, reduce the viscosity of blood, and prevent damage from cold agglutinins.

Emergency alarm

Site a large red panic button on the wall above each trolley to call for help. The best buzzer is one with an urgent repeating sequence that can be heard throughout the operating theatres, rest rooms, and changing rooms. To prevent these being accidentally activated, design them to pull on rather than push on. Identify them with large clear signs. Test them daily.

Emergency trolleys (crash carts)

Keep trays or trolleys *(carts)* set up nearby, and ready to use for the management of anaphylaxis, malignant hyperthermia, emergency airway care, emergency bronchoscopy, insertion of thoracic drains, minor surgical procedures, and vascular access. Each needs its own set of protocols attached to it. It helps to have a large, clear colour photograph of each setup so that the trays can be checked quickly, and are always put together the same way. Photos enable you to tell quickly what is missing.

Fire control equipment

Fit fire control equipment, and smoke detection devices in the recovery room (see page 421). Appoint staff as fire monitors, and take their photographs. Display their names, photographs, and duties, in case of emergency, at the entrance to the recovery room. Every one working in the recovery room should have a written instruction on the back of their identification labels about to what to do in the case of fire, or other emergencies requiring evacuation. Hold evacuation practices twice a year.

Monitors

At least one patient physiology monitor is needed for every bay. Most have a number of features such as ECG, pulse oximetery, end expired carbon dioxide, inspired oxygen concentration, blood, and other pressure modules, parameter trending, and non-invasive blood pressure monitoring. For the district hospital physiology monitoring you will need, at least, a pulse oximeter for each patient. ECG and non-invasive blood pressure monitors can be shared between two, or three bays as necessary (see page 394).

Refrigerator

A refrigerator for storing heat labile drugs, and other items such as ice used for testing the efficacy of local blocks. Always keep blood, blood products, and vaccines in a special thermostatically controlled refrigerator. This refrigerator should have a clock-chart, and alarm to warn if its temperature has risen or fallen outside set limits even when the recovery room is unattended. If this happens you may need to discard the biological products (see page 353).

Respirometers

Respirometers (anemometers) measure the volume of air moving in or out of the lungs (see page 411).

Screens

Some means of screening each patient for privacy, or if problems arise.

Sharps disposal

Sharps disposal is a major issue; especially with the increasing risk of HIV, and Hepatitis B, and C transmission due to needle stick injuries. Immediately after use, sharps such as needles, and empty ampoules, must be put into rigid sharp puncture proof containers. Do not overfill these containers. When they are full, seal them, and send them to be incinerated. Before handling the containers, check that no needle points are sticking through the walls of the container. Most hospitals now have formal programs for safely dealing with and disposing of sharps.

Trolleys

A minimum of three patient transport trolleys will be needed for each working theatre; one for attending to the patient in theatre, one for the patient in recovery room, and one for transporting the patient back to the ward. There are special International Standards for the design of these trolleys.

Ventilator

A mechanical ventilator with a humidifier, and all the necessary sterile tubing and connections.

Warming cupboard

A warming cupboard for warming blankets, and other items.

1. Nightingale F. (1863). *Notes on Hospitals,* page 89, Publishers: Longman, Roberts and Green.

23. Staffing and Management

Management's Responsibility To Recovery Room

It is the hospital management's responsibility to ensure that adequate nursing personnel, support staff and the appropriate drugs and equipment are available. Support staff include administrators, clerical staff, engineering staff, pharmacists and technicians. Before taking responsibility for the care of patients, the staff must be assessed as competent to carry out their duties. It is negligent to leave unstable postoperative patients in unskilled hands. Many countries such as the UK, USA and Australasia have special *standards* drawn up by professional bodies to lay down an acceptable standard of care for the patient in recovery room. It may help to consult the nursing or medical professional associations in your area.

Sir Robert Macintosh, the first Professor of Anaesthetics at Oxford University, said in 1970 that he regarded recovery rooms as one of the greatest advances in anaesthesia. Coroners, throughout the world, affirm the recovery room as the most important room in the hospital, for it is here the patient is at the greatest risk of coming to harm.

During normal office hours most work is with patients having elective operations. Work in the recovery room starts at the beginning of the operating lists, and finishes an hour or two after the last operation. Emergencies are usually dealt with at the end of day's routine operating and at night. Most recovery rooms are properly staffed during the day, but it is important to maintain proper staffing after hours too. The hospital's management needs to be reminded that emergency patients operated on after hours are often those most in need of highly specialised care.

Nursing Staff

Maintain a flexible ratio of experienced nurses to patients. The American Society of Post Anaesthetic Nurses (ASPAN) suggests sensible criteria for the allocation of nurses in the recovery room.

Class I. Uncomplicated patients who are conscious and stable require one trained nurse for three patients.

Class II. Uncomplicated paediatric patients who are stable and conscious, or patients who have undergone major surgery, or adult patients who are stable and unconscious, require one trained nurse for two patients.

Class III. Patients requiring life support care need one trained nurse for each patient.

There should always be two nurses in the recovery room, even if there is only one patient. One of these should be an experienced recovery room nurse. Nurses without sufficient recovery room experience need direct supervision, and should not be left on their own.

High dependency patients, such as those following neurosurgery, thoracic, vascular, or emergency trauma surgery need more nursing care than those undergoing more minor surgery. Lists with large numbers of short cases will require extra nurses.

Nursing banks

Nursing banks are organized by many hospitals to provide relief personnel to cover illness, holidays and times of peak activity. Many nurses prefer part time work. Sometimes it may be necessary to employ temporary staff from nursing agencies. These nurses may not have adequate experience in recovery room and will require extra supervision.

Orderlies or technicians

Orderlies or technicians are needed to lift, transport, and position patients, and help with equipment. Have at least one strong, competent orderly always available.

Training

Staff who know what they are doing are impressive, and it is training and experience that make them competent. Recovery room nursing is a skilled and demanding task. Training requires a structured post-graduate course, assimilating both operating theatre techniques, and intensive care nursing. It can be reinforced by rotating the recovery room staff through areas such as intensive care, high dependency units, and coronary care units. Establish a structured continuous education program to keep staff up to date.

MEDICAL STAFF

In most operating theatres the anaesthetist responsible for the anaesthetic is also responsible for the recovery room care of the same patient.

*For safety and efficient management
there must be enough trained staff.*

ADMINISTRATION

The recovery room is usually supervised by, either the Medical Director of Anaesthesia, or the Nursing Director of the Operating Theatre Suite. An experienced recovery room nurse should manage the area. Clerical staff are needed to answer phones, keep track of supplies, run errands and so on.

Planning

Planning is often delegated to an *operating theatre committee* composed of nurses, medical staff, and administrators. Some tips to make this committee run smoothly are that it should:
- be small, with no more than six members;
- hold regular meetings;
- have defined written responsibilities;
- have an agenda circulated some days before the meeting.

When confronted with a task to plan the committee should:
- define the task to be accomplished;
- provide appropriate resources to accomplish the task;
- establish people to be responsible for each phase;
- appoint someone to co-ordinate, and follow-up the task;
- set deadlines;
- keep good records.

Rosters

Rosters are best made up at least a fortnight in advance.

Policy manuals

Policy manuals help standardize protocols, procedures, and lines of communication. Write them in collaboration with all the staff in the operating theatres. It is the job of the operating theatre committee to organise this task.

Protocols and guidelines

Protocols are designed to be followed precisely, while *guidelines* allow latitude for common sense. *Policies* lay out a course of action for the future. Protocols ensure everyone does things the same way. Most administrative and clinical situations recur, and every hospital has its own routine and ways of coping with these situations. It is not easy to transplant routines from one hospital to another, so develop your own protocols, and guidelines about to what to do in given circumstances. Develop routines so that everyone approaches these recurring problems in the same way. Protocols and guidelines make audits easy.

Develop and keep nursing and medical protocols together, because it needs an informed and willing team to provide good holistic patient management. Nursing care has five elements: assessment, nursing diagnosis, development of a care plan, its implementation, and evaluation of the plan. This takes into account relevant preoperative emotional, psychosocial, and safety needs. Medical care includes the recognition of ordered, and the diagnosis of disordered, physiology and biochemistry of the patient, and their therapeutic management. The doctor is responsible for the overall physical, and mental welfare of his patient. This includes the duty of informing the patient of the risks of therapeutic intervention.

Review the guidelines and protocols regularly at unit meetings. You will need protocols for:
• checking of equipment and drugs;
• transfer of patient from operating theatre to the recovery room;
• handover of the patient from theatre staff to recovery room staff;
• observation and documentation of details about the patient;
• emergency procedures;
• discharge criteria and procedures;
• responsibilities of categories of staff.

Once routines are established errors are less likely to occur. Written guidelines help ward staff manage the more complex postoperative problems such as, management of epidural catheters, or airway problems after thyroidectomy.

Protocols need to be concise, clearly written and helpful. Keep them in the unit where they can be consulted. Do not make them too wordy or no one will read them. A successful policy, protocol and guideline book will soon look well thumbed and dog-eared.

Library

A library for reference is particularly useful after hours. Do not lock the books away. You never know when you may have to look up something urgently. References could include books on topics such as nursing, practical pharmacology, a synopsis of anaesthesia, and techniques of local anaesthesia. Collect useful articles from journals.

Message books

A message book is useful to pass on messages to staff on later shifts. Use it to keep track of equipment lent to other parts of the hospital, and to follow up ideas, new techniques, staff with special roster requests and so on.

Maintenance books

Maintenance books ensure the weekly check of the defibrillator, and regular servicing of equipment have been done properly.

Weekly meetings

Weekly meetings are a part of the quality assurance programme. Establish regular meetings to discuss cases, and problems and to keep staff up-to-date with recent advances. Involve all staff in educational and peer review meetings.

Audits

Audits are part of a quality control process. They help you find potential problems, as well as revealing occasionally surprising information to help you improve patient care, and justify the resources needed in the recovery room. Once you think you have corrected a problem, repeat your audit to make sure it really has been solved. This check is called *closing the audit*. Audits are sometimes a tedious chore, but do make a huge difference in the quality of care.

Do not attempt to review every patient at every audit. For example, take a homogeneous sample of ENT patients. Prepare a simple list of problems that arise in day-to-day routines, such as, restlessness after nasal surgery, sore eyes, or vomiting. These problems delay the discharge of patients. Survey the incidence of these problems for a month, and then use the results to find trends that will help improve efficiency and patient care. Perhaps you may find a high incidence of sore eyes and trace the cause back to the skin preparation used by one particular surgeon; there may be a delay in getting the patients back to the ward at the end of the morning. Staggered lunch breaks for the orderlies might solve this problem.

Errors, incidents, and accidents[1]

Errors, incidents, and accidents are bound to occur. Some errors are trivial and others disastrous, but error is unfortunately a part of every human activity. Accidents do happen, and not all errors are blameworthy. Normal people, under normal circumstances do not make mistakes on purpose. It is easy to be wise in hindsight.

Document them accurately including written reports from all the staff involved. The statements must contain facts only—do not try to interpret what happened. If there are likely to be medico-legal consequences ask the administrators in your hospital to help you prepare these statements.

Understanding why incidents occur is the first step in crisis management, and their analysis is useful to prevent them occurring again. The staff, the patients, their diseases, and the technology used in recovery room is a complex dynamic system, and those familiar with *Chaos theory* will know that a minor incident can set up a chain reaction of a series of subtle, and possibly undetected events coming together to explode as a catastrophe. Collect a record of incidents with sufficient detail to allow you to identify events and their contributing factors. Note what went wrong, and who was involved, what happened, and when, why and how it occurred. Include contributing factors such as fatigue, rostering problems, power failures and so on.

1. Runciman W. B., Sellen A., *et al.* (1993). *Anaesthesia and Intensive Care*, 21: 506–19

24. Drugs Used in the Recovery Room

This section is not intended to be a definitive pharmacopoeia. It is a guide to commonly used drugs. If you are not entirely familiar with a drug, its actions, side effects, contraindications and dose; then check the manufacturer's recommendations. Drug doses are being continually revised and new side effects recognized, so check with your hospital pharmacist if you are unfamiliar with a drug. The correct dose of drug will achieve the maximum effect. The right dose is enough, and increasing the dose will only increase the chances of toxicity.

Most drugs are very potent,
small amounts cause a big effect.

The drugs are listed alphabetically and include most of those used in the recovery room. Some are drugs only used in specialist units, and are included for information only.

WEIGHT

1000 micrograms = 1 milligram

1000 milligrams = 1 gram

or 1 gram = 1000 milligrams = 1 000 000 micrograms

Note: μ is the symbol for micro. μg = microgram

m is the symbol for milli. mg = milligram

Since 1 millilitre of water weighs 1 gram, a milligram is tiny amount, and a microgram would weigh as much as one millionth of 1 ml of water.

Drug	Use and action	Dose	Comments
Acetominophen	(see paracetamol)		
Adenosine[1] 'Adenocor'	Regular broad complex and narrow complex tachy-cardias arising in SA node. Depresses SA node. Purinergic receptor agonist.	Increments of 0.05 mg/kg every 1–2 min up to max of 0.25 mg/kg. Half life 10–30 sec	Effective Side effects: Last 2–20 seconds • flushing • dyspnoea • chest pain • hypotension • nausea Effects dangerously enhanced by dipyridamole.
Adrenaline In USA called epinephrine	Cardiac stimulant used for: • asystole • fine VF (see page 294) • anaphylaxis (see page 142) • normovolaemic shock (see page 288)	1 ml of 1/1000 IV or 0.1 ml/kg of 1/10,000 IV Infusion of 1–20 µg/min.	Monitor with ECG. Give 100% oxygen. Tachycardia, increased blood pressure. 1 ml of 1/1000 or 10 ml of 1/10000 = 1 mg of adrenaline
Alcuronium 'Alloferin'	Long-acting muscle relaxant Effects may persist into recovery room.	Variable dose, see literature	Only for use in ventilated patient.
Alfentanil 'Rapifen'	Short-acting opioid. (see page 190)	30–50 µg/kg IV Onset: 30–60 sec Lasts: 5–10 min	Only for use in ventilated patient. Good for out-patient anaesthesia.
Amiodarone 'Cordarone X'	Prolongs myocardial repolarization. Blocks fast sodium channels. Used in: • WPW syndrome. • Broad complex tachycardias.	Loading dose: 25 µg/kg/min for 4 hr Maintenance: 5–15 µg/kg/min (see page 248)	Slow acting, but well tolerated. Infuse into central vein. Hypotension and vasodilation. Need to reduce dose of warfarin and digoxin.
Aminophylline	Bronchodilator sometimes used in	Loading dose: 5 mg/kg IV over at	Toxic drug causing tachyarrhythmias

Drug	Use and action	Dose	Comments
	asthma. (see page 335)	least 20 minutes. (do not load if patient already taking theophylline)	Nausea, vomiting and convulsions.
	100 mg aminophylline = 80 mg theophylline		Monitor with ECG.
		Maintenance dose: 7 mg/kg/day by infusion.	For intravenous use only. I/M injection causes massive tissue necrosis.
Aprotinin 'Trasylol'	Plasmin and kallikrein inhibitor		Occasionally causes hypersensitivity reactions.
	Used with open heart surgery to reduce blood loss.	Loading dose 2 000 000 units then 500 000 units per hr.	
	Counteracts hyperplasminaemia during the mobilization of some tumours.	Loading dose 500 000 units then 200 000 units per hr.	
Aspirin	Nonsteroidal anti-inflammatory drug.	Up to 15 mg/kg 4 hrly orally.	Avoid in children under age of 15 years.
	Effective analgesic (see page 204)		Antiplatelet activity impairs blood clotting.
			Aggravates asthma.
			Decreases renal function especially in elderly.
Atenolol 'Tenormin'	Cardioselective beta adrenoceptor blocker. Used for supraventricular arrhythmias.	0.05 mg/kg give every 5 minutes until a response (max. 4 doses)	Monitor with ECG. Give oxygen.
			May precipitate cardiac failure and bradyarrhythmias.
			Similar to propanolol
Atracurium 'Tracium'	Medium acting muscle relaxant. Effects may persist into recovery room.	Variable dose – see literature	Only for use in ventilated patient.
Atropine	Blocks muscarinic nerve endings.	0.3–1.2 mg IV over 30 seconds.	Monitor with ECG. Give oxygen.

		Sinus bradycardias. (see page 252)	or 0.02 mg/kg IV.	
Benztropine 'Cogentin'		Used for treatment of drug induced muscle spasms and oculogyric crises. (see page 228). tachycardia.	0.02 mg/kg stat IV Repeat after 15 minutes if necessary.	Sedation, May exacerbate glaucoma.
Bicarbonate² NaHCO₃ HCO₃⁻ Sodium bicarbonate		Severe acidosis compromising cardiac function. Use only if pH<7.00 (see page 320)	0.2–0.5 mmol/kg intravenously only. Give over 3–5 minutes and reassess with blood gases if possible.	Extravasation causes massive tissue necrosis. Incompatible with most drugs and some IV fluids.
Bretylium tosylate 'Bretylate'		Ventricular arrhythmias resistant to other treatment.	5–10 mg/kg over at a minimum of 10 minutes. Maintenance infusion of 1–2 mg/minute	Monitor blood pressure and ECG. Hypotension Do not use I/M.
Bupivacaine 'Marcain'		Long-acting local anaesthetic agent. (see page 198)	Infiltration: up to 40 ml of 0.25% Epidural: up to 20 ml of 0.5%	More than 2 mg/kg in any 4 hr period is toxic and may cause fitting.
Calcium chloride		see Calcium gluconate	Safer to use the gluconate.	About 5 times as potent as calcium gluconate.
Calcium gluconate		Cardiac arrhythmias with: • overdose of calcium channel blockers. • hyperkalaemia • hypocalcaemia Citrate toxicity (see page 363)	10 ml of 10% solution IV. Inject only into large vein, extravasation causes tissue necrosis. 10 ml of 10% solution slowly IV over 1 minute.	Use in asystolic cardiac arrest is controversial. Do not give in same line as bicarbonate. 10 ml of 10%= 1 g Works as quickly as calcium chloride³.
Captopril		Angiotensin converting enzyme (ACE) inhibitor used in hypertension	Oral drug	Do not use NSAIDs in patients taking ACE inhibitors.

Drug	Use and action	Dose	Comments
Carboprost 'Hemabate'	Prostaglandin F_2 alpha used for postpartum haemorrhage. (see page 98)	250 µg deep I/M	Causes asthma, nausea, vomiting, chills, headache, and flushing. May cause pulmonary oedema. Reduces renal perfusion and exacerbates glaucoma.
Clonidine 'Catapres'	Centrally acting adrenergic blocker. Increasingly used as an adjuvant for analgesia (see page 219).	5 µg/kg IV	Often causes blood pressure to rise before fall.
Cocaine	Vasoconstriction of mucous membranes	Maximum dose is 1.5 mg/kg in fit adults.	Avoid in porphyria. Dangerous to use with adrenaline. Toxic • hypertension • cardiac arrhythmias
Codeine	Opioid analgesic used for mild to moderate pain.	0.5 mg/kg orally 4 hrly.	Usually used in combination with paracetamol.
Cortisone	See Hydrocortisone		
Cyclizine 'Valoid' 'Marezine'	Antihistamine used for nausea and vomiting. (see page 227)	0.4 mg/kg I/M 4–6 hrly	Mildly sedating.
Dalteparin 'Fragmin'	Low molecular weight heparin used for prevention of venous thromboembolism. Does not need laboratory monitoring.	2500 units 2 hr before surgery and then 2500 units every 24 hr. For high risk patients use 2500 units every 12 hr	Contraindicated in peptic ulcer, recent cerebral haemorrhage, severe hypertension, severe liver disease especially if oesophageal varices.
Dantrolene	Prophylaxis and treatment of malignant hyperthermia. (See page 159)	Prophylaxis: 5 mg/kg IV given in 24 hr before anaesthesia.	Thrombophlebitic Side effects: • dizziness • weakness

	Relaxes skeletal muscles.	Management of acute MH. Loading dose: 2.5 mg/kg repeat every 5 min to max of 10 mg/kg.	• hyperkalaemia
Desflurane 'Suprane'	Fast acting volatile anaesthetic agent.	Dose variable. Requires vaporizer.	Irritant causing coughing and laryngospasm.
Dexamethasone 'Decadron'	A steroid used in • anaphylaxis • acute allergy • cerebral oedema due to tumour	0.5–20 mg IV or 0.1–0.25 mg/kg IV, repeat in 6 hr	Takes 6–8 hr to reach peak effect
Dextrose 50%	Hypoglycaemia	Adult dose: 20–50 grams IV Child dose: 0.5 g/kg IV	Inject into a large vein because of risk of thrombophlebitis
Diazepam 'Valium' Diazamul is another preparation.	Long-acting benzodiazepine Used for: • sedation • convulsions • sedative for cardioversion.	Adult dose: 2–15 mg IV or up to 0.2 mg/kg IV	Give oxygen Causes pain when given in peripheral vein. Diazamuls are less painful.
Diamorphine Heroin Available in UK only.	Opioid analgesic used for severe pain.	0.1 mg/kg I/M or IV Onset 12–20 min Action 3–4 hr	Said to cause less nausea and vomiting than morphine.
Diclofenac 'Voltaren' 'Votarol' (see page 206)	A non-steroid anti-inflammatory drug. Anti-rheumatic, anti-pyretic.	Tablets 75–150 mg daily in divided doses. Suppositories 100 mg useful after minor orthopaedic and gynaecological surgery.	Takes 1 hr to work. Gastrointestinal bleeding, exacerbation of asthma, deterioration of renal function.
Digoxin (see page 249)	Cardiac glycoside • anti-arrhythmic • ionotrope • delays A-V conduction	Loading dose: 3.5–10 µg/kg IV slowly over 20 minutes Adult maintenance: 0.125–0.5 mg/day	Serum potassium should be > 3.8 mmol/l Use lower dose range in elderly.

Drug	Use and action	Dose	Comments
			Must be done with ECG control
		Therapeutic blood level: 0.8–2 nanograms/ml	Avoid using in: • bradyarrhythmias • heart block • WPW syndrome
Dipyridamole 'Persantin'	Anti-platelet drug. Used in ischaemic heard disease.	See literature	Dangerously potentiates adenosine
Dobutamine 'Dobutrex' (see page 286)	Derivative of dopamine. Useful as an ionotrope when arrhythmias are a problem.	3–15 µg/kg/min	No effect on renal vasculature.
		Increase dose by 1 µg/kg/min to get desired effect	Causes less tachycardia than dopamine.
			Infuse only into central veins.
Dopamine 'Inotropin' (see page 286)	Noradrenaline precursor.	Renal vasodilation 3 µg/kg/min	Useful cardiac ionotrope.
	Cardiac ionotrope Renal vasodilation	Cardiac β effect 5–15 µg/kg/min	Effects blocked by butyrephenones and metoclopramide.
		Alpha effect causing peripheral vasoconstriction > 15 µg/kg/min	Best effect in a normovolaemic patient.
			Infuse only into central veins.
		Increase dose by 1 µg/kg/min. to get desired effect.	
Dopexamine 'Dopacard' (see page 287)	β₂ agonist and ionotrope	500 nanograms/ kg/min which can be increased by 1 µg/kg/min to a limit of 6 µg/kg/min in steps at 10 minute intervals,	Useful following cardiac surgery.
	Peripheral vasodilator.		May cause excessive tachycardia if the patient is in atrial fibrillation.
			Infuse only into central veins.
Doxapram 'Dopram'	Non-specific respiratory stimulator. Not an opioid antagonist.	1–1.5 mg/kg IV over at least 30 seconds. Repeat in 1 hr if needed.	Contraindicated in • epilepsy • severe asthma • hypertension

Droperidol 'Droleptan' 'Inapsine'	Butyrephenone. Sometimes used as anti-emetic. (see page 229)	0.015 –0.03 mg/kg IV.	Can cause dystonia. Catatonic state most unpleasant for normal unsedated patient.
	Larger doses cause psychomotor retardation in restless patients.	5–10 mg IV.	Contraindicated in patients taking lithium,
Enflurane 'Ethrane'	Volatile anaesthetic vapour.	Dose is variable. Requires a vaporizer.	May precipitate epilepsy.
Ephedrine	Adrenergic vasopressor used in supporting blood pressure after spinal or epidural anaesthesia. (see page 214)	3–5 mg intravenously. Repeated after 2 minutes as necessary	Monitor with ECG. Give oxygen.
Ergometrine (see page 98)	Causes uterine contraction • caesarean section • normal delivery	Up to 10 mg intravenously	Hypertension, nausea and vomiting.
Esmolol 'Brevibloc' (see page 248)	Ultra short-acting $\beta 1_1$-selective (cardioselective) adrenergic blocking agent.	Loading dose: 500 µg/kg/min given over one minute.	Dilute in 5% dextrose (glucose). Hypotension ++
	Supraventricular tachycardias.	Maintenance dose: 50–200 µg/kg/min. for 40 minutes. Works within 5 minutes.	Irritates veins. Contraindications: • heart failure; • bradycardia; • heart block; • hypotension • concurrent use with verapamil.
Enalapril	see Captopril		Avoid using NSAIDs
Enoxaparin 'Clexane'	Low molecular weight heparin.	High risk patients: 40 mg s.c. 12 hr preoperatively and thence once daily.	High risk includes orthopaedic and pelvic surgery.
	Prevention of thrombo-embolic disorders of venous origin in surgical patients.	Moderate risk: 20 mg s.c. 2 hr preoperatively.	Contraindicated in peptic ulcer, recent cerebral haemorrhage, severe hypertension, severe liver disease especially if
	Does not need laboratory monitoring.	Treat for 7 to 10 days	oesophageal varices

Drug	Use and action	Dose	Comments
Etidocaine 'Duranest'	Long-acting local anaesthetic agent. Not available in many countries.	Dose must not exceed 4 mg/kg in any 4 hr period.	May cause fitting and hypotension.
'EMLA' (Eutectic mixture of lignocaine and prilocaine)	Topical anaesthetic agent used for numbing skin.		Slow onset. Takes 60–90 minutes to work.
Fentanyl 'Sublimaze'	Short-acting opioid acting for about 30 minutes. (see page 195)	1–1.5 µg/kg. Larger doses are often used in anaesthesia.	Respiratory depression, which may be delayed for hrs especially in elderly.
Flumazenil 'Anexate' (see page 78)	Benzodiazepine antagonist. Reverses diazepam, midazolam, and others.	5 µg/kg IV over 15 seconds then repeat at 60 second intervals. Maximum dose 40 µg/kg Infusion: 2–10 µg/kg/hr IV	Short-acting drug. May wear off before diazepam and other longer acting benzodiazepines. May precipitate epilepsy in susceptible patients.
Furosemide	see Frusemide		
Frusemide 'Lasix'	Potent diuretic. Used in treatment • renal failure; • cardiac failure.	5–40 mg slowly IV. in adult. or 0.1 to 0.5 mg/kg IV. High doses sometimes used.	Nephrotoxic and ototoxic. Potentiates damage caused by gentamicin and other aminoglycosides.
Gallamine 'Flaxedil'	Long-acting muscle relaxant used in anaesthesia. Effects may persist into recovery room.	Dose is variable.	Patient must be ventilated. Tachycardia. Needs reversing. Excreted only by kidneys.
Gentamicin	Aminoglycoside antibiotic which inhibits protein synthesis in susceptible bacteria.	Loading dose: 3–5 mg/kg on first day. Dose at 12 hrly intervals. Maintenance dose: 1 mg/kg depending on serum creatinine	Nephrotoxic, ototoxic. This is exacerbated by diuretics. Inactivated by penicillins.

Glycopyrrolate 'Robinul'	Longer acting than atropine. Useful substitute.	Dose is 200–400 µg or 4–8 µg/kg to max of 400 µg	Causes less tachycardia than atropine. Monitor with ECG.
Glyceryl trinitrate (Nitroglycerine) (GTN)	Short-acting vasodilator. Hypertension, acute myocardial ischaemia.	Infusion, tablets, or paste absorbed through skin.	May cause headache. Monitor with ECG during infusion. Do not use PVC containers because they reduce its potency.
Haloperidol 'Serenace'	Powerful tranquillizer. Useful for demented patients.	Dose: 5–10 mg will last about 8 hr	Psychomotor retardation.
Halothane 'Fluothane'	Volatile anaesthetic vapour.	Dose is variable and requires a vaporizer.	Very potent.
Hydralazine 'Apresoline' (see page 243)	Vasodilator used for hypertension.	Dose: 5–20 mg by slow injection over 10 minutes.	Causes a tachycardia. Do not use if patient has fixed cardiac output.
Hydrocortisone	Steroid essential for maintenance of blood pressure. Used in • anaphylaxis • allergies • adrenal failure	2–4 mg/kg IV at 6 hrly intervals.	Used prophylactic-ally in patients who have been receiving steroid therapy.
Hyoscine 'Buscopan'	Anti-cholinergic agent used to treat smooth muscle spasm especially in gut or ureters.	5–20 mg slowly intravenously.	Causes sedation and tachycardia.
Indomethacin 'Indocid'	NSAID, used as an analgesic especially by suppository.	Rectal suppository 200 mg.	Aggravates asthma, may affect renal function especially in elderly.
Ipratropium 'Atrovent'	Atropine derivative used in treatment of chronic asthma.	20 µg/dose by metered inhaler 6 hrly	Not usually used in acute asthmatic attack.
Isoflurane 'Forane'	Volatile anaesthetic vapour.	Dose is variable, and requires a vaporizer.	Respiratory depression.

Drug	Use and action	Dose	Comments
Isoprenaline (Isoproteranol in USA) 'Isuprel' 'Saventrine'	β_1 sympathetic cardiac stimulant used for treatment of asystole or heart block.	Infusion of 0.5–20 µg per minute. Increase dose by 0.01 µg/min to get desired effect.	Monitor with ECG. Bronchodilator. Give supplemental oxygen during infusion. Maximum effect in 3 minutes.
Ketamine 'Ketalar'	Dissociative anaesthetic with good cardiovascular and respiratory stability.	1–1.5 mg/kg IV. 5–10 mg/kg I/M. May be given by infusion.	Emergence delirium may be very disturbing and frightening for patient.
Ketorolac 'Toredol' (see page 206)	NSAID analgesic.	20–30 mg I/M.	Recent reports of renal damage especially in sick or elderly. Aggravates asthma.
Labetalol 'Trandate'	α and β adrenoceptor block	0.1 mg/kg IV over at least 1 minute; repeat in 5 minutes if needed. Maximum dose 0.3 mg/kg.	Reduces cardiac output and causes vasodilation. Monitor ECG and blood pressure.
Lignocaine (lidocaine in USA) 'Xylocaine'	Local anaesthetic agent. Topical 10% spray. Treatment of laryngospasm . Ventricular premature beats.	Infiltration of up to 5 mg/kg. 10 mg/squirt. 1.5 mg/kg IV. Bolus dose of 1.5 mg/kg followed by infusion of 1–4 mg/minute.	Be careful with dose. Monitor with ECG when giving intravenous lignocaine. Overdose causes fitting, and cardiac arrhythmias.
Magnesium sulphate	Anti-arrhythmic Multiple atrial ectopics Torsades de pointes	5 ml of 49.3% solution = 10 millimol. Give 10 mmol IV slowly over 5 min.	If injected too fast causes cutaneous vasodilation and hypotension.
Mannitol 'Osmitrol'	Osmotic diuretic used for forced diuresis in haemolytic transfusion reactions, ophthalmic surgery, raised intracranial pressure.	0.5–1 g/kg by IV infusion.	Works in minutes and lasts for 3–4 hours. May cause fluid overload.

			Extravasation causes tissue damage.
Meperidine	see Pethidine (also see page 193)		
Metaraminol 'Aramine'	Synthetic sympathetic amine which increases force of contraction of heart, heart rate, and blood pressure. Used for treatment of normovolaemic hypotension.	0.5–1 mg IV Repeat as necessary. Infusions cause tachyphylaxis after a few hours.	Give supplemental oxygen. Monitor with ECG.
Methohexitone 'Brietal'	Short-acting oxybarbiturate used for induction of anaesthesia.	Approximately 1 mg/kg.	May precipitate fitting in epileptics.
Methoxamine 'Vasoxine'	Direct acting vasoconstrictor used for increasing blood pressure.	15–30 µg/kg or 1 mg IV slowly at one minute intervals.	No effect on cardiac output. Can make cardiac failure worse by increasing cardiac pressure work.
Methoxyflurane 'Penthrane'	Volatile anaesthetic agent. Obsolete. Sometimes used for analgesia in trauma.	Variable dose. See literature.	Slow to act. May cause renal damage if used for more than an hr or so.
Metoclopramide 'Maxolon' 'Metramid' 'Parmid' 'Reglan' (see page 229)	Anti-emetic. Used to control nausea and vomiting.	10–20 mg intravenously or intramuscularly.	Avoid in children as it may cause rigidity and oculogyric crises. This can be treated with benztropine. Sedation may prolong recovery.
Metoprolol 'Betaloc' 'Lopressor' (see page 248)	Cardioselective beta adrenoceptor blocking drug for control of supraventricular tachycardias.	5 mg injected IV at rate of 1–2 mg/min. May be repeated in five minutes. Total dose should not exceed 15 mg.	Monitor with ECG. Give oxygen. May precipitate cardiac failure and bradyarrhythmias. Exacerbates asthma.

Drug	Use and action	Dose	Comments
Mexiletine 'Mexitil'	Membrane stabilizing anti-arrhythmic similar to lignocaine.	Loading dose: 5 mg/kg IV over 15 minutes then 5–20 µg/kg/min.	No use in SVT, Relatively low efficacy in ventricular ectopics. Toxic side effects. Will exacerbate heart block.
Midazolam 'Hypnovel'	Short acting benzodiazepine inducing sedation, and useful antegrade amnesia.	Sedation: 1–5 mg IV Start with lower dose and increase by 1 mg increments at 1 minute intervals.	Will exacerbate myasthenia gravis, acute glaucoma and COAD. Risk of respiratory depression, apnoea, hypotension. Use a pulse oximeter.
Milrinone 'Primacor'	A phosphodiesterase III inhibitor. Positive ionotrope and vasodilator with minimal effects on heart rate. Congestive cardiac failure not responding to other therapy.	Loading dose: 0.37–0.75 µg/kg/min. Effective in 5–15 min. Half life about 2 hr	Monitor with ECG. Reduce dose in renal failure. Precipitates with frusemide.
Misoprostol 'Cytotec'	Synthetic prostaglandin derivative with anti-secretory properties used in therapy of peptic ulcers.	Prophylaxis: 200 µg 2–4 times daily.	May cause hypotension. Increases uterine tone, thus not for use in pregnancy
Mivacurium 'Mivacrom'	Short-acting non-depolarizing muscle relaxant	See literature	
Moclobemide 'Aurorix'	Anti-depressant with reversible inhibition of mono-amine oxidase.	Short-acting with 1–2 hr elimination 1/2 life.	Cease 16 hr before surgery to clear drug from system.
Morphine (see page 192)	Opioid analgesic drug.	0.15–0.3 mg/kg.	Respiratory depression.

Nalorphine 'Lethidrone' (see page 198)	Partial opioid agonist used for reversing opioid induced respiratory depression.	Titrate to 0.15 mg/kg slowly IV over 3 minutes. Lasts 2–3 hr	Overdose may exacerbate respiratory depression.
Naloxone 'Narcan' (see page 198)	Potent pure opioid antagonist.	0.04–0.4 mg slowly IV over 3 minutes. Lasts about 35 minutes.	May plunge patient into severe pain with dangerous rise in blood pressure. Recurrence of respiratory depression.
Naltrexone	Long-acting opioid antagonist.		
Neostigmine 'Prostigmin' (see page 173)	Cholinesterase inhibitor used for reversing effects of non-depolarizing muscle relaxants eg. tubocurare pancuronium, alcuronium, vecuronium	0.5–2.5 mg IV. Give with atropine 0.4–1.2 mg IV to prevent bradycardia, salivation and bronchospasm.	Lasts for about 40 minutes. Causes bronchospasm Potentiates the effects of suxamethonium. Contributes to post operative nausea and vomiting.
Nifedipine (see page 242)	Slow-channel calcium blocking agent used for control of hypertension.	10 mg orally. Takes 2–3 minutes to work if capsule pieced with pin.	Useful if patient has angina or tachycardia. Monitor with ECG. Causes bradycardia if patient taking beta blockers.
Nimodipine 'Nimotop'	Calcium channel blocker for management of cerebral vasospasm following intracranial surgery.	Initial dose: 15 µg/kg/hr for 2 hr If BP remains stable, then increase to 30 µg/kg/hr.	Hypotension, bradycardia and decrease in renal blood flow.
Nitric Oxide[3] **NO** Previously known as endothelium derived relaxant factor. (EDRF).	Inhaled it is a selective pulmonary vasodilator. Neurotransmitter in CNS. Involved with immune response.	Given by inhalation. 0.06–80 ppm* (0.00006–0.08 ml) added to 10 litre per minute volume. * ppm = parts per million.	Requires special equipment for administration. Broken down by haemoglobin. Toxic. Hypotension.

Drug	Use and action	Dose	Comments
Nitroglycerine	see Glyceryl trinitrate		
Nitroprusside 'Nipride' (See page 244)	Very short acting vasodilator administered only by infusion. Used for acute hypertension.	Dose: 0.5–10 µg/kg/min. Dose increments = 20 µg. The average dose is about 100 µg per minute. Maximum effect seen in 3 minutes.	Decomposes rapidly if exposed to bright light, or heat so protect infusion with black paper or aluminium foil. Cyanide toxicity may occur[5]. Nausea, sweating, apprehension, headache, muscle twitching. Monitor with ECG and intra-arterial pressure line.
Noradrenaline 'Levophed'	Sometimes used in treatment of acute septic shock. Direct acting Vasoconstrictor causes increase in blood pressure, but decreases tissue perfusion especially in kidneys and gut.	Dose: 1–30 µg/minute. Increase dose by 1 µg per minute to get desired effect.	Administer only by a central venous catheter. Extravasation causes tissue necrosis. Monitor with ECG. Needs arterial pressure monitor.
Ondansetron[6] 'Zofran' (see page 230)	5-HT$_3$ receptor antagonist for the treatment of postoperative nausea and vomiting.	8 mg I/M 8 hrly.	Constipation, headache, blurred vision.
Oxytocin 'Syntocinon'	Synthetic oxytocin used for stimulating uterine contraction during and after . labour	Used after delivery 5–10 units IV slowly. May need infusion of 5–10 units/hr.	Hypotension, tachycardia and ECG changes.
Pancuronium 'Pavulon'	Long-acting muscle relaxant used in anaesthesia.	Variable—see literature.	Patient must be ventilated. Unsuitable for use in infants, neonates and in renal failure because of its slow elimination.

Paperveretum 'Omnopon' 'Pantopon'	Mixture of purified opioid alkaloids used for premedication or severe pain.	0.015–0.03 mg/kg IV or I/M	
Paracetamol 'Panadol' 'Tylanol'	Centrally acting prostaglandin inhibitor. Mild analgesic	15 mg/kg 4 hrly oral or PR.	Slow to work in immediate post-operative period.
Pethidine (Meperidine-USA) 'Pethoid' (see page 193)	A synthetic opioid analgesic. Used for patient controlled analgesia	Loading dose: 1–2 mg/kg I/M 0.5–1 mg/kg IV	Respiratory depression, nausea, vomiting, hypotension, sedation, sweating
Phenoperidine 'Operidine'	A synthetic opioid analgesic. Short-acting—about 40 minutes. Sometimes used for settling patients 'fighting' a ventilator.	0.01–0.03 mg/kg IV or I/M Up to 0.1 mg/kg IV can be used if a patient is being ventilated.	Respiratory depression. Cardiovascular stablity.
Phentolamine 'Regitine'	Short-acting alpha adrenoceptor blocker. A vasodilator used for hypertension,	Loading dose: 0.1 mg/kg IV Infusion: 5–50 µg/kg/min IV	Tachycardia Hypotension
Phenylepherine	Indirect acting sympathetic amine used for the treatment of acute hypotension	1.5–7 µg/kg.	Tachycardia Hypertension
Phenytoin 'Dilantin' 'Epinutin' (see page 125)	Anti-epileptic	Loading dose: 15–20 mg/kg IV over 1 hr Maintenance: 2 mg/kg IV 12 hrly.	Sedation Paediatric doses are variable. Consult literature.
Physostigmine	A cholinesterase inhibitor which crosses the blood brain barrier Used to reverse the delirium caused by scopolamine and other anticholinergics.	0.02 mg/kg IV every 5 minutes to a maximum of 0.2 mg/kg. (see page 154)	Short half life. If symptoms persist infuse at 1–10 µg/kg/min

Drug	Use and action	Dose	Comments
Prilocaine 'Citonest'	Local anaesthetic agent, less toxic than lignocaine.	Dose: Up to 5 mg/kg	Methaemo-globinaemia simulates cyanosis, and may produce hypoxia.
Procaine 'Novocaine'	Local anaesthetic, not as effective as lignocaine, but safer.	Dose: Up to 12 mg/kg Infiltration lasts 30–60 minutes.	Probably safe in patients with malignant hyperthermia.
Procainamide 'Pronestyl'	Membrane stabilizing anti-arrhythmic similar to lignocaine.	Loading dose: 3–6 mg/kg IV over 15 min Maintenance: 20–80 µg/kg/min	
Prochlorperazine Stemetil'	A centrally acting phenothiazine antiemetic agent used for control of postoperative vomiting.		Occasionally causes muscle rigidity, and nystagmus especially in children and young adults. This can be treated with benztropine, May cause prolonged sedation in elderly.
Promethazine 'Phenergan'	A centrally acting phenothiazine sedative and antiemetic agent.	0.5 mg/kg I/M 6–8 hrly.	Sedation marked. May cause confusion in elderly.
Propanolol 'Inderal'	Non-cardoselective beta-blocker used for control of tachycardias.	0.001–0.03 mg/kg IV. Repeat in 10 minutes if necessary.	Bradycardia, hypotension. Aggravates asthma.
Propofol 'Diprivan'	Short acting anaesthetic induction agent.	1–3 mg/kg stat.	Sometimes used as infusion. In patients over 50 years proceed cautiously, as hypotension is a risk.
Protamine	Used to reverse anticoagulant effects of heparin.	1 mg reverses 100 units of heparin. 1 mg/kg IV over 10 minutes.	Hypotension which may be severe. Flushing Bradycardia

Drug	Description	Dose	Notes
Ranitidine 'Zantac'	H_2-receptor antagonist which reduces gastric acid output.	Prophylaxis of acid aspiration: orally 150 mg 2 hr before theatre; or intravenously 50 mg by slow IV injection 45 minutes before theatre.

Prophylaxis of NSAID induced duodenal ulcers 150 mg twice daily. | Reduce dose in renal and hepatic disease, and during pregnancy or breast feeding.

High doses may rarely cause arrhythmias.

Ritrodine |
| **Rocuronium** 'Zemuron' 'Esmeron' | Non-depolarizing neuromuscular blocking agent. | Variable—see literature. | Patient must be ventilated. |
| **Ropivicaine**[7] | Long-acting local anaesthetic agent similar to bupivacaine. | | Less toxic than bupivacaine.

Slow onset. |
| **Salbutamol** 'Ventolin' | B_2 adrenoceptor stimulant used as bronchodilator (see page 336) and as a tocolytic agent (see page 97) | Metered inhaler 100 µg/puff. or 1 µg/kg IV at 2 min intervals until tachycardia becomes a problem

Max effect in 5 min Lasts: 3–4 hr | Safe drug.

Tachycardia Anxiety Headache |
| **Sevoflurane** | Volatile anaesthetic agent. | Dose variable. Requires a vaporizer. | |
| **Sotalol** 'Sotacor' (see page 248) | Beta adrenoceptor blocker which lengthens cardiac action potential duration.

Useful drug for: Atrial fibrillation Paroxysmal ventricular tachycardia Ventricular ectopics. Ventricular tachycardia. | Dose: 20–60 mg over 2–3 minutes using ECG monitoring. | Usually little effect on cardiac function.

Occasionally causes serious side effects:

• Sinus bradycardia • Torsade de pointes

Dangerous if hypokalaemic |

Drug	Use and action	Dose	Comments
Sufentanil[8]	Opioid analgesic	0.1 µg/kg Bigger doses sometimes used. Onset: 1–4 min Lasts: 30–60 min	Powerful respiratory depressant BP stable.
Suxamethonium (Succinyl choline) 'Scoline' 'Anectine'	Depolarizing muscle relaxant used for rapid intubation.	1–2 mg/kg IV Onset: 10–30 sec Lasts: 1–5 min	Store at 4°C Second dose causes severe bradycardia. Occasionally causes prolonged relaxation.
Tacrine 'THA'	Anticholinesterase which can pass the blood–brain barrier. Occasionally used as a respiratory stimulant.	0.25–1 mg/kg IV	Potentiates the effects of suxamethonium.
Temazepam	Short-acting oral benzodiazepine.	10–20 mg orally	Useful amnesic used in premed.
Thiopentone 'Pentothal'	Short-acting barbiturate used for induction of anaesthesia.	3–5 mg/kg IV	Hypotension
Tranexamic acid 'Cyklokapron'	Antifibrinolysin which inhibits plasminogen activation. Useful in bleeding after prostatectomy and dental surgery.	0.5–3 g slowly IV	Nausea, vomiting, hypotension.
Tubocurare 'Tubarine' 'Jexin'	Long-acting muscle relaxant. Effects may persist into recovery room.		Only for use in ventilated patient.
Vecuronium 'Norcuron'	Long-acting muscle relaxant. Effects may persist into recovery room.		Only for use in ventilated patient.
Verapamil 'Isoptin' 'Cordilox' 'Anpec'	Calcium antagonist used for supraventricular tachyarrhythmias.	Loading dose: 0.1–0.2 mg/kg over 10 minutes.	May cause: • bradycardia, • hypotension • heart block.

Maintenance:
5 µg/kg/min.

Monitor
- blood pressure
- ECG

Do not inject into
patient recently
treated with β
blockers because of
the danger of
hypotension and
asystole.

Avoid in
- Wolff–Parkinson–
  White syndrome
- broad complex
  tachycardias.

INFUSIONS

Some drugs need to be administered at a constant rate for a number of hours or longer. This is best achieved by an infusion. A solution is prepared with a known concentration of drug. This is delivered at a rate calculated to keep the blood concentration of the drug at a fairly constant level. A loading dose is needed for most drugs. The advantages of an infusion are that the effect of the drug is smoother, a lower overall dose is required and the need for repeated injections is eliminated.

There are two ways of administering an infusion.

1. Syringe drivers (see page 401) give small volumes of concentrated drug through a catheter placed in one of the large central veins such as the superior vena cava. The drugs are usually so concentrated that they will injure smaller peripheral veins and may cause severe tissue damage if extravasation occurs.

Never infuse concentrated drugs
through peripheral veins.

2. Infusion pumps (see page 401) give larger volumes of fluid. Generally the drugs are less concentrated and often it is possible to safely infuse them into smaller peripheral veins.

Prepare written protocols for each drug used. In them, set down the dose of the drug and the required pump or syringe drive settings. Include details of the expected effects, complications and management of these complications. Staff should be familiar with all the effects and expected problems before the infusion starts. Establish clear written instructions about limits of the parameters of blood pressure, pulse rate, respiratory rate and other variables. These are best set out on a whiteboard mounted on the wall near the head of the patient so that all staff can easily see them.

Each potent drug needs its own dedicated separate intravenous line. It is unwise to use one catheter for infusion a number of drugs. Do not 'piggy back' lines by using multi-entry ports or plug infusions into intravenous lines carrying other intravenous infusions. For safety potent drugs should be infused through a multilumen central venous catheter, with each lumen carrying only one drug.

For safety infuse only one drug
through each intravenous line.

Be careful of the *dead space* in lines and catheters. Unfamiliarity with the concept of dead space can cause dangerous problems. Prime (that means 'fill-up') the lines with the solution containing the drug. This prevents a delay in the drug reaching the patient. Unless properly primed it will take time for the drug solution to fill the volume of the tubing. This volume is called the dead space. Beware of inadvertently flushing this dead space because the patient may get a large dose of unwanted drug. For this reason, never injected anything into a line through which concentrated drug is being infused.

To prevent errors, the drug concentration and the rate of infusion must always be checked independently by two separate trained staff who understand the equipment and how to use it.

In the doses recommended below, the concentration of drug has been chosen so that the pump settings in millilitres per hour represent some simple numerical function of the drug dose in units per hour. For example if morphine is to be given then a setting of 4 ml/hour will give a dose of 4 mg/ hour.

Attach an intravenous additive label to bags, flasks, or syringes containing drugs.

Patient's name..   Unit record number ....

Ward...........   Date....................   Time prepared ....

Prepared by ....   Checked by

....

DRUG AND DOSE ADDED

Concentration...........   Duration of infusion ....
                                    Time to finish...........................

Fig 24. Label for infusions and dilutions

Important Notice

Most of the following drugs are highly concentrated and will cause severe thrombophlebitis and tissue necrosis if infused into peripheral veins. So infuse them into central veins only through a central venous catheter.

When infusing vasoactive or cardiac drugs always monitor cardiac rate and rhythm with an ECG and continuous record blood pressure preferably an intra-arterial blood cannula.

Patients receiving infusions need constant monitoring and careful nursing care. Patients must never be left unattended. Everyone needs to be familiar with the pharmacology of the drugs, their actions, and side effects. Written protocols are needed and patient cardiovascular and other parameters need to be carefully specified.

Note: Further information on these drugs and their actions is available in the table at the beginning of this chapter.

Drug	Dilution	Dose
Adrenaline Epinephrine in USA 1 ml of 1/1000 = 1 mg 10 ml of 1/10,000 = 1 mg	Adrenaline 3 mg Make up to 50 ml in 5% dextrose	1 ml/hr = 1 µg/min 1–30 µg/min. Increase dose by 1 µg/min until desired effect.
Amiodarone	Amiodarone 300 mg in 50 ml of 5% dextrose. (Not stable in saline), No need to use glass syringes.	Loading dose: 25 µg/kg/min for 4 hr May be given at 5 mg/kg over 20 min if urgent Maintenance: 5–15 µg/kg/min

Dopamine	Dopamine 300 mg
	
	Make up to 50 ml in 5% dextrose
		1 ml/hr = 100 µg/min
		
		Increase dose by 1 µg/kg/min until desired effect.
		
		Renal dose:
		  3–5 µg/kg/min
		Beta effect:
		  5–25 µg/kg/min
		Alpha effect:
		  > 25 µg/kg/min

Dobutamine	Dobutamine 250 mg Make up to 41.5 ml in 5% dextrose	1 ml/hr=100µg/min 2.5–15 µg/kg/min
Dopexamine	Dopexamine 10 mg Make up to 41.5 ml in 5% dextrose	1 ml/hr = 4 µg/min 0.5–60 µg/kg/min

Frusemide Furosemide in USA	Frusemide 100 mg	1 ml/hr = 2 mg/hr
	Make up to 50 ml in normal (0.9%) saline	Loading dose: 0.5 mg/kg Maintenance dose: 0.1–1 mg/kg/hr
		Protect from light.
Glyceryl trinitrate 'GTN' 'Nitroglycerine'	Glyceryl trinitrate 100 mg	1 ml/hr = 40 µg/min
	Make up to 41.5 ml in 5% dextrose	Maintenance dose: 1–5 µg/kg/min Increase dose by 2–40 µg/min
Heparin 1 mg = 100 units.	Heparin 25 000 units make up to 25 ml in 5% dextrose.	1 ml/hr = 1000 units/hr
		Low dose: 75 units/kg stat then 10–15 units/kg/hr
		Full heparinization: 200 units/kg stat then 15–30 units/kg/hr
Insulin	Insulin 50 units	1 ml/hr = 1 unit/hr
	Make up to 50 ml in 5% dextrose.	
Isoprenaline	Isoprenaline 3 mg	1 ml/hr = 1 µg/min
	Make up to 50 ml in 5% dextrose.	1–20 µg/min
		Increase dose by 1 µg/min until desired effect.
Lignocaine Lidocaine in USA 'Xylocard'	Lignocaine 1000 mg Make up to 41.5 ml in 5% dextrose.	1 ml/hr = 0.5 mg/min Run at: 8 ml/hr for 1st hr 6 ml/hr for 2nd hr 4 ml/hr for next 24 hrs
Milrinone	Milrinone 30 mg	1 ml/hr = 10 µg/min
	Make up to 50 ml in 5% dextrose	Min. 0.37 µg/kg/min Av. 0.5 µg/kg/min Max. 0.75 µg/kg/min
Morphine	Morphine 50 mg	1 ml/hr = 1 mg/hr
	Make up to 50 ml in 5% dextrose.	Loading dose: 0.1–0.5 mg/kg
		Normal requirements 0.02–0.1 mg/kg/hr

Drug	Dilution	Dose
Nimodopine		Initial dose: 15 µg/kg/hr for 2 hr. If BP remains stable, then increase to 30 µg/kg/hr.
Nitroglycerine	see Glyceryl trinitrate	
Nitroprusside 'Nipride'	Nitroprusside 50 mg	1 ml/hr = 20 µg/min
	Make up to 41.5 ml in 5% dextrose	0.5–10 µg/kg/min
	Do not exceed dose of 10 µg/kg/minute.	The average dose is 1.5 µg/kg/min
		Max effect seen in 3 minutes. Dose increments: 0.5 µg/kg
Noradrenaline Norepinephrine in USA	Noradrenaline 3 mg	1 ml/hr = 1 µg/min
	Make up to 50 ml in 5% dextrose	1–30 µg/min
		Increase dose by 1 µg/min until desired effect.
Pethidine	Pethidine 500 mg	1 ml/hr = 10 mg/hr
	Make up to 50 ml in 5% dextrose.	Loading dose: 0.75–1.5 mg/kg
		Maintenance dose: 0.1–0.4 mg/kg/hr
Procainamide	Procainamide 1000 mg	1 ml/hr = 0.5 mg/min Run at:
	Make up to 41.5 ml in 5% dextrose.	8 ml/hr for 1st hr 6 ml/hr for 2nd hr 4 ml/hr for next 24 hrs
Protamine	Use undiluted 500 mg in 50 ml	1 ml/hr = 10 mg/hr
		Dose: Take previously administered heparin dose (units/hr) and divide it by 100.

| **Verapamil** 'Cordilox' | Verapamil 50 mg | 1 ml/hr = 1 mg/hr |
| | Make up to 50 ml in 5% dextrose. | Loading dose: 1 mg/min up to 10 mg (10 ml of 10% calcium gluconate may be needed to control hypotension) **or** 0.1–0.15 mg/kg IV over 10 minutes. |

Drug names in Australasia, United Kingdom and United States

Australasia and UK	United States
Adrenaline	Epinephrine
Benzyl penicillin	Penicillin G
Ergometrine	Ergonovine
Frusemide	Furosemide
Hydrallazine	Hydralazine
Isoprenaline	Isoproteranol
Lignocaine	Lidocaine
Nitroglycerine	Nitroglycerin
Noradrenaline	Norepinephrine
Paracetamol	Acetaminophen
Pethidine	Meperidine
Hyoscine	Scopolamine
Suxamethonium	Succinylcholine
Thiopentone	Thiopental

1 Linker NJ. (1992) *British Journal of Hospital Medicine*, 47: 565-6.
2 Cooper J. (1994) *Australian Anaesthesia*, 1994, Editor J. Kenealy. Published Australian and New Zealand College of Anaesthetists, Melbourne, Australia.
3 Finfer, S., Hobbes A. (1994) *Australian Anesthesia 1994* pp. 187–95 Published by the Australian and New Zealand College of Anaesthetists, Melbourne, Australia.
5 Leader, (16/9/1978). *British Medical Journal*, p. 704.
6 Alon E, Himmelseher S, (1992). *Anaesthesia and Analgesia*, 75: 561–5.
7 Katz JA, Brindenbough PO, (1990). *Anaesthesia and Analgesia*, 70: 16

25. USEFUL DATA

Standardization

Over the years countries have developed their own units of measurement; for instance the Europeans measured liquid volume in litres, the UK in imperial gallons, and the US in a different gallon. The Systeme Internationale d'Unites (SI system) was developed to overcome these difficulties. It has become standard to measure length in metres, mass in kilograms, and time in seconds, pressure in pascals, work in joules, volume in cubic metres and so on. Non-standard units are still widely used and include millimetres of mercury, litres, and degrees Fahrenheit. It will be many years before one drinks 0.180×10^{-3} cubic metres instead of a tumbler (or glass) of water, or say today's temperature is 300°K.

Factors

FACTOR	PREFIX	SYMBOL
10^6	mega	M
10^3	kilo	k
10^{-1}	deci	d
10^{-2}	centi	c
10^{-3}	milli	m
10^{-6}	micro	μ
10^{-9}	nano	n
10^{-12}	pico	p

Temperature

SI unit is the degree Kelvin, but Celsius is the usual notation Centigrade means the same as Celsius.

$C° = (F° - 32) \times 5/9$

$F° = (C° \times 9/5) + 32$

C°	F°	C°	F°	C°	F°
30	86.0	35	95.0	38	100.4
32	87.8	36	96.8	39	102.2
34	93.2	37	98.6	40	104.0

Length

SI unit is the metre
1 metre = 100 centimetres = 1000 millimetres
1 foot = 30.48 cm = 304.8 mm
1 inch = 2.54 cm = 25.4 mm

Volume

SI unit is the cubic metre
1000 millilitres = 10 decilitres = 1 litre
1 teaspoon = 4.5 ml
1 tablespoon = 15 ml
1 teacup = 120 ml
1 tumbler = 240 ml
1 pint = 568 ml
1 fluid ounce = 28.42 ml

Conversion table for solution strengths

By definition a 1 per cent solution contains 1 gram of substance in every 100 ml of solution. This can also be written as 1:100 or 10 mg/ml.

DILUTION	SOLUTION	MG/ML
1:200 000	0.0002%	0.002 mg/ml
1:100 000	0.001%	0.01 mg/ml
1:10 000	0.01%	0.1 mg/ml
1:5000	0.02%	0.2 mg/ml
1:1000	0.1%	1.0 mg/ml
1:500	0.2%	2.0 mg/ml
1:200	0.5%	5.0 mg/ml
1:100	1.0%	10.0 mg/ml
1:50	2.0%	20.0 mg/ml
1:10	10.%	100.0 mg/ml

Pressure

SI unit is the pascal. A kilopascal is 1000 pascals. Some places measure pressures in kilopascals (kPa), whereas others measure it in millimetres of mercury (mmHg).

7.6 mmHg = 1 kPa
1 mmHg ≈ 13 Pa
Occasionally pressure is measured in centimetres of water
10 cmH_2O = 1.36 mmHg

SI UNIT	OLD UNIT	OLD TO SI	SI TO OLD
kPa	mmHg	× 0.133	× 7.60
	cm H$_2$O	× 0.098	×10.20
	lb per inch^2	× 6.894	× 0.145

mmHg	kPa	mmHg	kPa	mmHg	kPa	mmHg	kPa	mmHg	kPa
1	0.13	21	2.76	41	5.39	61	8.03	81	10.66
2	0.26	22	2.89	42	5.52	62	8.16	82	10.79
3	0.39	23	3.03	43	5.65	63	8.29	83	10.92
4	0.53	24	3.16	44	5.79	64	8.42	84	11.05
5	0.66	25	3.29	45	5.92	65	8.55	85	11.18
6	0.79	26	3.42	46	6.05	66	8.68	86	11.32
7	0.92	27	3.55	47	6.18	67	8.82	87	11.45
8	1.05	28	3.68	48	6.32	68	8.95	88	11.58
9	1.08	29	3.82	49	6.45	69	9.08	89	11.71
10	1.32	30	3.95	50	6.58	70	9.21	90	11.84
11	1.45	31	4.08	51	6.71	71	9.34	91	11.97
12	1.58	32	4.21	52	6.84	72	9.47	92	12.11
13	1.71	33	4.34	53	6.97	73	9.60	93	12.24
14	1.84	34	4.47	54	7.11	74	9.73	94	12.37
15	1.97	35	4.60	55	7.24	75	9.87	95	12.50
16	2.11	36	4.73	56	7.37	76	10.00	96	12.63
17	2.24	37	4.87	57	7.50	77	10.13	97	12.76
18	2.37	38	5.00	58	7.63	78	10.26	98	12.89
19	2.50	39	5.13	59	7.76	79	10.39	99	13.03
20	2.63	40	5.26	60	7.89	80	10.53	100	13.16

Weight

1 000 000 microgram = 1000 milligram = 1 gram = 0.001 kg

1 ounce (oz) = 28.35 g

1 pound (lb) = 0.4536 kg

1 stone = 14 lb = 6.35 kg

26. ABBREVIATIONS

Abbreviations are frequently used by medical and nursing staff. They are sometimes specific to a particular area, and are a mystery to outsiders, but many are in common use. To avoid errors and mishaps use only abbreviations approved by your hospital. Even approved abbreviations can be misunderstood if they are not written clearly, and clear script is not a virtue of many doctors. Always explain abbreviations if there is the possibility they have more than one meaning, for example, DOA could mean dead on arrival, or date of admission; ARF could mean acute respiratory failure or acute renal failure; and Cx could mean cervical spine or cervix. This is a list of common abbreviations used in many hospitals.

Never act on an abbreviation
unless you are absolutely sure what it means.

a.c.	before food is given; it applies to medication.	ASAP	as soon as possible
		Assist	assistants
AC	alternating current	ATLS	advanced trauma life support
ABG	arterial blood gases	AUC	area under curve
ACE	angiotensin converting enzyme	AV shunt	arteriovenous shunt
ACLS	advanced cardiac life support	AV node	atrioventricular node
ADT	any damn thing	AXR	abdominal x-ray
AED	automatic external defibrillator	BA	bowel action
AF	atrial fibrillation	BCC	basal cell carcinoma
AIDS	acquired immune deficiency syndrome	BCLS	basic cardiac life support
		b.d.	twice daily
a.m.	before noon	BF	breast fed
AMI	acute myocardial infarction	BIP	bisthmus iodine paste
ANS	autonomic nervous system	BKA	below knee amputation
APACHE	acute physiology and chronic health evaluation	BP	blood pressure
		B.S.	blood sugar
APS	acute pain service	BUN	bound urinary nitrogen
APTT	activated partial thromboplastin time	BVM	bab valve mask unit
		Bx	biopsy
ARDS	adult respiratory distress syndrome	Ca	carcinoma
ARF	acute renal failure	Ca^{2+}	calcium ion

CaO$_2$	arterial oxygen content	DPG	diphosphoglycerate
CABG	coronary artery bypass graft	DOA	dead on arrival
CAN	cardiac autonomic neuropathy	DO$_2$	oxygen supply
CAD	coronary artery disease	DOB	date of birth
CAPD	ambulatory peritoneal dialysis	dTC	tubocurare
CAVDH	continuous arterio-venous haemodialysis	DUT	diabetic urine tests
		Dx	diathermy
CCF	congestive cardiac failure	D5W	dextrose 5% in water
CDH	congenital dislocationof the hip	EACA	epsilon amino caproic acid
		ECF	extracellular fluid
CE	continuing education	ECG	electrocardiograph
CETT	cuffed endotracheal tube	ED	emergency department
CK	creatinine kinase	EKG	electrocardiograph
CKMB	creatinine kinase isoenzyme—muscle band	ELISA	enzyme-linked immunosorbent assay
Cl-	chloride ion	EMB	early morning breakfast
cm	centimetre	EMLA	eutectic mixture of local anaesthetics
CMV	cytomegalovirus		
CNS	central nervous system	ENT	ear, nose and throat surgery
CO$_2$	carbon dioxide	E/o	excision of
COAD	chronic obstructive airway disease	ER	emergency room
		ERSF	end stage renal failure
COPD	chronic obstructive pulmonary disease	ESWL	extracorporeal shock wave lithotripsy
CPAP	continuous positive airway pressure	ESU	electrosurgical unit (diathermy in the UK)
CRF	chronic renal failure	ETA	estimated time of arrival
CRI	cardiac risk index	ETT	endotracheal tube
CSF	cerebrospinal fluid	EUA	examination under anaesthesia
CT	computographic scan	FB	foreign body
CVA	cerebrovascular accident	FBC	fluid balance chart
CVC	central venous catheter	FBE	full blood examination
CVP	central venous pressure	FDA	Federal Drug Authority—an USA agency
CvO$_2$	mixed venus oxygen content		
CWMS	colour,warmth, movement, sensation	FDP	fibrin degredation products
		FEV$_1$	forced expiratory volume in one second
Cx	cervix		
Cx	cervical spine	FF	free fluids
C5	fifth cervical vertebra	FHx	family history
CXR	chest x-ray	FI	for investigation
DDAVP®	desmopressin,	FIO$_2$	fractional concentration of inspired oxygen
DB&C	deep breath and cough		
DC	direct current	FNAB	fine-needle aspiration biopsy

FNH	febrile non-haemolytic reactions		ICF	intracellular fluid
FRC	functional residual capacity		IDDM	insulin dependent diabetes mellitus
FS	frozen section		IgA	immunoglobin A, (others are M, E.and G).
FSH	follicle stimulating hormone			
FVC	forced vital capacity		IHD	ischaemic heart disease
FWD	full ward diet		IMV	intermittent manditory ventilation
FWT	full ward test of urine			
G	gauge		INR	International normalized ratio (see PTT)
GA	general anaesthesia			
GABA	gamma aminobutyric acid		IPPV	intermittent positive pressure ventilation
GAMP	general anaesthetic, manipulation and plaster		ISQ	in status quo (meaning 'unchanged')
GCS	Glasgow Coma Scale		I.U.	International units
GGT	gamma-glutamyltransferase		IUD	intrauterine device
GFR	glomerular filtration rate		IV	intravenous
GTN	glyceryl trinitrate		IVI	intravenous injection
Gyn	gynaecology		JVP	jugular venous pressure
Hb	haemoglobin		K^+	potassium ion
HCO_3	bicarbonate ion		KCl	potassium chloride
HFV	high frequency ventilation		kg	kilogram
HIC	head injury chart		kPa	kilopasacal
HITs	heparin induced thrombocytopaenia		LA	local anaesthesia
			Lac	laceration
HIV	human immunodeficiency virus		LBBB	left bundle branch block
			LDH	lactic dehydrogenase
HNPU	has not passed urine		LIF	left iliac fossa
HOCUM	hypertrophic obstructive cardiomyopathy		LMA	laryngeal mask airway
			LOC	loss of consciousness
HPV	hypoxic pulmonary vasoconstriction		LP	lumbar puncture
			LUQ	left upper quadrant
hrly	hourly		LVF	left ventricular failure
HSV	herpes simplex virus		L3-4	interspace between 3rd and 4th lumbar vertebrae
Htn	hypertension			
HT	hypertension		m^2	square metre
HTR	haemolytic transfusion reactions		mane	in the morning
			MAC	minimum anaesthetic concentration
HTLV	human T cell lymphotrophic virus		MAC	monitored anaesthetic care
Hx	history		MAHA	micro-angiopathic haemolytic anaemia
i.d.	internal diameter			
I/M	intramuscular		MAO	mono-amine oxidase
ICC	intercostal catheter			

MAOI	mono-amine oxidase inhibitor	nocte	at night
MAP	mean arterial pressure	NO	nitric oxide
MAR	medicine administration record	NOF	neck of femur
MAT	multifocal atrial tachycardia	NPA	nasopharyngeal aspiration
MBA	motor bicycle accident	N/S	normal saline
MCA	motor car accident	NTG	nitroglycerine (see GTN)
MEAC	mean effect anaesthetic concentration	NSAID	non-steriodal anti-inflammatory drugs
mcg	microgram	NYO	not yet ordered
Mg^{2+}	magnesium ion	N_2O	nitrous oxide
mg	milligram	O	oral
MH	malignant hyperthermia	O_2	oxygen
MI	myocardial infarction	O/A	on admission
MIC	minimum inhibitory concentration	O/call	on call
		OD	overdose
min	minute	OPD	out-patients department
mm	millimetre	OR	operating room
mmHg	millimetre of mercury pressure	Ortho	orthopaedics
mmol	millimol	OSA	obstructive sleep apnoea
mosmol	milli osmol	OT	operating theatre
ms	millisecond	OXI	pulse oximetery
MS	multiple sclerosis	P	partial pressure as in PO_2
MSOF	multisystem organ failure	$PaCO_2$	partial pressure of carbon dioxide in the arterial blood
MRSA	multiple resistant Staphylococcus aureus	PACU	post-anaesthetic care unit
MTBF	mean time between failures	Paed	paediatrics
mV	millivolt	PaO_2	partial pressure of oxygen in the arterial blood
MVA	motor vehicle accident		
MVPS	mitral valve prolapse syndrome	PA	pulmonary artery
Na^+	sodium ion	PAP	pulmonary artery pressure
NAD	nothing abnormal detected	PAT	paroxysmal atrial tachycardia
NBP	non-invasive blood pressure	PAWP	pulmonary artery wedge pressure
NIBP	non-invasive blood pressure		
Neg	negative	P.C.	after meals
NFO	no further orders	PCA	patient controlled analgesia
NFR	not for resuscitation	PCEA	patient controlled epidural analgesia
N/G	nasogastric		
NIDDM	non-insulin dependent diabetes mellitus	PCTA	percutaneous transluminal angioplasty
NMBD	neuromuscular blocking drugs	PD	peritoneal dialysis
NMDA	N-methyl-D-aspartic acid	PDE	phosphodiesterase
NMS	Neuroleptic malignant syndrome	PDQ	pretty damn quick
		PEA	pre-emptive analgesia

PEEP	positive end-expiratory pressure	resps	respiration
		RIA	radio-immuno assay
PERLA	pupils equal and reacting to light and accommodation	RIB	rest in bed
		RIF	right iliac fossa
pH	inverse logarithm of the hydrogen ion activity	ROP	retinopathy of prematurity
		RPAO	routine post anaesthetic orders
PHx	past history	RUQ	right upper quarrant
p.m.	after midday	RVF	right ventricular failure
PM	post-mortem	SA node	sino-atrial node
PND	paroxysmal nocturnal dyspnoea	SAP	systemic arterial pressure
		S/B	seen by
PONV	post operative nausea and vomiting	SBE	subacute bacterial endocarditis
		sec	seconds
PORC	postoperative residual curarization	S/C	subcutaneous
		SG	specific gravity
POP	plaster of Paris	SIADH	syndrome of inappropriate antidiuretic hormone secretion
Pos	positive		
PORC	post-operative residual curarization	SLE	systemic lupus erythematosus
		SMR	submucosal resection
PPF	plasma protein fraction	SNP	sodium nitroprusside
ppm	parts per million	SOF	shaft of femur
PR	per rectum	SOOB	sit out of bed
PRBC	packed red blood cells	Sp/A	spinal anaesthesia
premed	premedication	SR	sinus rhthym
PRN	when necessary (pro re nata)	SSG	split skin graft
PT	prothrombin time (also see INR)	Stat	statum (immediately)
		STD	sexually transmitted disease
PTH	post transfusion hepatitis	STOP	suction termination of pregnancy
PTSD	post traumatic stress disorder		
PTTK	activated partial thromplastin time (see APPT)	STP	sodium thiopentone
		STP	standard temperature and pressure
PUO	pyrexia of unknown origin		
PV	per vagina	Sux	suxamethonium chloride
PVB	premature ventricular beat	SVR	systemic vascular resistance
PVC	polyvinyl chloride	SVT	supraventricular tachycardia
PVC	premature ventricular contraction	SWMA	systolic wall movement abnormality
PVR	pulmonary vascular resistance	tabs	tablets
QD	once daily (use of this is discouraged)	TAH	total abdominal hysterectomy
		TB	tuberculosis
QID	four times daily	TCP	transcutaneous pacemaker
®	registered name	tds	three times a day
RBBB	right bundle branch block		
RBF	renal blood flow		

TENS	transcutaneous nerve stimulation	#	number
THR	total hip replacement	5-HT	5 hydroxytryptamine (also called serotonin)
TIA	transient ischaemic attack	$[Na^+]$	concentration of sodium ion
TMOA	too many obscure abbreviations	$[X]$	concentration of X
TOF	train-of-four with a nerve stimulator	<	less than
TOP	termination of pregnancy	>	greater than
TPN	total parenteral nutrition	«	much less than
TPR	temperature, pulse and respiration	»	much greater than
TRLI	transfusion related lung injury	/	per or each (breaths/min)
Ts&A	tonsillectomy and adenoidectomy	%	per cent
TTN	transient tachypnea of the newborn	@	at
TURP	transurethral resection of prostate	°C	degree centigrade
T_3	tri-iodothyronine	°F	degree fahrenheit
T6	sixth thoracic vertebra	®	registered name
U&E	urea and electrolytes	©	copyright
URTI	upper respiratory tract infection	™	trade mark
UTT	up to toilet	α	greek letter, alpha
UWSD	under-water sealed drainage	β	greek letter, beta (pronounce bee-ta)
V	volt	γ	greek letter, gamma
VC	vital capacity	δ	greek letter, delta
VEs	ventricular extrasystoles	Δ	greek letter upper case delta used to describe differences
VF	ventricular fibrillation	ε	greek letter, epsilon
VO_2	oxygen consumption	μ	greek letter, mu (pronounced mew)
VPBs	ventricular premature beats	π	greek letter, pi (pronounced pie)
VT	ventricular tachycardia		
VVs	varicose veins		
WEL	weekend leave		
WHO	World Health Organization		
WNL	within normal limits		
WPW	Wolff–Parkinson–White syndrome		
WYSWYG	What you see is what you get (a computer term)		
X-match	cross-match blood		
XDP	fibrin d-dimer		
#	fracture		

INDEX

A-a gradient 306
abbreviations 467
ABCD of resuscitation 146
abdominal lipectomy 82
abdominal surgery 82
abduction pillows 101
abortions 96
acetaminophen *see* paracetamol 204
acid base balance 315
acid base disorders, management of 320
acidosis 320
   and acidaemia 317
   in haemorrhage 352
activated partial thromboplastin time 365
acupressure for vomiting 230
acute diastolic dysfunction 285
addiction to opioids 191
addicts 123
adenosine 247
admission
   assessment of patient 14
   monitoring 15
   to recovery room 10
adolescents 70
adrenal suppression, after steroid therapy 136
adrenaline
   dose regime 285
   use in anaphylaxis 142
   infusion 460
adrenergic receptors 234
adult respiratory distress syndrome 118
after fall, temperature 167
aged, definition 71
AIDS 119
air embolism 140
   obstetric 96
airway, patent 6
airway obstruction 328
   burns 84
   causes and management 331
   children 62
   in obesity 130
   signs 330
airways
   floppy 71
   oropharyngeal 393
airways disease, chronic obstructive 338
ALA synthetase 132
alcoholics - nerve damage 170
alcoholism 119
alcuronium 439
alfentanil 190
alkalosis 320
Allen's test 374
allergy
   penicillin 144
   see anaphylaxis 142
alpha adrenergic agonists 234
alveolar air equation 306
aminophylline 335
   toxicity 336
amiodarone 248
   infusion 460
ammonia toxicity 112
amnesia 78
   due to opioids 192
amphetamine abusers 124

anaemia 120
anaemic patients, management 120
anaesthesia, regional 207
anaesthetist, responsibilities in day surgery 76
analgesia
   in smokers 136
   multimodal 194
   pre-emptive 193
anaphylactoid reaction 142
anaphylaxis, due to blood transfusion 354
   management 142
anesthesia, *see* anaesthesia
angina 276
angiography 113
anti-D immunoglobulin 368
anti-emetics 226
anticoagulants
   dalteparin 131
   enoxaparin 445
   oral 360
antigen 142
aortic surgery 114
apnoea, neonatal 66
aprotonin 354
Aramine, *see* metaraminol 448
ARDS, adult respiratory distress syndrome 117
   following trauma 137
arrhythmias, diagnosis of 250
arterial injection, accidental 378
arterial punctures, bruising 146
ASA grading of fitness 117
aspiration
   after trauma 137
   children 65
   risk in obesity 130
aspiration pneumonitis 336
   prevention of 98
aspirin 204
asthma, diagnosis and management 335
asystole 271
atenolol 247
atracurium 440
atrial
   premature beats 253
   fibrillation 259
   flutter 258
   tachycardia 254
atrioventricular blocks 261
atropine 252
   use in bradycardias 253
audit 436
autoclaves 40
autonomic neuropathy 122
awareness 145

baroreceptors, carotid surgery 116
base deficit/excess 318
batteries 393
benzamide drugs 228
benztropine 228
β blockers 247
   hypoglycaemia masked 121
   in Paget's disease 131
   in renal disease 134
Betadine, *see also* poviodine 360
bicarbonate 320
bigeminy 267

biliary pain   126
bleeding, *see* haemorrhage   349
    after nasal surgery   92
blindness, after urological surgery   111
    transient   157
blood
    brown with bubbles   355
    infected   355
    whole   367
blood clotting   366
blood colloids   370
blood filters   358
blood gases   373
    how to interpret   321
blood loss, mammoplasty   91
blood patch   214
blood pressure
    equipment   377
    frequency of measurement   15
    how to measure   375
    importance of   234
blood pressure monitors, types   394
blood products   367
blood sugar, management of   121
blood transfusion   347
    disease transmitted by   356
    filters   358
    massive   352
    reactions   353
blood volume
    newborn   50
    signs of depletion   52
blood warmers
    in line   8
    types   394
blue bloaters   313
body fluids
    physiology   50
    potential infection   37
body mass index   129
Bohr effect   309
brachial plexus blocks   208
bradycardia
    hypoxic in children   67
    sinus   252
brainstem surgery   95
branch blocks
    left   262
    right   262
breast binders   83
breast feeding   145
breast surgery   83
breathing   302
    abnormal patterns of   322
    control of   303–4
    noisy   6
    patterns of   322
breathing bags   411
breathing exercises   17
bretylium tocylate   441
bronchoscopes   395
bronchoscopy   84
bronchospasm, anaphylaxis   143
brown fat   69
bruising, after venipuncture   146
bupivacaine
    how to add adrenaline   208
    pharmacology   215
buprenorphine   198
burns
    airway obstruction   84
    bleeding   86
    fluid balance   85
    monitoring   84

postoperative care   84
septicaemia   86

Caesarean section, *see* obstetric patients   96
    air embolism   140
calcium chloride   69
calcium gluconate   69
Campbell ventilator   415
cannula, insertion of intravenous   57
cannulas   359
capnography   378
captopril   241
carboprost, for post partum haemorrhage   98
cardiac
    electrophysiology   244, 298
    index   379
    infarction   274
    ischaemia   274
    drugs used   279
    nicotine   136
    output   379
    pressures   380
    standstill   271
    tamponade   287
    terminology   295
cardiac arrest
    ABCD   290
    management   289
    paediatric   292
cardiac arrhythmias
    in quadraplegics   128
    management of   246
cardiac failure   281
    heart sounds   283
    low output   284
    postoperative fluids   60
    ventricular dysfunctions   282
cardiopulmonary catheters   379
cardioversion
    atrial fibrillation   258
    children   293
    damage pacemakers   171
    dose   272
carotid endarterectomy   115
Catapres   219
cataracts   87
catheters
    suction   413
    urinary   33
caudal blocks   207
central venous cannulas
    pacemakers   171
    purchase of   395
central venous lines   380
central venous pressure
    complications of   384
    use in bleeding   383
    what it means   238
cerebral aneurysm   94
cerebral oedema, head injury   94
cerebral vasospasm, nimodipine   94
cervical sutures   97
Charnley pillow   101
chemoreceptors   303
chest pain   276
    causes   146
Cheynes-Stokes breathing   322
children
    crying   8
    laryngeal spasm   63
chlorpromazine
    core hyperthermia   162
    hiccough   158

circulation
  fluid depletion 54
  fluid overload 54
  times in elderly 72
citrate toxicity 363
cleaning equipment 39
cleft palate 86
clocks 395
clonidine 219
  epidural use 219
clotting cascade 365
clotting factor deficiency 361
clotting studies, how to interpret 364
COAD 338
coagulopathy - dilutional 356
cocaine 442
  abusers 124
codeine 442
Cogentin 228
collapse, management 148
colloids 59
coma position 6
confusion 153
  after hip replacement 101
  after urological surgery 112
  elderly 73
conversion table
  solution strengths 465
  pressures 465
convulsions
  causes and management 148
  children 69
  congestive heart failure 31
  management of fitting 125
  toxaemia of pregnancy 99
cor pulmonale 313
core balance 427
coroner's clot 332
cough 149
  in smokers 136
  suppressed by opioids 149
coughing exercises 17
cricothyroid puncture 334
cross infection 423
  prevention of 38
cross matching 357
croup 64
crying patient 149
crystalloids 59
curarization, residual postoperative 172
CVP, see also central venous pressure 238
cyanide toxicity 244
cyanosis 150
  after urological surgery 112
  anaphylaxis 143
cyclizine, an antiemetic 227

dalteparin 131
Dalton's law of partial pressures 306
dantrolene 159
  treatment of malignant hyperthermia 161
day surgery 75
  discharge criteria 78
  driving after 80
  organization 76
  pain relief 77
  step down procedure 77
  street fitness 78
DDVAP, see desmopressin
dead space 302
deafness 150
death in recovery room 151
deep vein thrombosis
  after orthopaedic surgery 103

risk in multiple sclerosis 128
risk in myeloma 127
risk in obesity 131
defibrillator 396
delayed emergence 152
delirium 153
  after hip replacement 101
  in elderly 73
  scopolamine 160
dental surgery 86
desflurane 443
desmopressin
  hypophysectomy 95
  pharmacology 354
  von Willebrand's disease 138
dexamethasone 443
dextrans 371
dextrose 123
  treatment of hypoglycaemia 165
  50% dextrose 443
diabetes
  postoperative care 121
  nerve damage 170
diamorphine 195
diazepam 443
  treatment of local anaesthetic toxicity 210
DIC, disseminated intravascular coagulation 362
diclofenac 206
diffusion hypoxia 71
digoxin, digitalization 249
dipyridamole 444
discharge criteria 23
discharge
  to intensive care 25
  day surgery 79
  from recovery room 22–3
disseminated intravascular coagulation 362
  in fat emboli 103
diuretics 346
dobutamine 286
  infusion 460
dopamine 286
  effects on the kidney 342
  infusion 460
dopexamine 287
  infusion 460
Dopram, see doxapram 175
Down's syndrome 123
Dragermeter 391
  use in extubation 22
drains 27
  closed 27
  concertina 28
  pleural 28
  pleural, insertion of 30
  pleural, milking 30
  pleural, suction 30
  pleural, water seal 29
  principles of care 27
  simple 27
  sump 27
driving, after day surgery 80
dromperidone, an anti-emetic 229
droperidol, an anti-emetic 229
drug
  decay curves 43
  dosing 43
  incompatibility 41
  names 463
drug addicts 123
drug dosages 47
  in elderly 47
  in obesity 130
  in paediatrics 45

drugs
  precautions with patients   41
  prevention of accidents   41
  toxic effect on kidney   344
dural puncture   213
DVT, *see* deep vein thrombosis
dysphasic patients   128
dyspnoea   322
  after urological surgery   110
  causes of   155
  J receptors   303
  toxaemia of pregnancy   99

ear surgery, postoperative care   87
Eaton-Lambert syndrome   128
ECG, *see* electrocardiography   300
  changes in ischaemia and infarction   277
  changes with potassium disturbance   55
  indications for   385
  interpretation   300
  J wave   168
  prolonged QT interval   363
  trace components   299
edrophonium   106
elderly   71
  delirium   73
  drug doses   47
  NSAIDs causing bleeding   48
  oxygen requirement   72
  oxygen transfer   71
  physiology and anatomy   71
  problems with joints   73
  skin   73
electrical protection devices   427
electrical safety   421
electrocardiogram, purchase of   396
electrolytes disorders, treatment of   56
embolism
  air   140
  fat   102
  pulmonary   339
emergence   6
  delayed   152
emergency
  alarm   429
  trolley   397
EMLA   446
emphysema
  subcutaneous   178
  surgical   178
endotracheal tubes, description   397
enoxaparin   445
ephidrine   214
  an antiemetic   230
epidural anaesthesia   212
epidural
  lumbar   218
  care of lines   214
epilepsy   124
equipment
  cleaning of   39
  for isolated hospital   417
  servicing   419
  sterilization of   39
ergometrine, for postpartum haemorrhage   98
escharotomy, burns   85
esmolol   248
  in phaeochromocytoma   164
esophagectomy, *see* oesophagectomy
ethylene oxide   40
exercises on admission to recovery room   17
extradural, *see* epidural
extrapyramidal syndrome   176
  description   228

extravasation
  drugs   155
  nerve damage   170
extubation procedure   21
eye surgery   87
eyes
  foreign bodies   156
  red, nasal surgery   92
  redness of   156

face masks   407
facial surgery   88
facial swelling
  facial surgery   91
  in children   70
faciomaxillary surgery   88
factors   464
fat embolism   102
febrile non-haemolytic reaction (FNH)   355
fentanyl   195
  as a cause of itch   169
  description of   195
  epidural use   217
  in elderly   48
  in renal disease   133
fever   159
FFP, fresh frozen plasma   369
fibrin degradation products   365
fibrinogen, levels   366
fibrinolysis   363
filters, used in blood transfusion   358
fingernails   157
fire
  equipment   429
  safety   421
fitting *see* epilepsy   124
  toxaemia of pregnancy   99
floppy airways   71
fluid balance, burns   85
fluids, maintenance
  adults   59
  after surgery   60
  children   59
flumazenil   78
FNH, *see* febrile non-haemolytic reaction   355
formulary   41
FRC, *see* functional residual capacity   302
fresh frozen plasma   369
frusemide   346
  heart failure   344
  infusion   460
  renal failure   344
  renal toxicity   344
full stomach   137
functional residual capacity   302

gas embolism   140
gases, piped   428
gas transfer, lung   304
gastric distension, acute   60
gentamicin   446
geriatrics, drug doses   47
Glasgow Coma Scale   93
glaucoma   157
  caused by ketamine   157
glucose   123
glucose meters   398
glyceryl trinitrate   242
glycine toxicity   112
glycopyrrolate   447
golden rules   5
gynaecology   88

Haemaccel	371
haemoglobin	
glycolysated	121
oxygen dissociation curve	309
saturation	309
haemoglobinometers	399
haemoglobinuria	355
haemophilia	126
pseudo	138
haemorrhage	
causes of continuing bleeding	360
clinical signs	349
pathophysiology	348
postpartum	97
renal disease	134
retrobulbar	157
von Willebrand's disease	138
Wegner's granulomatosis	138
hair	157
hand surgery	89
hand washing	38
in recovery room	427
handover to ward staff	25
Hartmann's solution, composition	58
HbA₁C	121
headache	158
after hypotension	105
after liposuction	90
after spinal anaesthesia	110
after urological surgery	110
caused by dural tap	213
in day surgery	76
head boxes	408
head injury, cerebral oedema	94
heart block	
second degree	264
third degree	265
heart failure	282
heart rate	
maximum acceptable	255
normal in paediatrics	67
heart sounds, cardiac failure	283
Hemabate	98
hemoglobin see haemoglobin	309
hemorrhage, see haemorrhage	
Henderson equation	318
heparin	360
infusion	461
hepato-renal syndrome	126
heroin	124, 195
Hess's test	367
hiatus hernia, in obesity	130
hiccups	158
hip surgery	101
HIV	119
humidification, tracheostomy	109
humidifiers, types	399
hydralazine	242
hydrocortisone, see also steroids	447
in malignant hyperthermia	162
in thyroid storm	163
hydrogen ion	316
hydromorphone, description of	195
hyoscine	447
hypercoaguability	159
hyperglycaemia	121
hyperkalaemia	55
hyperosmolar crisis	121
hyperperfusion syndrome	116
hyperpyrexia, malignant	160
hypertension	
acute	240
after vascular surgery	113
following carotid surgery	115
in quadraplegics	128
management	241
neurosurgery	93
in neurofibromatosis	128
in Parkinson's disease	132
physiology	240
postoperative	5
toxaemia of pregnancy	99
hyperthermia	159
core, in obesity	131, 162
malignant	160
infants	69
hypertonic	
fluids	52
saline	53
hypocalcaemia in infants	69
hypofibrinogenaemia	363
hypoglycaemia	165
in alcoholics	119
a cause of delayed emergence	153
dangers of	121
infants	68
in liver disease	126
hypokalaemia	55
hypomagnesaemia	
cause of bigeminy	267
oesophagectomy	100
hyponatraemia after urological surgery	111
hypophysectomy	94
hypotension	
in amphetamine abusers	124
anaphylaxis	143
causes of	237
epidural anaesthesia	214
management of	239
neurosurgery	93
postural in diabetes	122
refractory, steroids and	137
urological surgery	109
after vascular surgery	113
hypotensive anaesthesia, causing headache	105
hypothermia	165
after neurological surgery	109
in alcoholics	119
assessment of acid-base balance	375
burns	85
due to transfusions	351
in elderly	72
infants	69
J wave on ECG	168
space blankets	412
vascular surgery	114
hypothyroidism	126
hypoventilation	302
in heroin addicts	124
in obesity	130
signs of	325
hypovolaemia	
effects on the kidney	341
neonates and infants	67
paediatric	293
hypoxia	
after hip replacement	101
anaphylaxis	143
causes in recovery room	169
classification	307
dangers with opioids	197
in obesity	130
physiology	301
postoperative	71, 327
signs of	324
transient as a cause of delirium	153
hypoxia and hypoventilation, management of	326
hypoxia and hypoxaemia, description	301

ibuprofen   206
immunosuppression
  due to blood transfusion   356
imprest system   427
incompatibility   41
incubators, neonates   70
indomethacin   447
infants, shivering   166
infection, sources of   37
infection control
  contaminated spills   36
  staff exposure to body fluids   36
  universal precautions   35
infusions   458
  labels   459
  protocols   458
  pumps   401
injections, how to give them   44
INR, see international normalized ratio   365
insulin
  in surgical patient   122
  infusion   461
  treatment of hyperkalaemia   55
intercostal blocks   207
intra-articular local anaesthesia   209
intracranial haemorrhage, infants   68
intracranial pressure, rising, signs of   93
intrapleural blocks   208
intravenous, cannulas   57, 359
intravenous additive labels   57
intravenous fluids, additives   56
intubated patients, care of   18
iontophoresis   195
ischaemia, demand and supply   275
ischaemic heart disease, see cardiac ischaemia
ischaemic limbs   85, 113
isolated hospital, equipment for   417
isolation transformers   427
isoprenaline   448
  infusion   461
isotonic solutionsm composition   58
itch   169
  anaphylaxis and   142
  produced by opioids   191

jaws – wired   88
junctional rhythms   260

ketamine   448
  delirium   153
  use in violent patient   154
ketarolac   206
kidney, see also renal   340
Krogh cylinder   311
Kussmaul's breathing   322

labetalol   242
laparoscopy, gynaecological surgery   89
laryngeal masks   401
  contraindicated in obesity   130
laryngeal nerve damage   158
laryngeal oedema   333
  due to anaphylaxis   143
laryngoscopes   404
laryngospasm   331
  after nasal surgery   91
  in children   63
Lasix, see frusemide   346
laundry   428
leg exercises   17
length, measurement of   465
library   435
lignocaine   97
  dose for arrhythmias   249

in ventricular tachycardias   269
  infusion   461
limb ischaemia, burns   85
limb perfusion
  following orthopaedic surgery   113
  following vascular surgery   113
lipectomy   82
liposuction   90
liver, function in elderly   72
liver disease   126
loading dose, theory of   197
local anaesthetic agents
  properties of   211
  toxicity of   211

macroshock   426
magnesium, use in arrhythmias   255, 267
magnesium sulphate
  antiarrythmic   448
  toxaemia of pregnancy   99
malar fractures, postoperative care   90
malignant hyperthermia   160
mammoplasty, postoperative care   91
Manley ventilator   415
mannitol   448
  in malignant hyperthermia   162
Mapleson C circuit   411
Marcain, see bupivacaine
masks, face   407
Maxolon, see also metoclopramide   229
mediastinoscopy   91
Mendelson's syndrome   222, 336
meperidine, see also pethidine   193
message books   436
metabolic effect of surgery   122
metaraminol   448
methadone   195
  equivalence with morphine   124
methaemoglobinaemia   151
methohexitone   449
methoxamine   449
methylene blue   151
metoclopramide, an antiemetic   229
metoprolol   248
micro-atelectasis   305
microshock   426
midazalam   450
  in day surgery   78
migraines, after carotid surgery   116
milrinone   450
  infusion   461
mismatch   305
mitochondria   311
  production of energy   316
Möbitz type blocks   264
moclobemide   450
monitoring   373
morphine   192
  compared with pethidine   194
  epidural use   217
  in renal disease   133
  in smokers   136
  infusion of   461
  receptors   188
  pharmacology   192
mouth, dryness of   154
multiple myelomatosis   127
multiple sclerosis   128
multisystem organ failure, MOSF   137
muscle, regaining power   7
muscle relaxants
  sensitivity in muscle disease   127
muscle rigidity   176

muscle twitching
  in children — 69
  toxaemia of pregnancy — 99
muscle weakness
  carcinoma — 128
muscular dystrophy — 127
myaesthenia gravis
  lung problems — 128
  thymectomy — 106
myocardial ischaemia — 274
  vascular surgery — 113

nalorphine — 198
naloxone — 198
  in day surgery — 78
  pharmacology of — 198
  use in itch — 167
naproxen — 206
Narcan, see naloxone
nasal surgery — 91
nasogastric tubes — 32
nasopharyngeal airways — 404
nausea
  after urological surgery — 109, 110
  definition — 219
  in day surgery — 76
  management of — 225
needle sizes — 45
needle stick injury, procedure — 37
neonate
  apnoea — 66
  shivering — 166
neostigmine — 173
nephrotoxins — 345
nerve stimulators — 387
nerves. damage to — 170
neurofibromatosis — 127
neuroleptic malignant syndrome — 164
neurological damage
  causing delayed emergence — 153
neurosurgery
  postoperative care — 92
  postoperative fluids — 60
neutral thermal environment — 70
newborn, care after delivery — 95
nifedipine — 242
nimodipine — 451
  infusion — 461
nitric oxide — 451
nitroglycerine, see glyceryl trinitrate — 460
  description — 242
  infusion — 243
nitroprusside — 242, 244
  toxaemia of pregnancy — 99
  infusion — 462
nodal rhythms — 260
nomedopine — 94
non-steroidal anti-inflammatory drugs — 202
noradrenaline — 285
  infusion — 461
normal saline — 58
NSA, normal serum albumin — 370
NSAIDs
  adverse effects — 205
  precautions in breast feeding women — 145
nystagmus — 228

obesity — 129
  drug doses — 46
  morbid — 130
obstetric surgery — 96
obstructive lung disease — 322
oculogyric crisis — 228

oedema
  burns — 85
  pulmonary — 281
oesphagectomy — 100
oliguria, management of — 344
Omnopon — 192
ondansetron, an anti-emetic — 230
Ondine's curse — 189
  spinal cord surgery — 95
Operidine, see phenoperidone
opioid abusers — 124
opioids
  blood pressure — 7
  cause of nausea and vomiting — 190
  continuous infusions — 202
  danger of hypoxia — 197
  dose used in patient controlled
    analgesia — 200
  effect on vestibular nerves — 224
  effects on respiratory centres — 325
  epidural — 217
  in infants and neonates — 197
  intrathecal — 217
  intrathecal use — 219
  pharmacology — 188
  receptors — 188
  reduce dose in myxoedema — 137
  reduced dose in muscular dystrophy — 127
  resistance to — 71
orthopaedic surgery — 100
  hips — 101
oxygen
  concentrators — 406
  cylinders — 406
  supply to tissues — 307
  toxicity — 313
oxygen delivery
  devices — 407
  in renal disease — 133
oxygen dissociation curve — 309
oxygen extraction failure — 311
oxytocin — 452
  for post-partum haemorrhage — 98

pacemakers
  in heart block — 261
  cardiac — 171
packed cells — 368
paediatric
  cardiac arrhythmias — 68
  cardiovascular physiology — 66
  drug doses — 45
  heart rates — 67
  intramuscular injections — 45
  maintenance fluids — 59
  respiratory physiology — 62
Paget's disease — 131
pain — 182
  assessment — 186
  assessment in children — 187
  burns — 84
  clinical points — 184
  components — 183
  harmful effects — 182
  management principles — 185
  pleuritic — 322
  treatment plan — 196
pain relief
  in day surgery — 77
  in smokers — 136
  nasal surgery — 91
pain scale, visual analogue — 186
pallor, causes — 171
papaveretum — 195

paracetamol 204
  in breast-feeding women 146
paraesthesia 170
  with plasters 102
parallax 376
parathyroidectomy 106
paravertebral blocks 208
Parkinson's disease 132
paroxysmal supraventricular tachycardia 256
patient controlled analgesia 199
  protocols 200
patient controlled epidural anaesthesia 218
PCA, patient controlled analgesia 199
PCA devices, description of 409
penicillin allergy 144
penile blocks 209
pentastarch 371
peptic ulceration 132
  caused by NSAIDs 205
perfusion status 236
perineal operations 104
persantin 444
petechiae 367
pethidine 193, 462
  compared with morphine 194
  dangers of in renal disease 133
  epidural use 217
  hypotension 190
  in breast feeding women 145
  in smokers 136
  pharmacology 193
pH, definition 316
phaeochromocytoma 163
  as a cause of fever 160
pharmacodynamics 44
pharmacokinetics 43
pharmacology, in elderly 48
phenoperidine 195
phentolamine 163
phenylephrine 453
phenytoin 125
physostigmine 154
Pickwickian syndrome 130
pink puffers 313
pins and needles 170
  with plasters 103
plaster check 101
plastic surgery 104
platelet, deficiency 361
platelets, transfusion of 368
pleural drains, emergency insertion of 31
pleural drain tubes, clamping 105
pleuritic pain 322
pneumonitis, aspiration 98
pneumothorax 339
  after insertion of CVP 384
  after trauma 137
  infants 65
policy manuals 434
polygeline 371
polyuria, hypophysectomy 95
PONV, postoperative nausea and vomiting 24
PORC, see residual curarisation
  postoperative 172
porphyria 132
post traumatic stress disorder 145
postoperative
  care 105
  fluid maintenance 60
  hypoxia 71
postpartum haemorrhage 97
potassium
  hyperkalaemia 55
  hypokalaemia 55

poviodine 360
power, emergency 426
premature ventricular contractions 266
prescriptions, illegible 43
pressure 465
pressure care 17
pressure infusion bags 409
prilocaine 454
Primacor 450
procainamide
  in ventricular tachycardias 269
  infusion 462
procaine 454
prochlorperazine, an antiemetic 228
promethazine, an antiemetic 228
propofol
propylthiouracil, dose 163
prostaglandins, effect on kidneys 205
Prostigmin, see neostigmine
protamine 462
protective clothing 38
prothrombin time 365
protocols for recovery rooms 434
psychiatric disease 132
pulmonary embolism 339
  after orthopaedic surgery 104
  and ritrodrine 97
pulmonary fibrosis, respiratory rate 135
pulmonary flotation catheters, pacemakers 171
pulmonary oedema 281
  due to blood transfusion 355
  high pressure 118
  laryngeal spasm 65
  low pressure 118
  management 283
  toxaemia of pregnancy 99
pulse oximeters 388
  purchase of 410
  sources of errors 389
pulse rate 236
pulsus alternans 235
pulsus paradoxus 235
pupils
  dilated 172
  unilateral 92, 172
pyrexia 159

QT interval, prolonged 55
quadraplegics 128

ranitidine 455
receptors
  osmoreceptors and volume 50
recovery
  after day surgery 77
  patient's perceptions 13
  phases 15
  staff perceptions 13
  position 11
recovery room
  administration 434
  adolescents in 70
  audits 436
  death in 152
  discharge from 22
  drugs used in 438
  flooring 427
  function 1
  length of stay 23
  lighting 428
  location and design 423
  obstetric unit 96
  plan of day surgery 75
  procedures 17

rostering	434
safety in	421
scoring systems	16
staffing	432
standard equipment	423
untoward incidents	436
red eyes	156
refrigerator	430
regional anaesthesia	207
caudal	207
precautions	209
renal function	
in elderly	72
vascular surgery	114
renal blood flow	340
renal disease	133
drug dosage	133
renal failure	
due to hypovolaemia	343
high output	343
oliguric	342
postoperative fluids	60
residual curarization	172
respiration monitors	390
respiratory centres	303
respiratory definitions	315
respiratory depression	
caused by epidural opioids	218
due to opioids	189
in children	65
respiratory failure	323
respiratory function	328
respiratory muscle failure	325
respiratory symbols	314
respirometers	411
restlessness	5
restrictive lung disease	322
resuscitation ABCD	146
resuscitation bags	411
retrobulbar haemorrhage	157
Reye's syndrome	206
rhabdomyolysis	55
rheumatoid arthritis	134
rigidity in muscles	176
Ringer's lactate, composition of	58
ritrodrine	97
ropivacaine	211, 455
ruler test for street fitness	79
safety in the recovery room	421
salbutamol	336
use as a tocolytic	97
saline depletion	53
saline loading	51
salivary glands, enlargement in child	70
scopolamine, an anti-emetic	227
scoring systems in recovery room	16
sedation, produced by opioids	190
see-saw breathing	323
septicaemia	
after urological surgery	112
burns	86
sevoflurane	455
shaking	173
sharps	
disposal	430
disposal of contaminated	36
shivering	173
danger in hepatic disease	126
due to hypothermia	166
shock	
blood pressure	5
cardiogenic	288

catecholamines used in management	285
classification	176
signs of	52
shunting	305
sickle cell syndromes	135
sinus	
arrhythmia	250
bradycardia	252
tachycardia	251
sleep apnoea syndrome, obesity	130
slings - arm	90
smokers	136
snoring	178
sodium bicarbonate	292
sodium iodide	163
sore throat	178
sotalol	248
space blankets	412
how to use	166
specimens, transport of contaminated	36
spinal anaesthesia	24
spinal cord surgery	95
spirit level	412
sputum retention	178
squints, vomiting	87
staff	
medical	433
nursing	432
standard bicarbonate	318
standardization	464
standards	424
starches	
esterified for use in blood replacement	371
steam autoclave, bacteria and	40
Stemetil	228
step down procedure	77
stereotactic surgery	94
sterilization of equipment	39
sterilizers	
maintenance of	40
types of	40
steroids, withdrawal	136
stethoscopes	413
stir-up exercises	17
street fitness	78
stress, response to	233
stridor	
in anaphylaxis	144
children	65
management after thyroidectomy	107
stroke	
due to air embolism	141
following carotid surgery	115
postoperative management	128
suction	
catheters	413
pharyngeal	17
specifications for	413
tracheobronchial	17
sufentanil	190
suprapubic catheters, indications for	34
surgeon, responsibilities in day surgery	77
surgical emphysema	178
suxamethonium	455
Swan Ganz catheters	379
sweating, causes and management	179
syringe driver	401
dilutions	459
systolic dysfunction, acute	281
T-piece	408
use of	22
T waves, peaked	55

tachycardia
  sinus   251
  summary of treatment   273
  supraventricular   255
  ventricular   268
tacrine   455
teeth   179
telephones   428
temazepam   455
temperature   464
  low temperature measurement   414
  measurement of   390
  monitors   390
Tensilon test   106
terbutaline, use as a tocolytic   97
thermocouples   390
thiopentone   455
thoracotomy   105
three way taps   382
throat, sore   178
thrombophlebitis   9
  causes of   58
  danger in renal disease   134
thymectomy   106
thyroid disease   137
thyroid storm   162
  as a cause of fever   160
thyroidectomy   106
tissue grafts   105
tobacco smokers   136
tocolytic agents   97
tolerance to opioids   191
tongue sutures   88
tonsillectomy   107
torches   414
Torsade de pointes   270
tourniquets   101
toxaemia of pregnancy   99
tracheostomy   108
tranexamic acid   354
transformers, isolation   427
transfusion related lung injury, TRALI   355
transport
  of the obese patient   131
  to recovery room   11
  safety   25
  trauma patients   138
Trasylol, see aprotinin
trauma   137
trolleys, description   414
twitching, toxaemia of pregnancy   99

universal precautions   35
urinary catheters   33
  blocked   34
  continuous irrigation   34
urinary retention, due to opioids   191
urological surgery   109
urticaria
  caused by transfused blood   355

  due to blood transfusion   355
  useful data   464

vaginal surgery   89
valves, non-reflux   405
valvular heart disease   288
vascular surgery   113
Vasoxine   449
venous admixture   305
ventilation
  in pulmonary disease   133
  indications for   327
ventilators   415
ventilatory volumes   390
ventricular
  contractions, premature   266
  fibrillation   270
  tachycardia, polymorphic   270
verapamil   249, 462
  dangers   272
violent patient   154
visitors to recovery room   13
vocal cord paralysis   334
voice, hoarse   158
Voltaren   206
volume   465
volume meters, respiratory   390
vomiting
  caused by drugs   224
  centres   222
  clinical hints   231
  definition   219
  ear surgery   87
  eye surgery   87
  management of   225
  physiology of   223
  squints   87
Von Recklinhausen's disease   127
von Willebrand's disease   138

warfarin, pharmacology   361
warming blankets   416
warming infants   69
water depletion   52
water intoxication, after urological surgery   110
water loading   51
water overload   53
Wegner's granulomatosis   138
weights and measures   466
wheeze
  causes   180
  toxaemia of pregnancy   99
  treatment   335
whole blood coagulation time   364
Wolff–Parkinson–White syndrome   257
Wright's Respirometer   391
  use in extubation   22

X-ray   391
  power outlets for   429